Next Generation NCLEX-PN Study Guide 2024-2025

Complete Review + 725 Questions and Detailed Answer Explanations (5 Full-Length Exams)

Printed in the United States of America

Table of Contents

Introduction

Exam Administration

The exam is administered through computerized adaptive testing that uses measurement theory and computer technology. Each candidate receives a customized test in real time based on their aptitude and prior responses. Items are chosen from a pool organized by test plan type, difficulty, and clinical judgment processes. After each response, the computer estimates the candidate's ability and selects the next item as appropriate. This process continues until a pass/fail judgment is determined.

Passing Criteria

The exam is administered by the National Council of State Boards of Nursing. The NCSBN-appointed professionals determine the passing criteria. In cases where the candidate's performance is near the passing standard, the computer continues to ask questions until a definitive result is obtained. If time constraints lead to the premature termination of the test, the computer will evaluate the candidate's performance based on the most recent 85 questions. Candidates who consistently surpass the passing score are deemed successful. Those who only achieve or fall below the passing score are considered unsuccessful.

Review the Responses

The computer screen displays one exam item at a time. Each question has no time restriction, which allows candidates to modify their responses if necessary. Once the answer is confirmed, the candidate cannot return to previous items. If unsure of the correct response, the candidate should make their best guess and proceed to the next question.

Register for the Test

The initial step in the registration process is to apply to the state board of nursing in your desired state for licensure. Once the board confirms that you meet all the prerequisites, you can register for the NCLEX test with Pearson Vue. There are three registration options: phone, US mail, or online.

Adherence to the registration guidelines and completion of the registration forms is essential. Failure to follow these steps or provide the correct payments may delay your test. Keep in mind that there is a test fee.

The Day of the Exam

It is required that you arrive at the testing location at least 30 minutes before the scheduled exam start time. Failure to do so may lead to cancellation of your exam appointment and additional expenses. We recommend that you visit the location a few days before the exam to familiarize yourself with any potential roadblocks, traffic, or parking issues.

On the day of the test, ensure you have the Authorization to Test (ATT) and a valid, current form of identification with your photo and signature to be eligible for the exam.

Chapter 1: Coordinated Care

Advance Directives Information

Advance directives provide guidance for medical decisions should patients become gravely ill or unable to vocalize their preferences.

Types of Advance Directives

1) Durable power of attorney: This designates a proxy who has the authority to make medical decisions that fall in line with the patient's values and intentions.

2) Living will: This legal document specifies how patients wish to be treated if they cannot make decisions about emergency care.

Without an advance directive, a patient's state of residence laws will determine who has the authority to make medical decisions. If the patient's children are adults, the authority may be given to them, a partner, or a spouse. When no relatives are available, some states permit a close friend who understands the patient's wishes to assist.

Although healthcare providers and proxies will try to follow a patient's advance instructions, there may be situations where they cannot, or a healthcare professional could choose not to comply with the directives for specific reasons.

Medical Orders

1) Do not resuscitate (DNR).

The DNR is an order made by a physician when a patient expresses a wish to be allowed to die if they experience cardiac or respiratory arrest. The patient or their legal agent must offer informed permission for the DNR status. The DNR order must be properly worded so that other therapies not denied by the patient are continued. It must be regularly reviewed, and all healthcare providers must know whether a patient has a DNR order. Healthcare providers must make every attempt to resuscitate a patient if they do not have a DNR order. DNR procedures may differ from state to state, so nurses must know their state guidelines.

2) Out-of-hospital DNR.

If the patient is not in the hospital, emergency responders will be informed of the person's preferences for CPR.

3) Do not intubate order.

This order indicates the patient refuses hospital or nursing home ventilators.

Advocate for Client Rights and Needs

Patient advocacy is a vital aspect of healthcare. It safeguards patient rights, maintains high care standards, respects human dignity, promotes patient equality, and empowers individuals to decide on health-related matters.

Advocacy entails advocacy for patients' issues. Medical professionals must listen to their needs, worries, and requests.

Roles of an Advocate

- Engage the legal system on the patient's behalf.
- Communicate with relatives.
- Facilitate communication between patients and medical professionals.
- Present arguments against medical theories.
- Provide clarification or object to advice or therapy.
- Explain medical terminology or procedures.
- Review care schedules.
- Uphold moral principles and ethics.
- Ensure quality treatment.

Who Can Be a Patient Advocate?

Everyone in the medical industry should advocate for patients' rights, but nurses are often seen as primary patient advocates due to their close interactions with them.

Promote Client Self-Advocacy

Some ways to assist with client self-advocacy include:

1) Request clear communication.

Inform patients about their right to understand their treatment, which includes the option to request a language interpreter.

2) Choose a medical team.

Encourage patients to research healthcare providers they are comfortable with.

3) Create a medical summary.

Explain the value of a summary that contains medication dosages, allergies, and medical issues. Provide sample summaries as models.

4) Assist patients to access services.

Help patients access services within and outside the hospital, such as financial aid, support groups, and other resources.

5) Be present.

Stay with patients during significant events, such as doctor rounds or discussions about their diagnosis or progress, and encourage them to ask questions.

6) Educate patients.

Inform patients about their condition, advancements, setbacks, and coping strategies. Use simple language to explain complex medical terms and encourage the patients to learn more about their condition through the use of reputable sources.

Assign Client Care and Related Tasks

Nurses must assess each patient's competence to make choices and obtain consent for care. Nursing evaluations gather and analyze patient data to determine their needs. Based on the evaluation, planned care involves evidence-based nursing treatments to address identified requirements.

The patient's circumstances, characteristics, and desires must be emphasized when treatment is planned. The individual should be included in decision-making for a person-centered approach.

VIPS is an acronym used to define what should and should not be considered in person-centered care.

1) Values people: Values and promotes the patient's rights regardless of age or cognitive capacity.

2) Individual's needs: Provides personalized treatment.

3) Perspective: Understands care from the perspective of the patient.

4) Supportive social psychology: Aids in the resolution of the patient's psychological requirements, which include mental, emotional, and spiritual needs.

Involve the Client in Decisions about Care

Patients have the right to make decisions, and healthcare staff should respect their choices. The patient's consent authorizes the healthcare professional to provide care. Consent can be expressed or implied.

Expressed consent occurs when written or spoken approval is given for a specific procedure. The patient is informed about the disease and treatment choices and can accept or decline therapy.

In a medical emergency, consent for essential treatment to sustain life or restore health is presumed unless evidence suggests the patient would reject the intervention.

The patient should understand the healthcare provider's advice. Informed consent relies on patients to ask questions when unsure, consider their options carefully, and be open and honest with their healthcare providers about their values, concerns, and reservations about a particular recommendation.

Healthcare practitioners should inform patients about their medical condition, goals, choices, potential outcomes, and risks associated with suggested therapy.

Adult patients are presumed competent to make medical choices unless a court rules otherwise.

Update Each Client's Plan of Care

After the patient's requirements are evaluated, the next step is to carefully plan how to address the identified and anticipated difficulties. Documentation in various forms, such as digital, handwritten, or preprinted care plans, is always necessary for effective communication.

Care Planning Stages

Step 1: Identify issues.

Identify the patient's needs and prioritize them with the patient's permission. Categorize the needs as high, intermediate, and low to establish the correct objectives.

Step 2: Determine goals.

Short-term objectives may be met quickly, and long-term goals could take days, weeks, or months to complete. Nurses can use the acronym S.M.A.R.T. to develop Specific, Measurable, Achievable, Realistic, and Timebound objectives.

Step 3: Implement interventions.

These are procedures or treatments based on clinical judgment that aim to achieve the objectives established at the previous care level.

There are three types of interventions: those launched independently by nurses, those reliant on a physician or other healthcare professionals, and those dependent on the expertise, abilities, and knowledge of numerous professions.

Independent nursing interventions are planned and carried out by nurses without the guidance of any other healthcare experts. Other healthcare professionals frequently direct dependent nursing interventions. Interdependent interventions are often collaborative care plans that must be agreed upon by all parties engaged in multidisciplinary meetings.

Step 4: Perform an evaluation.

The outcomes of the intervention are reviewed to determine its success. This may be a continuous process, and the evaluation plan should define the frequency and length of the assessment.

Participate as a Member of an Interdisciplinary Team

An interdisciplinary team is composed of experts from different fields who collaborate to treat a patient with various physical and psychological needs. They complement each other's expertise and work together to achieve common treatment objectives.

Nurses and physicians are often part of multidisciplinary teams that collaborate to deliver healthcare in a single place, and they must effectively communicate about the treatments they deliver.

Patients often have initial interactions with nurses either alone or with a medical practitioner. As a result, nurses usually spend more time with patients than many other healthcare providers.

The role of nurses extends beyond mere caregiving. They act as conduits of information within the healthcare system. Their observations and judgments are pivotal in future care planning. Furthermore, nurses often become patients' voices, echo their preferences, and facilitate an approach rooted in patient-centered care.

Ward nurses provide direct care to assigned patients throughout the day. They often identify the deterioration of a patient's health before other health workers and physicians.

Individuals with complicated physical challenges, limited mobility, or neurological disorders, such as stroke patients, must be moved frequently to prevent pressure ulcers. Moreover, gradual movement is often part of a patient's stroke recovery regimen. Nurses are trained in how to move and handle patients safely.

Additionally, nurses may learn about the patient's home environment. This is critical to plan discharge for stroke patients, as communication impairments may hinder their ability to convey information.

Moreover, for patients who live alone or have minimal family support, home nursing services or telemonitoring technology may be necessary. This assistance can mitigate injury risks and provide a means for individuals to promptly signal emergency services if they suffer a fall or experience a stroke.

Recognize and Report Staff Conflict

Conflict resolution in nursing is essential to promote a productive and secure workplace, refocus time and effort on patients, lower stress levels, and enhance the workplace for staff and patients.

Identify a Conflict

1) Interpersonal conflict.

Conflict may arise when people have different personalities or communication styles. Positive traits like cooperation, adaptability, and patience can help resolve issues. However, conflicts can sometimes involve coworkers who act as bullies. In such cases, a mediator can help resolve the issue. Nurse managers and human resources representatives are usually the ones to settle the disagreement.

2) Values conflict.

This type of conflict may arise when nurses have different personal values. A mutually beneficial change based on common interests should be the goal of dispute resolution.

3) Task-based conflict.

This conflict occurs when two medical experts disagree on a particular method. Each organization probably has established procedures for all nurses to follow, but that doesn't mean there won't be disagreements on how to proceed in different situations.

Conflict Management

1) Evaluate the situation.

Take a moment to determine if the problem really needs resolution and how it impacts you and the work atmosphere.

2) Resolve the conflict.

Act as quickly as you can.

3) Speak with the other party.

Arrange a private conversation away from patients and colleagues for an honest, positive discussion.

4) Listen actively.

Pay close attention to the other person's viewpoint as they may offer a fresh perspective. Ask questions if you need additional details or clarification.

Participate in Staff Education

In-service programs are essential for nurses and staff to stay updated on the latest advancements in healthcare practice. Effective instructional strategies include feedback, interaction, clinical simulations, and case-based learning.

Passive teaching methods like lectures have little impact on learning results. Continuous learning in workplace environments leads to better outcomes.

Computer-based learning is an affordable and equally effective alternative to live instruction. Effective strategies result in improved knowledge, skill outcomes, and clinical practice behaviors, although the link between continued professional education and clinical results is not explicit.

Use Data from Various Credible Sources to Make Clinical Decisions

Data-driven clinical decisions are necessary to integrate disease tests, symptoms, and diagnoses. The goal is to optimize patient care.

Provide Evidence-based Patient Care

Experienced nurses can quickly identify small changes in a patient's state and determine care requirements. They base decisions on the effectiveness of interventions or therapies.

Higher-quality research-based knowledge is available through research accessible on organizational intranets, electronic publications, and printed resources like Clinical Evidence and Evidence-based Medicine. Nurses use these sources for clinical practice and also rely on their peers for research expertise.

Evaluate Written Sources

Nurses cross-reference sources with ward-based records and other resources. They note publication dates, citations of related studies, resource types, and clinical focus.

Consult Colleagues

Clinical nurse specialists with research-based resources, business networks, and personal development techniques are valuable.

Monitor Activities of Assistive Personnel

Nursing assistants (NAs) are vital team players who work under the direction of licensed professional nurses (LPNs). Registered nurses (RNs) direct NAs and LPNs.

The Five Rights of Delegation—proper person, situation, task, monitoring and assessment, and communication—should be followed when tasks are assigned.

All care provided by assistive nursing staff must be assigned and overseen by an RN, aligned with the patient's care plan and the staff member's skill set.

Tasks for assistive nursing staff can be categorized into basic and secondary skill sets. Basic skills include tasks that support feeding, cleanliness, daily living, and assisting expert nursing evaluations. Secondary skills require extra training and proficiency.

Maintain Client Confidentiality

In the healthcare system, confidentiality ensures that the patient's personal information remains private. The nurse-patient relationship demands that information shared is not disclosed to anyone not directly involved in the patient's care. Medical professionals should avoid disclosure of patient information to unauthorized individuals, such as friends or family, without explicit patient permission or a legal/ethical need.

Medical information should be stored to maintain patient confidentiality through the use of secure procedures and tools such as antivirus software, firewalls, passwords, and encryption. When professionals confer online, they should use secure apps, platforms, and networks to avoid unprotected or public devices.

Both electronic records and paper documents should be properly disposed of.

Provide for Privacy Needs

Respect for patients' privacy fosters a positive relationship with the medical staff.

Patients' physical privacy requires respect for personal space, permission for procedures, and appropriate introductions to ward staff. Courteous acts such as a knock on a patient's door are also imperative.

Psycho-mental privacy, on the other hand, demands respectful dialogue, clear instructions upon discharge, avoidance of ridicule, correct usage of patients' names, and respect for their values and beliefs.

Ensure physical distance in busy areas like emergency departments to prevent inadvertent disclosure of patient information to nearby individuals.

Follow Up with Clients After Discharge

Nurses must reach out to patients to assess their progress. This practice aims to maintain a positive nurse-patient relationship, address concerns, clarify doubts, perform further evaluations, and adjust treatments as needed. During follow-up, inquire about the patient's preferences on how they receive information about their diagnosis, treatment side effects, blood and imaging tests, etc.

Forms of Follow-Up

1) Calls.

Help patients understand discharge instructions, be aware of follow-up visit dates, exchange information, provide health education and counseling, manage symptoms, identify issues early, and reduce wait time for medical consultations.

2) Home Visits.

Home visits provide assistance with illness and injury prevention as well as treatment.

3) Appointments.

Patients and practitioners meet at predetermined times and locations for health education, counseling, diagnosis, treatment, and clinical support.

Who Follows Up?

Who follows up on a patient is determined by the communication objective.

1) Primary care doctors may conduct follow-ups for difficult cases.

2) Nurses and medical assistants may check blood pressure and blood glucose levels, discuss healthy habits, assess medication adherence, and explain test findings patients have received in the mail.

3) Pharmacists may follow up with patients about their medications.

4) Additional office personnel may schedule appointments, ensure follow-up on recommendations, and provide patients with community resource information.

Participate in Discharge or Transfer

Work with patients to plan their discharge, discuss their condition and next steps in therapy, and prevent complications. Patient assessments, education, and post-discharge care all contribute to lower readmission rates.

Patient Medical Transfer

Patient medical transfer involves the movement of a client from one unit to another. Transfers are used for cases that require less intense nursing care, to save healthcare expenses, or for specialized treatment in life-threatening emergencies. The procedure entails the relocation of the patient and their belongings, coordination with the destination unit, creation of a transfer summary, and communication with the patient and their family.

Patient Release and Discharge

Discharge refers to the end of care from a healthcare organization, and preparation for it starts at admission. This incorporates room sanitation requests, a summary of the client's health status, aid for client departure, business office notification, discharge instruction completion, procurement of medical directives, verification of home healthcare eligibility, home self-care discussions, goal setting with the patient, and evaluation of healthcare necessities.

Provide and Receive Reports

Nursing reports are written accounts of a patient's condition provided to the next shift's nurse by the current nurse. The reports cover patient data, recent changes in symptoms, pain management, level of consciousness, allergies, dietary restrictions, medication details, reason for admission, and medical history. Additional information may include wounds, required care, upcoming medical tests, discharge instructions, mobility assistance, IV fluids, catheter use, isolation needs, and oxygenation requirements.

Report Presentation

1) Problem.

This includes the patient's current medical problems, medical background, and personal details.

2) Assessment.

The report should include evaluations performed by the patient's medical team or specialists.

3) Changes.

Recent or anticipated adjustments to the patient's requirements or medications, such as lab tests, visits, or prescriptions, should be documented in the report.

4) Evaluation.

The patient's treatment plan objectives and any progress achieved should all be documented.

How to Write a Nursing Report

1) Organize information clearly.

Structure the report to help the next nurse easily find the patient data they need. Consider the creation of a digital template that can be quickly adapted for multiple patients.

2) Review recent orders.

Certain patients, like those in the ICU, may experience rapid changes in symptoms, which require specific orders from healthcare providers.

3) Be explicit in your wording.

Write concise and accurate reports that use precise language.

4) Collect pertinent information during your shift.

To prepare for your shift report, keep track of any changes or updates to your patients' conditions and medical needs throughout the day.

Organize and Prioritize Care Based on Client Needs

Prioritize short-term acute patient care demands and issues over longer-term chronic needs. Focus on actual needs over wellness, potential risks, and health promotion.

Maslow's Hierarchy of Needs is a useful framework to prioritize patient needs:

1) Physical and biological needs.

Address essential needs like personal care, sleep, and nourishment.

2) Safety and psychological needs.

Ensure comfort, emotional support, and a secure environment.

3) Love and belonging.

Address the need for affection, community, and acceptance.

4) Self-esteem.

Recognize and appreciate the value of oneself and others.

5) Self-actualization.

Encourage patients to realize their fullest potential and abilities.

6) ABCs.

Prioritize the assessment and management of the patient's airway, breathing, and cardiovascular conditions.

Manage Time Efficiently and Practice Ethically

Nurses should have a strategy to manage time, minimize distractions, and help others without compromising patient care priorities.

Adherence to the Code of Ethics for Nurses is essential, as noncompliance could lead to the loss of one's nursing license and potential malpractice lawsuits.

The Nursing Practice Act

Each state has a Nursing Practice Act that outlines the norms and legislation applicable to licensed nurses who practice in that state, which includes restrictions and training requirements. If a nurse encounters a scenario beyond their qualifications, they must seek guidance from a physician or another nursing authority. Failure to do so could cause the nurse to lose their license and face legal action, either individually or against the healthcare organization or hospital.

Nursing Code of Ethics

1) Autonomy.

Autonomy means respect for an individual's right to self-determination.

2) Nonmaleficence.

Nonmaleficence involves a commitment not to harm others.

3) Beneficence and paternalism.

Beneficence aims to promote well-being.

4) Justice.

Justice involves equal distribution of potential benefits and responsibilities when patient care orders are determined.

5) Truthfulness.

This involves the commitment to truthful communication.

6) Fidelity.

Fidelity is an obligation to fulfill promises made.

Participate in the Client Consent Process

Client consents are legal documents that express a patient's authorization for a procedure and permission to share information with third parties. Consents also include expressed comprehension of treatment risks and benefits, the consequences of not undergoing the procedure, treatment options, and the identity of the healthcare practitioner who will perform the surgery or procedure.

Before any operation or treatment, patients must have their queries addressed. The patient should sign the consent form freely, without fear, and with a witness present. The patient needs to be intellectually and emotionally competent. Patients who have been administered sedatives or drugs that impair cognitive capacity should not be asked to sign a consent form. If a patient is mentally or emotionally incompetent, the next of kin, a court-appointed guardian, or a durable power of attorney can consent. Competent patients above the age of 18 can sign a consent form.

Types of Consent

1) Admission agreement: Acquired at admission, this outlines the healthcare agency's obligations to the patient.

2) Vaccination consent: This may be necessary before certain vaccines are administered and ensures that patients are informed of the advantages and hazards of immunization.

3) Permission for blood transfusion: This provides information about the benefits and risks of the transfusion and acknowledges religious views that may prohibit the procedure.

4) Surgical consent: This type of consent is obtained for any surgical or invasive operations or invasive diagnostic tests. It discusses the process, its risks, advantages, and feasible alternatives.

5) Research consent: This signed form consents to a patient's participation in a research project, fully aware of the potential risks, effects, and rewards.

6) Special consent: This consent pertains to specific situations like the disposal of body parts after surgery or postmortem organ donation.

Minors' Consent

As defined by state law, a minor is below the legal age of majority, usually younger than 18. Before a minor can receive treatment, it is essential to obtain consent from their legal guardian or parent. However, in certain situations, such as emergencies, treatment can be initiated without parental or legal guardian consent. Examples of such situations include substance abuse treatment, HIV testing and AIDS treatment, and sexually transmitted infections treatment.

Use Information Technology in Client Care

Patient data should only be accessible to healthcare staff. Confidentiality can be protected through the use of unique, regularly updated computer access codes/passwords to restrict personnel access to computer systems. Information provided by patients during research must not be disclosed in any way that identifies the patient or be shared with anyone outside the research team.

Ways Healthcare Executives Can Use Data to Prompt Change

1) Structural indicators measure the qualifications, specialization, and experience of healthcare professionals, as well as the type of resources available for patient care.

2) Process indicators track the interaction between patients and healthcare providers, such as the time taken for patient admission after a doctor's visit, the adherence to clinical guidelines, and the timeliness and completeness of provided services.

3) Outcome indicators evaluate a patient's health status due to healthcare, such as the rate of recovery, patient satisfaction, or the occurrence of postoperative infections.

4) Balance metrics assess the equilibrium between different components within the healthcare system, such as the trade-offs between quality improvement and cost control.

5) Leaders can use data as a catalyst for change. Analyze patient data to devise strategies for the reduction of surgical infections or implementation of data-driven approaches to minimize hospital stays.

Examples

- One approach might involve specialized staff training to care for individuals with dementia. Enhancement of the physical environment of nursing homes, increased staffing ratios per shift, and the provision of more opportunities for residents to engage in activities can also be beneficial.

- Quality improvement initiatives in nursing homes may address factors like organizational culture and pressure ulcer management. High rates of pressure ulcer formation can raise concerns about other aspects of quality care in nursing homes.

Verify Healthcare Provider Orders

Healthcare provider orders are the primary communication between doctors and the multidisciplinary hospital team. They form the basis for patient care and action. These orders, both in paper and computerized formats, guide treatment decisions and impact various healthcare aspects, which include payment, patient safety, utilization, and quality standards.

Although studies highlight the positive impact of computerized physician orders and electronic reminders on patient care, paper-based methods facilitate multidisciplinary integration and precise communication. Technological advancements have enhanced the flexibility and adaptability of preprinted physician orders. This allows swift adjustments to hospital procedures, patient needs, and available services.

Preprinted Physician Orders

Preprinted physician orders play a pivotal role in the improvement of healthcare systems, elevation of the standard of treatment, and improvement of patient outcomes. These steps should be taken to ensure the effectiveness of these orders:

1) Compliance.

Properly manage order modifications with regular updates to ensure the most recent versions are accessible. This minimizes misunderstandings, unwanted variations, and errors.

2) Education.

Provide doctors, staff, and patients with timely guidance on best practices and patient safety. This may include indicators for appropriate antibiotic usage, a list of eligible formulary drugs and doses, reportable core measurements for specific conditions, and evidence-based algorithms to aid treatment and decision-making.

3) Engineering.

- Recommendations for drug safety ensure clear and consistent prescription information or instructions for all aspects of doctor orders.
- Format considerations include appropriate space for handwritten input, white space, point size, and font.
- Content should be organized to ensure orders are accurate, comprehensive, and cover all relevant information.

Recognize Self-limitations of Tasks and Seek Assistance When Needed

In nursing, self-reflection is essential to high-quality patient care. Self-reflection involves awareness of limitations, critical evaluation of actions, and consideration of different perspectives to guide future patient interactions.

Conscious Attention

Authenticity is characterized by undivided mental focus and the acceptance of one's true feelings and thoughts. This can help professionals better understand ethical and unethical nursing practices and develop a thorough awareness of their behaviors and responsibilities in nursing tasks.

Contextual Attention

Contextual attention is about the interpersonal factors that influence each situation. This includes one's temperament, prejudices, and emotions during nurse-patient interactions.

Professional Sensibility

Professional sensibility involves the identification of how one's behaviors and actions impact patients, their families, and other healthcare professionals.

Personal Attention

Personal attention requires introspection into one's ideas, emotions, strengths, weaknesses, and their effects on one's overall well-being and relationships with others.

Nursing Self-care

Nursing self-care is vital for well-being. The incorporation of self-care into daily routines can be made more accessible if nurses:

1) Seek assistance.

Awareness of when to ask for professional help is important, especially when nurses find it a challenge to care for themselves. Support from coworkers, mentors, superiors, qualified counselors, and therapists can make a significant difference.

2) Practice self-compassion.

Self-compassion can reduce stress, sadness, burnout, and secondary traumatic stress.

3) Create a self-care plan.

Nurses should take note of personal pressures, triggers, and symptoms and develop a plan to enhance self-care practices.

4) Diversify self-care practices.

Nurses should incorporate a variety of stress-reduction and well-being-enhancement techniques into their daily lives.

Respond to the Unsafe Practices of a Healthcare Provider

Unsafe practices can encompass intentional violations of practice standards and codes and repeated practice violations. This causes an unacceptably high risk of emotional, psychosocial, or physical harm to patients, families, or others.

Efforts to address unsafe practices focus on early reporting, reinforcement of professional standards and codes of conduct, and the creation of a no-blame culture.

Healthcare providers may be subject to complaints if they:

- Disrespect or act unprofessionally toward the patient.
- Fail to provide adequate information or limit the patient's decision-making ability.
- Provide insufficient care.

Complaints made to the Health Complaints Commissioner or health ombudsman help improve healthcare in the future by turning problems and mistakes into opportunities for growth.

Follow Regulations to Report Specific Issues

Children and Elder Abuse

Research has shown a link between childhood maltreatment and the development of physical and mental health issues that can persist into adulthood. Elderly individuals, especially those in poor physical condition, with functional limitations, or who reside in nursing facilities, are also at risk of abuse from staff or other residents.

Healthcare professionals have an ethical and legal duty to recognize and report abuse of children and vulnerable populations to the appropriate authorities. Neglect is often reported in the clinical context, such as medical, dietary, physical, or emotional neglect.

When suspected abuse cases are evaluated, healthcare professionals should take a comprehensive history, conduct a thorough physical examination, order relevant laboratory tests, and contact the appropriate authorities.

Infectious Illnesses

Certain infectious illnesses pose significant public health concerns, and there is a responsibility placed on healthcare professionals to report them for the benefit of the larger population.

Underreported infectious illnesses may be attributed to a lack of awareness about which conditions should be reported and uncertainty about the reporting process. An interprofessional approach can help identify reportable illnesses and reduce the likelihood of underreporting.

Reports of infectious illnesses are required for public health initiatives to control their spread and enable effective measures for their containment and elimination.

Provide Care within the Legal Scope of Practice

Nurses must possess knowledge of the rules and legislation that govern nursing care. Adherence to the nursing scope of practice is essential for nurses to maintain competence and deliver high-quality care.

Areas of Legal Risk

1) Assault.

This occurs when one person threatens another with harm.

2) Battery.

This involves deliberate contact with another person without their consent.

3) Invasion of privacy.

This includes the violation of confidentiality, invasion of the private affairs of patients or families, and disclosure of patient information to unauthorized individuals.

4) False imprisonment.

This arises when a patient is unjustifiably detained in a healthcare institution or when restraints are used without a valid clinical reason. If a patient declines treatment and is competent to make decisions, an Against Medical Advice form may be signed. Clear documentation in the medical record can prevent disputes.

5) Defamation.

This refers to false statements, whether spoken or written, that harm someone's reputation.

6) Fraud.

This involves intentional deception aimed at illegal gains.

Disciplinary Procedures

Nursing boards have legislative power to refuse, revoke, or suspend a nurse's license. Examples of reasons for disciplinary actions may include:

1) Unprofessional behavior.
2) Actions that may endanger public health and welfare.
3) Violation of patient confidentiality.
4) Failure to use appropriate knowledge, skills, or nursing judgment.
5) Physical or verbal abuse of a patient.
6) Assumption of responsibilities without adequate preparedness.
7) Delegation of nursing care to unlicensed personnel
8) Failure to maintain proper records for each patient.
9) Falsification of patient records.
10) Abandonment of one's nursing duties.

Participate in Quality Improvement Activities

Quality improvement initiatives are a systematic approach that pinpoints issues related to quality, implements improvement activities, and monitors outcomes to achieve desired results. These initiatives are used in hospitals to enhance patient care, streamline operations, and meet regulatory standards.

Quality improvement programs often involve changes to healthcare processes and policies, tools, and methodologies such as data collection and analysis, process mapping, and root cause analysis. Control charts may be utilized to graph events and assess their performance over time.

Quality can be measured in various ways, which include outcomes, processes, and balancing measures. When outcomes are analyzed, it is essential to focus on the immediate effects of service provision, such as mortality rates and patient satisfaction.

Service quality measurements are process metrics that focus on service delivery, such as when a doctor sees a patient or assesses the quality of a patient's medical records. To establish a fair and equitable balance between the needs of patients and providers, it is necessary to achieve a balanced approach to services.

Quality Improvement Methodologies

The most commonly used quality improvement approaches are the plan-do-study-act (PDSA), Six sigma, and lean techniques. In the widely used PDSA strategy, small-scale experiments are conducted before changes are made. These involve the formulation of hypotheses or the proposal of improvement ideas.

Apply Evidence-based Practice

Evidence-based practice (EBP) combines the best available research data and clinical expertise. To apply EBP effectively, clinicians must use accurate and relevant research summaries.

These steps often apply to the use of EBP principles:

1) Formulate a medical question.

Well-designed inquiries specify the outcome, comparison, intervention, and population to increase the likelihood that specific answers will be found in the medical literature.

2) Compile data.

Literature and reliable sources like ACP Journal Club or PubMed can provide a comprehensive selection of relevant research.

3) Assess the reliability and quality of the data.

Different types of research vary in scientific merits and legitimacy. The study's generalizability, internal validity, and timeliness (such as whether the research is recent or outdated) are essential to assess.

4) Apply findings to patient treatment.

Adaptation of findings from a randomized trial to a specific patient requires consideration of the person's preferences for aggressive or invasive tests and treatments and their tolerance for pain, risk, and uncertainty. The cost of tests and treatments may also impact decision-making for both healthcare practitioners and patients.

Evidence Levels

The highest-quality evidence is Level 1, which includes systematic reviews or meta-analyses of randomized controlled trials and excellent single randomized controlled studies.

Cohort studies are categorized as Level 2 evidence.

Level 3 evidence consists of case-control studies that have been systematically reviewed.

Case studies are considered Level 4 evidence.

Expert judgment derived from physiology, bench research, or fundamental concepts is classified as Level 5 evidence without critical evaluation.

Participate in Client Data Collection

Patient data collection is necessary as it forms the foundation for all future patient treatments. As patients may feel anxious in the hospital, the nurse must create a comfortable environment.

Data collected during the evaluation includes emotional, safety, psychological, cultural, physical, and environmental information.

Nurses employ proven techniques to gather objective and subjective data when patient assessments are conducted. Common data collection methods include patient interviews, physical examinations, and observation. A thorough examination of the patient addresses each bodily system and notes any anomalies, complaints, or concerns.

Patient interviews are purposeful and planned interactions to gather information, inform the patient's family and caregivers, offer support, assess changes, and identify any worries or issues.

It is important to differentiate between cues and inferences. Cues are indications provided by the patient or observed by the nurse, while inferences are the nurse's interpretations or conclusions drawn from the cues.

Participate in the Client Referral Process

Nurses refer patients to specialists, supplementary healthcare professionals, laboratories, and screening facilities. Consider these steps to ensure a smooth referral process:

1) Maintain professional connections.

Establish and maintain connections with professionals to whom patients are referred. This fosters effective communication and coordination of treatment. Avoid referrals to professionals who do not provide timely updates or fail to coordinate care.

2) Share essential information.

Do not rely solely on patients to communicate information. Share important details, such as the reason for the referral, medical records, and lab results, directly with the receiving office.

3) Ensure patients understand.

Make sure the patient fully comprehends the purpose of the referral. Provide a detailed explanation of the risks and benefits of screenings and address any concerns or anxieties.

4) Provide clear instructions.

Give clear and written instructions about the referral site and the complete referral process. Include information on how the nurse and the other clinician will exchange information and when the patient should return for follow-up.

5) Follow-up on referrals.

Follow up on the referral status and record the outcome in the patient's medical record. Ensure that the patient receives the results of any tests or screenings. Explain how the results will be utilized and address any obstacles if the patient does not complete the referral.

6) Monitor progress.

To regularly assess the referral process, randomly review a sample of referrals made in a given period. Track the proportion of patients whose referral results are documented in their medical records one month later.

Provide Cost-effective Care

Healthcare providers should adopt cost-effective care strategies that reduce treatment and operational costs and maintain the quality of patient care.

Patient-centered Nursing Techniques

Nurse practitioners can significantly reduce healthcare costs when they prioritize patients' health and implement proactive care practices. These nursing practices can enhance cost-effective care:

1) Remove barriers to care.

Many patients encounter obstacles such as remote living locations, absence of health insurance, or lack of transportation. These barriers hinder their ability to attend regular medical appointments. Nurse practitioners can assist these patients through the provision of essential primary care services in rural regions where primary care professionals are scarce.

2) Use an active care approach.

Nurse practitioners can conduct patient health risk assessments and design tailored programs to address their needs. These approaches are particularly beneficial for elderly individuals. They help assess frailty and maintain patients' everyday functions. Additionally, nurse practitioners can proactively visit seniors.

3) Coordinate care for patients with complex needs.

An increasing number of patients have multiple chronic health conditions. Effective communication among healthcare providers is vital to avoid unnecessary repetition or neglect of procedures. Nurse practitioners coordinate patient information among different providers. Regular preventive care visits by nurse practitioners ensure patients adhere to self-care routines, which reduces the need for hospitalization when chronic conditions are well-managed.

4) Assist healthcare facilities with cost management.

Nurse practitioners play an important role in the management of costs with a variety of tools and techniques, which include:

- Regular preventive care visits to prevent disease progression.
- Provision of holistic care to identify new health and environmental concerns and address nutrition and exercise requirements.

- Use of technological advancements like wearable technology, telemedicine, artificial intelligence, and virtual reality to enhance patient care.
- Establishment of online portals for interactions with nurses and assistants, refill requests, appointment scheduling, and medical record access.
- Electronic health records to track and document patient symptoms and progress effectively.

Chapter 2: Safety and Infection Control – Identify and Manage Client Allergies

Upon initial contact with the client, the nurse must determine known sensitivities to latex, radiocontrast used in diagnostic tests, foods, or drugs.

Medication Allergies

Nurses must be well-informed about the signs and symptoms of drug allergic reactions. All drug allergies must be documented in the drug administration record and the patient's medical file.

Common drug allergies, such as penicillin, sulfonamides, and cephalosporins, can be extremely harmful, even fatal. The first exposure to penicillin can sensitize the body and cause an anaphylactic shock upon subsequent exposure.

Radiocontrast Media Allergies

Ionic high osmolality and non-ionic low osmolality are two types of radiocontrast media that can trigger allergies in some individuals. Risk factors for radiocontrast media allergies include cardiac or kidney illness, female gender, older age, and use of beta-blockers.

Latex Allergy

Latex allergies manifest differently in individuals. Some may experience acute contact dermatitis, while others may have delayed contact dermatitis or a life-threatening allergic response. Patients with asthma, eczema, or immunosuppressive disorders like AIDS are at higher risk of latex allergies.

Identify Allergic Reactions

Signs of anaphylaxis and anaphylactic shock include rapid pulse, rash, respiratory distress, laryngeal edema, hypotension, and severe collapse of venules and arterioles in the circulatory system. Dermatitis due to latex presents with symptoms like skin itchiness, burns, and scales, which may spread to other body areas.

Interventions

When allergies are identified, the nurse must promptly report and document them. In cases of life-threatening anaphylactic shock, CPR and other life-saving measures may be necessary. Corticosteroids or antihistamines may be administered based on a doctor's prescription.

Standard Safety Measures

Standard safety measures encompass various practices to protect both patients and healthcare providers.

Hands should be washed between patient interactions, after contact with contaminated objects or equipment, and immediately after gloves are removed. Alcohol-based hand rubs may not be effective against specific pathogens like C. difficile spores but are suitable for regular hand decontamination when hands are not visibly soiled.

Masks, eye protection, or face shields should be worn when patient care tasks are performed that might lead to blood or bodily fluid splashes or sprays. Gowns should also be used if blood or bodily fluids are likely. After the gown is removed, the hands should be washed.

Use Transfer Assistive Devices

Assistive devices are essential tools to aid patients in their daily activities. Some commonly used assistive devices are:

1) Gait belts.

These provide a secure hold on unsteady patients when they move, which enhances stability and safety.

2) Slider boards.

These facilitate the supine movement of immobile patients from one surface to another.

3) Mechanical lifts.

This type of ceiling-mounted equipment transfers patients who cannot bear weight or need assistance due to medical conditions or unpredictable behavior.

4) Wedge pillows.

A triangular-shaped cushion made of sturdy foam is used for leg abduction after total hip replacement surgery.

5) Trochanter rolls.

These are used to prevent external rotation of the legs while the patient is supine. They can be made with a folded sheet or blanket that is placed lengthwise from the popliteal area's lower border to the femur's greater trochanter.

6) Trapeze bars.

A trapeze bar hangs from a firmly fixed overhead bar attached to the bedframe. It allows the patient to use their extremities to lift their trunk, assist the patient to move from the bed to a wheelchair and perform upper arm strengthening activities.

7) Side rails.

Side rails run the bed's length, which provides patient protection and enhanced mobility.

8) Sandbags.

These soft devices are filled with molded material that conforms to the body's curves. They immobilize the extremities and keep the body in a specific position.

9) Pillows.

Pillows offer support, elevate body parts, splint incisional areas, and alleviate postoperative discomfort from physical activity, coughing, or deep breathing. The size of the pillows should match the body part being positioned.

10) Hand-wrist Splints.

These are custom-made splints to keep the thumb in slight adduction and the wrist in mild dorsiflexion.

11) Hand rolls.

Hand rolls maintain slight finger flexion and function, with the thumb slightly adducted in opposition to the fingers.

12) Boots.

These boots are made of stiff plastic or heavy foam and flex the foot at the correct angle. They should be removed twice or thrice daily to check the skin's integrity and joint mobility.

13) Bed rails.

Plywood planks installed under the mattress's surface provide back support and body alignment.

Evaluate the Appropriateness of Healthcare Providers' Orders for Clients

There are several steps to determine if a client's healthcare provider's order is appropriate:

1) Review the order for accuracy and legibility.

2) Verify that the order suits the client's condition and aligns with their medical history.

3) Ensure the order follows the latest standards of care and does not conflict with other directives or medications the client takes.

4) Examine the order for potential side effects or interactions with other prescription drugs or medical procedures.

5) Provide healthcare services without discrimination based on race, religion, gender, national origin, or disabilities. This is to ensure that patients receive equal care and treatment.

6) Offer patients access to psychological, nutritional, and other counseling services. The option to participate in relevant clinical trials and access new treatments may improve a patient's prognosis.

Additionally, effective patient-healthcare provider communication can reduce anxiety and improve patient satisfaction. Provide essential information to patients about their condition, potential treatments, costs, clinician expertise, and potential outcomes. Patients should receive sufficient information in a language they understand. Healthcare professionals should be attentive to their reactions.

Participate in Preparation for Internal and External Disasters

Radiation Safety

- Avoid contact with loose implants.
- Keep all bedsheets and dressings in the patient's room until the implant is removed.
- Place patients with radiation implants in a separate space.
- Use a film badge to measure radiation exposure.

- Minimize time spent close to the radiation source, increase distance, and use shielding devices like lead aprons to prevent exposure.
- Properly label any potentially radioactive materials.
- Be familiar with the healthcare organization's procedures and standards.

Electrical Safety

- If a patient is electrically shocked, switch off the power before you handle them. Maintenance staff must inspect any electrical equipment patients bring to the healthcare facility.
- Always unplug equipment from the outlet before you clean it.
- Avoid the use of electrical equipment near bathtubs, sinks, or water sources.
- Never pull a plug by its cord, and always grip the plug firmly.
- Electrical wires should never be run under carpets.
- Keep extension cables to a minimum and securely tape them to the floor.
- Read warning labels.
- Avoid the overload of circuits.
- Check for exposed, frayed, or damaged electrical cables and outlet wires.
- Use a three-pronged electrical plug.
- Ensure electrical equipment is grounded and well-maintained to prevent hazards.

Fire Safety

- Bedridden patients can be transported in a fire with stretchers, beds, or wheelchairs. Proper transfer procedures, body mechanics, and ergonomics should be followed to prevent injuries. Specialized tools may be available for non-ambulatory patients.
- Ambulatory individuals should be directed to safe locations where they may help move patients who use wheelchairs.

- Use an Ambu bag to maintain a patient's breathing condition until they are moved away from the fire.
- Turn off appliances and oxygen in the event of a fire.
- Avoid elevators during a fire.
- Know the location of fire alarms, exits, and extinguishers. Familiarize yourself with the agency's fire drill, evacuation plan, and fire department phone number.
- Identify fire exits.
- Keep open areas free from clutter.

Poison Safety

Poisons can harm a person's health or cause death when ingested, inhaled, or absorbed. They can affect various systems in the body, such as the renal, gastrointestinal, hepatic, central nervous, circulatory, or respiratory systems. Young children, toddlers, and preschoolers must be especially protected from accidental poisoning. In older individuals, vision and memory issues can lead to unintentional poisoning or prescription medication overdose.

Specific antidotes or therapies exist for only a few types of poisons. The body's ability to recover from a toxin determines the reversibility of its effects. In case of suspected poisoning, immediately call the poison control hotline.

Interventions:

- Contact the poison control hotline before you take action, and call an ambulance if they advise that you take the poisoned individual to the emergency room.
- If the patient goes to the emergency room, send the container of the poisonous substance with them.
- Do not induce vomiting in unconscious victims or those who have consumed petroleum, grease, household cleansers, or lye compounds.
- If instructed, save the vomitus and take it to the poison control center.
- Identify the type and quantity of the poison consumed.
- Remove any visible poison immediately from the mouth, eyes, or body area.

Use Safe Client Handling Techniques (e.g., Body Mechanics)

Body Mechanics Principles

- Keep your back straight to prevent injuries.
- Maintain a wide base of support by spacing your feet.
- Bend from the hips and knees rather than the waist.
- Use your longest and strongest muscles.
- Utilize your body weight to assist when you push or pull.
- Avoid twists and turns with your entire body.
- Keep heavy objects close to your body.
- Whenever possible, push or pull and try not to lift.
- Ask for assistance when needed.
- Use rotating sheets and mechanical equipment whenever possible.

Transfer a Patient from the Bed to the Chair

Place the chair next to the bed, toward the foot of the bed, on the patient's stronger side. Stabilize and lock the wheelchair's wheels. Lower the bed and raise the head of the bed.

If the patient requires assistance:

- Put one arm under the patient's shoulders and the other around the patient's legs.
- Lift the patient's legs over the edge of the bed while they raise their shoulders off the bed.
- Allow the patient time to adjust and regain balance before they stand up.
- Use a sling or clothes to support the paralyzed arm during the transfer if needed.
- Place the patient's feet flat on the floor. Support the weak leg with your leg and foot if necessary.

- Position your arms under the patient's armpits, have them lean forward, and support their upper body.
- Use a broad support base, bend your knees, and lift the patient to a standing position by pivoting the feet, legs, and hips.
- Pivot until the patient is above the chair, then gently guide them into the chair.
- Secure the patient in the chair with the safety belt and place their feet on the footrests.
- Encourage the patient to assist in the transfer as much as possible.

Log Rolling with Turning Sheet

Log rolling with a turning sheet is essential to maintain a straight spinal column, such as after spinal surgery. This procedure requires two or more people.

- Raise the bed to its highest setting.
- Place the turning sheet under the patient.
- One person should stand on each side of the bed. The person facing the movement guides it with the turning sheet while the other applies gentle pressure on the patient's back in the direction of the movement, enabling the patient to roll.
- Place pillows at the patient's back and abdomen for support.
- Check the patient's alignment and comfort.
- Raise the side rails and lower the bed for safety.

Identify and Address Unsafe Conditions in Healthcare and Home Environments

Unsafe Healthcare Conditions

Nurses are often involved in patient care in nursing or retirement homes. Difficulties may arise due to health conditions, physical or cognitive disabilities, or the patient's inability to adapt to the environment. It can be difficult to monitor their health, especially for patients with limited movement caused by neurological disorders like Parkinson's or dementia.

Medication administration and preparation require adherence to instructions from pharmacists or manufacturer recommendations. Hospital pharmacists personnel work quickly to fulfill prescriptions for patients with various medical conditions, which increases the probability of human error. Drug administration or manufacturing mistakes can jeopardize patient health or life.

Additionally, nurses must understand the purpose of prescribed medications to monitor patients effectively after administration and document any changes observed. It is vital to follow the advice of both doctors and pharmacists to avoid errors and justify clinical actions. Effective and open communication allows nurses to ask questions and raise concerns, which fosters a strong working relationship.

Unsafe Home Conditions

1) Handrails.

For home-care clients with functional limitations, assistive hardware like grab rails, handrails, and elevated toilet seats is essential to ensure safety and reduce fall risks. Clients at risk for falls should wear warning devices, especially if they live alone.

2) Emergency escape plan.

Clients and family members must be informed about emergency escape routes in case of smoke, fire, or carbon monoxide inside the house.

3) Electrical safety.

Home inspections should check for frayed wires, functional smoke alarms, fire extinguishers, electrical objects near water, overloaded electrical outlets, and electrical items in proximity to water.

4) Sanitation and cleanliness.

Keep the home clean and pest-free to help safeguard clients against diseases.

5) Carbon monoxide.

Nurses must be able to recognize the symptoms of carbon monoxide poisoning. The appropriate medical authorities should be contacted immediately for treatment.

6) Food safety.

Clients, especially children, the elderly, and those with weakened immune systems, are at risk of food-borne infections. Proper food handling, cooking, and hygiene practices can prevent infections caused by bacteria like Escherichia coli and salmonella.

Follow Protocol for Timed Client Monitoring

Non-time-critical scheduled drugs: These medications can be administered early or delayed one to two hours without harm to the patient.

Planned drugs that must be taken on time: These medications include pancrelipase, alendronate, oral antidiabetic agents, or rapid-, short-, or ultra-short-acting insulins. They require administration within a specific time window to ensure effectiveness. Other examples include drugs that must be taken separately from others, immunosuppressive drugs, and opioids.

Scheduled drugs: All maintenance dosages given on a regular, recurring schedule (e.g., yearly, monthly, weekly, daily, BID, TID, QID, and q4h) are considered scheduled drugs.

Effective treatments to minimize acute care usage involve multiple components, such as forecasting health changes, prompt alarm response, individualized patient parameters, and improved patient self-management.

Implement the Timed Client Monitoring System

An interdisciplinary committee with sufficient nursing representation must convert recommendations into facility-specific policies and procedures.

1) Medications taken monthly, weekly, or daily.

Administer within two hours of the appointed time or immediately after. Consumption of these medications within a window of more than two hours is generally safe. However, keep the window within two hours before or after the planned time to avoid missed doses.

2) Medications given more than once but no more than every four hours.

Administer these medications within an hour of the planned time or later. Technology updates may be necessary to ensure timely medication administration.

3) Initial doses.

Hospitals should set specific deadlines for the initial doses of important drugs, such as IV antiepileptics, anticoagulants, or anti-infectives, where timeliness is required. Use procedures to facilitate administration time objectives.

4) Identify appropriate patients.

Patients with more severe diseases and a higher risk of readmission benefit most from less acute care.

5) Patients' readiness to self-monitor and perceived ease of illness management.

Patients with diabetes, asthma, and hypertension are more inclined to self-monitor, while those with rheumatism, migraines, and neurological conditions show less willingness.

6) Interventions with instructional components.

The intervention design may increase engagement and utilization. Consider the patient's social situation, as socially connected patients tend to have better results, possibly due to faster access to assistance.

Implement the Least Restrictive Restraints

Restraints are tools or methods that restrict a client's mobility and can be chemical or physical. They prevent falls, protect against harm to the client or others, and secure medically necessary tubes and catheters, such as tracheostomy tubes and intravenous lines.

Chemical restraints are medications used to control behavior or restrict the patient's freedom of movement and are not a standard treatment for the patient's medical or psychiatric condition. On the other hand, physical restraints involve manual techniques or devices attached to the client's body, like a vest or leather restraints, to prevent falls or unwanted movements. The least restrictive restraints aim to provide maximum freedom of movement while meeting the client's needs, such as the use of mittens to protect catheters and medically required lines.

Restraint Orders

Orders for restraint use must come from a doctor, except in emergencies when a certified nurse can apply restraints per a set procedure until the doctor's order is obtained. The application of restraints operates under multiple laws and rules. These may involve the observation and care of clients under restraint, the use of preventive strategies to minimize restraint use, and the assessment of a client's well-being.

Application of Restraints

Positive and negative reinforcement, stress management, relaxation strategies, behavior modification, and behavior management techniques can be employed to minimize the need for restraints that result from aggressive behavior.

Observe Restrained Clients

It is essential to conduct a thorough assessment when a restrained client is observed. This includes evaluation of the safe and appropriate use of the restraint, the client's reaction when the restraints are temporarily removed for treatment, their psychological and emotional state, and their physical condition. The latter includes mobility, hygiene, hydration, nutrition, injuries, and vital signs.

Acknowledge and Document Practice Error

Identify Practice Errors

To prevent injuries and accidents, a nurse must be able to recognize and document any treatment orders and prescriptions to ensure they do not pose any risks to the client. Treatments and procedures, especially invasive ones like surgery and diagnostic tests, carry higher risks and potential for practice errors.

Specific procedures, such as contrast media for diagnostic tests, mechanical ventilation, chest tubes, central venous catheters, peripheral venous catheters, intubation, cardiac catheterizations, and surgical procedures, pose higher risks during and after the process.

Competent nurses should:

- Manage patients under mild sedation during and after surgery.
- Provide preoperative, postoperative, and intraoperative care.
- Inform clients about procedures and therapies.
- Conduct careful assessments.
- Identify patterns and changes in client conditions and take appropriate action.
- Implement safety measures to prevent harm during surgery or diagnosis.

- Skillfully place, maintain, and remove stomach tubes, urine catheters, and peripheral intravenous lines.
- Collect various samples, such as wounds, feces, urine, and blood.
- Perform diagnostic tests like ECGs, oxygen saturation tests, and glucose monitoring.

Adherence to these guidelines and documentation of all aspects of care helps prevent practice errors and ensure client safety throughout the treatment process.

Document Practice Errors

All incidents must be reported per the rules of the healthcare institution to ensure the prevention of future occurrences. The data collected from these reports is analyzed, recorded, and monitored over time.

Nurses should report any issues related to client care to the charge nurse, supervisory nurse, risk management, or performance improvement department, accompanied by a written report.

There are different report variations, which include patient-specific, system-specific, and practitioner-specific. Patient variations are related to the patient, system variations pertain to the facility's care delivery, and practitioner variations involve the treatment given by a healthcare professional.

A formal incident report should include:

- The names of individuals involved.
- Details of medical attention and treatments given.
- Any harm caused.
- A clear description of the event and circumstances.
- The date, time, and location of the incident.

Ensure the Availability and Safety of Client Care Equipment

Proper education on equipment safety is necessary for healthcare providers and clients. Operators should be trained on equipment use to ensure safety. Healthcare professionals should seek guidance if they feel unqualified to handle specific equipment.

Safety inspections involve the examination of equipment for missing, broken, or frayed parts and documentation of preventive maintenance and safety inspections. Any equipment that raises slight safety concerns must be taken out of service immediately and sent for evaluation and repairs.

Educate Patients on the Proper Use of Medical Equipment

Clients and staff who need medical equipment for self-care at home should be educated about its safe use. Proper instructions should be provided for non-electrical equipment like canes or walkers, continuous passive motion devices, and electrical oxygen supplementation treatment. It is essential to perform preventative maintenance, even if the equipment appears to be in good condition.

Initiate and Participate in Security Alerts

Nurses are vital in the implementation of security plans and drills to evaluate their effectiveness and respond to security threats. Critical thinking and clinical decision-making skills are required to respond quickly and appropriately to security concerns, such as information theft, computer hacking, aggressive patients, or child abduction.

Healthcare facilities implement various security measures that include:

- Protocols for security dangers like active shooter situations or bomb threats.
- Electronic tools like mother-baby bracelets to prevent infant abductions.
- Specialized training to ensure quick responses to security breaches.
- Secure entryways.
- Closed-circuit monitoring.
- Alarm systems in high-risk areas.
- Identification badges for visitors and staff, and security alert systems like code pink for infant abductions.

Apply Principles of Infection Control

Infection control precautions are based on different transmission modes, such as contact, droplet, and airborne measures.

Contact Safety Principles

Infections can spread through direct contact when a patient touches a contaminated item and then touches their mouth or nose. Indirect contact transmission occurs when a contaminated item is used. Some infections that can spread through contact include:

- Wound or skin infections.
- Conjunctivitis.
- Multidrug-resistant organisms.
- C. difficile.

To prevent contact transmission, wear gloves and a gown when in contact with the patient and place the patient in a private room or with a cohort patient (one infected by the same organism). For C. difficile, additional precautions necessitate gloves and a gown while in the room, sanitization of hands with soap and water before departure, use of exclusive equipment for each patient, and room sanitation with chlorine to prevent infection spread.

Droplet Safety Principles

Diseases like adenovirus, pneumonic plague, pneumonia, pertussis, and parvovirus B19 can spread through droplets. Infected patients should be placed in a private room or with a cohort patient, and healthcare workers should wear masks when within three feet of the patient to prevent droplet transmission.

Airborne Disease Safety Principles

Tuberculosis, disseminated varicella-zoster, chicken pox, and measles are examples of diseases that can spread through airborne droplets. Airborne precautions necessitate the infected patient's placement in a single, negative-pressure room. The door must remain shut, and negative airflow and multiple air exchanges per hour must be maintained. The patient should wear a surgical mask when they leave the room. Healthcare professionals should also wear personal protective equipment (PPE), which includes respiratory masks with an N95 level or above.

Disposal of Contagious Waste

Handle contagious items with care and ensure proper labels. Dispose of waste in approved containers and designated areas. Sharps should be immediately disposed of in leakproof, closed, puncture-resistant containers that are labeled or colored appropriately.

Hand Hygiene

Hand hygiene includes surgical hand antisepsis, alcohol hand cleaner gel or foam, and washing hands with water and soap.

1) Soap and water versus alcohol hand sanitizer.

In most clinical settings, an alcohol hand cleaner is recommended for washing hands as it effectively reduces germs. However, water and soap should be used in certain situations:

- When hands are visibly contaminated.
- After contact with a patient known to have infectious diarrhea.
- After exposure to confirmed or suspected spores like Clostridium difficile or B. anthracis.

Use an alcohol-based hand cleaner during routine patient care, such as:

- Before you touch a patient.
- Before the use of invasive medical equipment or aseptic tasks like device insertion.
- After contact with the patient or their environment.
- Immediately after gloves are removed.
- When contact is made with contaminated surfaces with bodily fluids or blood.

Alcohol hand cleaner protocol:

- Apply the product and rub hands together for 20 seconds until dry.

Soap and water protocol:

- Wet hands with water, use the recommended amount of soap and rub hands together for at least 20 seconds.
- Dry hands with paper towels after you rinse them with water.
- Use the towel to turn off the tap.
- Avoid the use of hot water to prevent skin dryness.

2) Gloves.

- Use gloves if there is expected contact with blood, contaminated equipment, contaminated skin, nonintact skin, mucous membranes, or other potentially infectious materials. Gloves do not replace handwashing. Wash your hands before you wear gloves or come into contact with a patient or their surroundings. Immediately wash your hands after you remove the gloves.

- Change gloves if they are torn or contaminated with bodily fluids or blood during a procedure or when you move from a dirty site to a clean site on the same patient. Never use the same gloves for multiple patients. Remove gloves carefully to avoid hand contamination.

3) Surgical asepsis.

- Before you start the surgical hand cleanse, remove any jewelry. Clean the nails thoroughly under flowing water to remove dirt from underneath. During surgical procedures, perform a surgical hand cleanse either with antibacterial soap or alcohol hand cleanser.

- For an antibacterial soap hand cleanse, scrub forearms and hands for the time specified by the manufacturer, usually two to six minutes. Longer scrub times, such as ten minutes, are unnecessary.

- Ensure the forearms and hands are completely dry before you apply the alcohol solution. After you use the alcohol-based product as directed, allow the hands and forearms to dry thoroughly before putting on sterile gloves.

- Double gloving is recommended during invasive procedures with a higher risk of blood exposure. When you prevent bacteria from a surgeon's hands from entering the surgical area, this helps reduce the risk of wound infections. Antiseptic substances used in preoperative cleaning inhibit bacterial growth.

- If surgical gloves are punctured or torn during surgery, less skin flora on the surgical team's hands lowers the likelihood of germs in the surgical field.

4) Fingernail care.

- Even after hands are washed and an alcohol-based hand cleaner is used, bacteria may persist beneath fake fingernails. Healthcare professionals should avoid extensions or fake fingernails when they directly interact with patients at higher risk.

- Limit the length of fingernails to a quarter inch to maintain proper hand hygiene.

Chapter 3: Health Promotion and Maintenance

Provide Comprehensive Care for Newborns (Less Than 1 Month Old) and Infants or Toddlers (2 Years Old)

Neonatal Care

Essential Care:

1) Arrange necessary referrals.

2) Prevent infections.

3) Provide assistance with breastfeeding.

4) Ensure heat protection.

5) Offer immediate care during childbirth, early nursing, skin-to-skin contact, respiratory evaluation, drying, and delayed cord clamping.

Standard Physical Care:

1) Within 24 hours after birth, the neonate passes meconium and urine. Females may have slight vaginal bleeding and some labia edema. Males have present testes, rugae on the scrotum, and a urinary meatus at the tip of the penis.

2) Observe the tongue for tiny white cysts known as Epstein pearls. Ensure adequate tongue movements, symmetrical lips, and a closed oral palate. A tongue that protrudes may indicate Down's syndrome.

3) Check the fontanels for softness and flatness. Bulging may indicate elevated intracranial pressure. Depression may indicate dehydration.

4) Examine the neonate's skin for any cyanosis, jaundice, or blueness. The skin should be smooth with normal wrinkles. Unusual skin findings like nevus flammeus, purple-blue Mongolian spots, telangiectatic nevi, small red spots called milia, fine hair called lanugo, and Vernix caseosa (a thick cheesy substance) are usually temporary.

5) Ensure the newborn's ears are bilaterally positioned with strong, well-formed cartilage and the capacity to hear noises. Low-set ears may suggest Down syndrome.

6) Verify the presence of red and pupillary reflexes and ensure the size and shape of the eyes are bilaterally equal.

7) Examine the umbilical cord and site for any signs of infection, such as redness and pus, and observe the newborn's abdomen for proper movement during breathing. Bowel noises should be audible within a few hours after delivery.

8) The newborn's length should be between 18–22 inches, chest circumference between 12–13 inches, and head circumference between 12.6–14.5 inches.

The New Ballard Scale:

The New Ballard Scale assesses gestational age in neonates based on physical and neuromuscular maturity. It assigns a score from negative one to five, considering factors such as square window formation (neonate's wrist movement), scarf sign (arms crossed over the chest), heel-to-ear movement, posture, and arm recoil. This evaluation helps determine the neonate's level of morbidity and mortality.

Apgar Score:

The Apgar score evaluates newborns with five criteria: respiratory effort and rate, skin tone, reflexes, pulse, and appearance. Each factor receives a score between zero and two, and the assessment is conducted one minute after delivery, and again five minutes after delivery. Scores between seven and ten are considered satisfactory, four to six indicate moderate discomfort, and a score of less than four indicates severe distress, which requires immediate medical attention.

Infant Care

1) Infants have passive protection from their mothers but are still susceptible to illnesses due to their immature immune systems.

2) Infants are fed with formula or breast milk every two to four hours, with a daily consumption of 70–100 ml/kg.

3) Teething begins during infancy.

4) Infants begin to babble as they learn to communicate.

5) Infants begin to walk at around one year of age.

6) Infant height or length grows by approximately an inch every month for the first six months. Growth rate then decreases to about half an inch per month from six months to one year.

7) Head circumference increases by approximately half an inch per month for the first six months, and then by about one-quarter of an inch per month from six months to one year.

8) Infants experience significant growth. They gain five to seven ounces per week initially and will double their birth weight within the first year.

Toddler Care

1) Toddlers grow about three inches per year. By the age of two, most toddlers weigh approximately four times their birth weight.

2) Age-appropriate toys for toddlers should be big and vibrant and should not present a choking hazard.

3) Toddlers play with other children but may not interact in the same way as older kids.

4) Toddlers under three are susceptible to various hazards, such as asphyxia, car crashes, burns, aspiration, falls, and drowning.

5) Toddlers should have three meals a day. The recommended daily caloric intake is between 1,000 and 1,400 calories for children aged one to three years. Iron supplements may be required based on dietary intake and the healthcare provider's advice.

6) Toddlers have low tolerance thresholds for frustration and strangers.

7) Toddlers think in an imaginative and concrete manner. They have a short attention span, poor impulse control, and high curiosity and energy levels.

8) Toddlers are aware of parental restrictions and rules.

9) Toddlers communicate with succinct yet meaningful words.

10) Potty training is usually completed during the toddler stage.

Provide Care that Meets the Needs of Preschool, School Age, and Adolescent Clients Ages 3 Through 17 Years

Preschoolers

1) Preschoolers have a complete gender identity.
2) Preschoolers can speak in whole sentences.
3) Preschoolers engage in activities such as dress-up games, painting, and basic puzzles.
4) Preschoolers begin to actively play with others. They often ask questions to understand the reasons behind things.
5) Preschoolers need approximately 1,200 to 2,000 calories daily, dependent on age, gender, and level of physical activity, with snacks between meals.
6) Preschoolers can follow quick, straightforward, and specific instructions.
7) Preschoolers experience less separation anxiety. Common fears are fear of the dark and of physical harm.
8) Preschoolers show improved verbal communication skills.
9) Preschoolers' gross and fine motor abilities continue to develop.
10) On average, preschoolers grow two to three inches in height and gain four to seven pounds each year.

School-age Children

1) Suitable activities for school-age children include sports, board games, computer games, and pet care.
2) By the age of 12, children have almost completely mastered their native language and vocabulary and are in the concrete operations stage of cognitive development.
3) School-age children gain four to ten pounds in weight each year and experience growth spurts. Puberty begins, which leads to the development of secondary sex characteristics.

4) School-age children may experience fears of the unknown, self-mutilation, death, and failure.

5) School-age children prefer peers of the same gender.

6) School-age children begin to question and criticize their parents.

7) School-age children require approximately 1,600 to 2,500 calories per day for girls and 2,000 to 3,000 calories per day for boys, dependent on age, gender, and level of physical activity. They need a balanced intake of all essential vitamins and minerals, such as vitamins A and B, iron, and calcium.

Adolescents

1) Common dangers for adolescents include substance abuse, injuries from firearms, burns, car accidents, sexually transmitted diseases, and unintended pregnancies.

2) Adolescents reach sexual maturity at various ages, and while many may be attracted to people of the opposite gender, it's important to recognize that others may be attracted to people of the same gender or be bisexual.

3) Adolescents will often seek acceptance from their peers and can sometimes exhibit unpredictable behavior or challenge authority figures.

4) The muscular and skeletal systems grow and develop significantly during adolescence, which results in increased nutritional and calorie demands. Protein, calcium, and vitamins are important.

5) Females may require an iron supplement due to menstruation, but this is not a universal requirement. It is recommended to seek medical advice on individual dietary needs. Some teenagers may experience eating disorders such as anorexia nervosa and bulimia.

Provide Care That Meets the Needs of Adult Clients Ages 18 Through 64 Years

Young Adults

1) STDs, drug misuse, injuries from weapons, and car accidents are common incidents in this age group.

2) Physical development is complete in young adults.

3) Common pressures for this age group include learning to manage responsibilities, finances, career, and starting a family.

4) Young adults take ownership of their thoughts, feelings, views, ideals, and actions.

5) Young adults maintain constant connections.

Middle-aged Adults

1) Health checks for this age group include Dexa testing for osteoporosis and eye exams for glaucoma.

2) Calcium and vitamin D supplements are necessary to prevent osteoporosis, which may develop due to menopause in middle-aged females.

3) Changes such as erectile dysfunction in males, menopause in females, a decline in sexual desire, and a deterioration in muscle strength may occur in middle-aged adults.

Provide Care That Meets the Needs of Adult Clients Ages 65 and Over

Older patients are more likely to have physiological changes that increase their risk of accidents.

Genitourinary Changes:

- Increased nocturia and incontinence episodes.

Sensory Changes:

- Cataracts and decreased eyesight may occur.
- The transmission of cold and hot sensations is delayed.
- Hearing becomes impaired, so high-frequency tones are less audible.

CNS Changes:

- Both voluntary and autonomic responses are slowed.
- There is a reduced capacity to react to many stimuli.

- There is reduced tactile sensitivity.

Musculoskeletal Changes:

- Muscle strength and function deteriorate.
- Bones become brittle, and joints lose their mobility.
- There is a restricted range of motion and alterations in posture.

Patients' Fall Risk

Assessment of Fall Risk:

The assessment of fall risks includes the patient's perceptions of their fall risk factors and how they have adapted to them. Areas of concern may involve eyesight, balance, coordination, muscular strength, stability, and gait. Check for any environmental concerns, such as higher toilet seats, grab bars, throw rugs, and stairs. Inquire about any recent incidents. Review the patient's medications for any side effects that may increase their risk of falls.

Fall Prevention Steps:

- Minimize bathroom hazards and maintain the patient's consistent daily routine.
- Ensure adequate lighting, especially soft lighting at night.
- Remove any obstructions from the patient's room.
- Keep the patient's personal belongings within reach.
- Lock the wheels on all beds, wheelchairs, and stretchers.
- Adjust the bed to a low position. Adhere to state and agency laws and procedures that pertain to the use of side rails.
- Encourage the patient to ask for help when they get up.
- Place any patient who is susceptible to falls in a room close to the nurses' station.

Measures to Encourage Patient Ambulation Safety:

A gait belt may be used to maintain the midline of the center of gravity.

- Before walking, secure the belt on the patient.

- Place the belt around the patient's waist.
- Hold onto the belt's side or rear to prevent the patient from leaning to one side.
- If the patient experiences vertigo or becomes unstable, return them to bed or a nearby chair.

Assist with Care for Postpartum Clients

Take a Patient's History

- Ask about recreational drug usage, alcohol use, smoking, exercise, diet, and nutrition.
- Obtain contact information for the patient's partner and any other individuals involved in the baby's care.
- Inquire about any health issues the patient's spouse or other family members have that may significantly impact the patient's health and well-being, the strength of her support system, or the condition of her family and home.
- Ask about any risks and concerns related to the patient's employment.
- Inquire about herbal therapies, dietary supplements, and over-the-counter medications the patient may be taking.
- Ask about any past or present mental health issues, such as a history of mental illness, severe anxiety, or depressive or anxious disorders.
- Obtain the patient's medical, obstetric, and family histories. If necessary, review the patient's previous medical records, such as those from other healthcare professionals.
- At the first prenatal check-up or at an appropriate time when the patient is alone, ask about domestic violence in a polite and sensitive manner.

Risk Assessment

- Determine which patients require further care.
- Review and reevaluate the pregnancy care plan.
- Provide the patient with a safe environment and opportunities to discuss issues such as mental health concerns, birth anxieties, or domestic violence.

- Inquire about the patient's overall health and well-being.
- Add medications, examination results, test results, and historical information to the patient's prenatal records.

Pregnant Patient Information and Assistance

Information should be:

- Evidence-based and consistent.
- Positive and respectful.
- Personalized and thoughtful.
- Provided throughout the patient's care.
- Accessible through various formats such as Braille, easy-read, digital, or printed content.
- Supported by group discussions (including partners or patients only).
- Offered in one-on-one or paired sessions.

Information about prenatal care should include:

- Contact information for regional or international peer support programs during the first prenatal consultation.
- Support services and resources that are available for new and expecting parents.
- Safe use of prescription drugs, nutritional supplements, and herbal therapies during pregnancy.
- Measures to reduce the risk of illnesses, such as handwashing.
- Information on immunizations for flu, pertussis (whooping cough), and other illnesses (including COVID-19) during pregnancy.
- Anticipated changes in the patient's relationship with their partner and how they can support each other throughout the pregnancy.
- Physical, emotional, and mental changes that occur during pregnancy.

- What to expect at each stage of pregnancy.
- The baby's development during pregnancy.
- The importance and benefits of screening initiatives, available blood tests, and ultrasound exams.
- How to contact the maternity service for immediate concerns such as pain and bleeding.
- Who to contact for non-urgent guidance from the midwifery team.
- Which medical personnel will attend prenatal visits.
- The location and expected number of prenatal visits.
- The importance of prenatal care and its significance.
- Advice on the use of recreational drugs, smoking, alcohol consumption, physical exercise, and nutrition. Alcohol consumption during pregnancy may cause long-term damage to the baby. Emphasize that no safe amount of alcohol use during pregnancy is known, so it is safest to avoid alcohol completely to minimize risks to the unborn child.

Provide information after 28 weeks on:

- Postnatal mental health and awareness of mood changes.
- Pelvic floor exercises after a person gives birth.
- Newborn examination.
- Infant feeding options.
- Infant care.
- Preparation for labor and delivery, such as coping strategies for labor pains and birth plan considerations.

Monitor Clients in Labor

Initial Evaluation

The initial evaluation may be delayed until the patient enters active labor or when a risk factor is identified. Low-risk factors include no medical or obstetrical complications, vertex presentation, absence of meconium, Category I electronic fetal monitoring strip on admission, appropriate estimated fetal weight for gestational age, and 37–41 weeks gestation.

The physician's first assessment and record in labor and delivery should include:

- Delivery plans.
- Fetal status, such as interpretation of auscultation or electronic fetal monitoring strip. This must be done for any fetus who has reached 24 weeks or more of development. Record fetal heart rate and uterine contractions until the classification of fetal heart rate tracing is established.
- Description of fetal presentation, cervical dilation and effacement, membrane status, and uterine activity in the labor state.
- Patient's previous pregnancies.

Initial Phase of Labor

If the first fetal heart rate tracing shows a Category I trace and there are no risk factors, continuous fetal heart rate monitoring is not necessary.

During the active stage of labor, the fetal heart rate should be monitored and recorded at least every 30 minutes based on the patient's risk status. Fetal heart rate should be measured after a natural rupture of the membranes or right after an artificial rupture.

The fetal heart rate should be monitored continuously for patients over 42 weeks, those with significant vaginal bleeding, meconium-stained amniotic fluid, atypical second-stage labor, use of oxytocin, unsatisfactory fetal evaluation, multiple pregnancies, history of previous cesarean birth, or breech presentation.

Each patient assessment must include:

- Preparation for healthcare treatments and pain management.
- Description of vaginal exam results, such as progression since the previous exam, membrane status, fetal stage, and cervical dilation and effacement.

- Uterine contractions.

Second Stage of Labor:

Documentation must be time- and date-stamped and include:

- Evaluation of delivery strategy and progression.
- Fetal position and station.
- Uterine contractions.
- Fetal and maternal status, with fetal heart rate checked and recorded at least every 15 minutes based on the patient's risk status.

Delivery

Fetal monitoring should be set up in the room where the patient will give birth. Patients who will have a cesarean birth should be monitored for as long as possible until the abdominal region is ready for surgery.

In cases of concern about the fetal condition at birth, a double-clamped piece of the umbilical cord should be kept for possible arterial blood gas analysis if the Apgar score is low. Blood may be taken from the clamped cord shortly after delivery as long as it remains undisturbed.

Monitor Recovery of Stable Postpartum Clients

After delivery, the healthcare provider must thoroughly document all delivery-related events in the medical record. Once the patient is stable and the immediate (30-minute) postpartum period has passed, the clinician should return to the unit.

The postpartum period, which lasts for 12 weeks after childbirth, is important for both the patient and the infant's well-being. Early postpartum visits should assess for common postpartum medical issues as well as any pregnancy-related complications. The recommended postpartum visit schedule includes appointments at three days, 7–14 days, 6 weeks, and 12 weeks.

Postpartum Complications

1) Weight retention.

Postpartum weight loss can be facilitated through nutritional counseling or a combination of dietary changes and exercise.

2) Constipation and hemorrhoids.

Pushing during the second stage of labor may lead to hemorrhoids. Oral iron supplements during pregnancy might also play a role. Increased fiber and water intake, along with osmotic laxatives, are the initial treatments.

3) Urinary incontinence.

Pelvic floor muscle exercises, weight management, fluid regulation, and bladder training can alleviate symptoms of urinary incontinence.

4) Depression.

It is recommended to conduct one or more postpartum depression screening tests. Preventative counseling is also suggested for patients at high risk of prenatal depression, which includes those with healthcare or financial challenges, unintended pregnancies, relationship abuse, or a history of depression.

5) Thyroid disease.

Postpartum hyperthyroidism is temporary and usually does not require medical intervention. Hypothyroidism is treated with thyroid hormone therapy. Patients with a history of Graves' disease are more susceptible to postpartum relapses, which can be differentiated from postpartum thyroiditis by the presence of positive antibodies to thyroid-stimulating hormone receptors. It is essential to monitor the growth and development of breastfeeding babies whose mothers are receiving thyroid treatment.

6) Hypertension.

Follow-up blood pressure monitoring is vital, and any signs of end-organ damage should be investigated. Antihypertensive medications are prescribed, and in cases of end-organ damage, hospitalization and parenteral magnesium sulfate therapy may be necessary.

7) Thromboembolism.

Patients with a history of thromboembolism should receive anticoagulation medication for at least the first six weeks postpartum, and possibly longer if other risk factors are present. Warfarin is safe for nursing mothers as it is not excreted in breast milk.

8) Endometritis.

Patients who experience fever, tachycardia, vaginal discharge, or uterine pain during the postpartum period should be evaluated for endometritis. Risk factors include chorioamnionitis and prolonged membrane rupture. Intravenous antibiotics, such as gentamicin and clindamycin, are used for treatment.

9) Secondary postpartum hemorrhage.

Common causes of vaginal bleeding beyond 24 hours postpartum include infection and retained placental tissue. Ultrasonography is used to examine any remaining placental tissue, and treatment includes uterine curettage, uterotonic drugs, and antibiotics to address endometritis.

Identify Community Resources for Clients

Community resources have a significant impact on the health outcomes of individuals with complex needs. These clients require support in areas such as transportation, income, food security, and housing, which are beyond the scope of medical procedures. It is important to connect patients with relevant community services to address these needs effectively.

How to Identify Community Resources

1) Incorporate community resource recommendations into the clinical process through the use of automated clinician prompts.

2) Determine which team members will be responsible for introducing patients to local services, such as social workers.

3) Plan how referrals to neighborhood services will be funded. Utilize flexible funds or working relationships with payers to cover services outside the health system.

4) Prioritize collaborations with community resources that target the most important and prevalent issues in your area.

5) Engage patients and their families to identify critical social needs, create a list of local services, and select the most suitable options for them.

6) Follow up with patients to ensure they were able to access assistance. Update the list of local options based on their feedback.

7) Evaluate the requirements and support network of each patient to ensure eligibility and accessibility to referred resources based on their location.

8) Establish partnerships with community services to facilitate seamless handoffs.

9) Compile a comprehensive list of community resources in your area, such as address, phone number, and availability to share with patients.

Collect Data for Health History

A complete medical history can pinpoint important chronic conditions and past diseases that may not be actively treated but can have long-term effects on the patient's health.

The medical history includes questions about allergies, social background, family medical history, past surgical procedures, and current medications.

1) Tailor the questions for medical history based on the patient's age and gender. For instance, ask parents of newborns about birth, pregnancy, and immunization history, while age-appropriate inquiries for female patients should include their recent menstrual history and history of pregnancies (gravidity and parity).

2) Verify the patient's current medication to avoid drug interactions.

3) Patient allergies should be noted as they can have severe implications.

4) Inquire about the patient's social history, such as drug, alcohol, and smoking habits, as well as sexual behavior, interests, jobs, relationships, and mental and spiritual well-being.

5) Family history can provide insights into any hereditary predisposition to certain illnesses.

6) Include details of any past surgical procedures in the patient's history.

7) Thoroughly investigate the patient's medical conditions, such as current and previous illnesses, which may have an extended impact on their health.

Collect Baseline Physical Data

Before the start of any form of therapy, it is essential to gather baseline physical data to better understand clients' health status.

Initial Physical Data

1) Record the first vital sign readings, such as BMI, weight in kilograms, pulse oximetry on room air, blood pressure with an appropriate-sized cuff, pulse rate, respiration rate, urine output, and temperature in Celsius.

2) Assess the general psychological and emotional condition of the client.

3) Observe body and breath odor.

4) Evaluate personal hygiene.

5) Assess the patient's overall state of health.

Secondary Physical Data

1) Examine the skin for color (reddish, pale, cyanotic, jaundiced, mottled, flushed), warmth, coolness, diaphoresis, integrity, and turgor.

2) Inspect the skin for any signs of chronic wounds or breakdown.

3) Evaluate the neuromuscular system by assessing swallowing abilities, gait stability, regular extremities movement, pupil reactivity, speech, Glasgow coma scale, and level of consciousness.

4) Inquire about urinary health, such as any issues with catheterization, hesitation, frequency, painful urination, itching, rashes, history of hysterectomy, menopause, last menstrual cycle, vaginal hemorrhage, or discharge.

5) Check for abdominal scars, lumps, discomfort, vomiting, weight changes, hunger, consistency and type of stool, and bowel sounds. Use the stethoscope's diaphragm to listen for bowel sounds in each quadrant, moving clockwise from the lower right quadrant.

6) Assess respiratory symptoms such as dyspnea, chest symmetry, retractions, gasps, agonal breathing, shallow breathing, type of sputum, coughing, breathing patterns, and breath sounds.

7) Evaluate cardiovascular health by assessing pulse, heartbeat, cyanosis, edema, swelling, capillary refill time, and extremity temperature.

8) If applicable, assess for a thrill or bruit in the presence of a fistula for hemodialysis and note its presence or absence.

9) Be vigilant for any signs of abuse or mistreatment.

Identify Barriers to Communication

Communication barriers can arise due to various factors that prevent effective and clear communication between individuals.

Cultural Differences

Differences in cultures and traditions can lead to varied communication habits, which affect how people work, speak, eat, and dress. Respect for cultural diversity is important to overcome these barriers.

Physical Barriers

Environmental factors, such as communication tools that malfunction, locked doors, and noise, can create physical barriers to communication. The use of modern technology and effective tools can help mitigate these challenges.

Emotional Barriers

The emotions and mental state of both the sender and receiver can influence how a message is perceived and conveyed. Emotional intelligence plays a vital role in effective communication, and the management of emotions like irritation, humor, fear, and anger is essential.

Psychological Barriers

The receiver's mental state can affect how they interpret and respond to messages. Factors like low self-esteem, speech difficulties, phobias, and depression may hinder effective communication and require careful consideration and support.

Language Barriers

One significant communication barrier is the inability of the recipient to understand the sender's language. Even when both parties speak the same language, the use of specialized jargon or technical terms can cause confusion if the recipient is unfamiliar with it.

Identify Barriers to Learning

In any workplace, continuous learning is essential for employees to keep up with changes and progress in their careers. However, there are several barriers to effective learning:

1) Reluctance to learn.

Some employees may resist stepping out of their comfort zones to the point where they reject new skills and hinder their own growth and development.

2) Resistance to change.

When employees are required to take on new responsibilities, resistance to change can impede their willingness to embrace new knowledge and skills.

3) Lack of motivation.

Lack of motivation can arise from unimportant job tasks, lack of support from management, conflicts with superiors or colleagues, office politics, and inadequate compensation.

4) Lack of creativity.

Stale and unoriginal learning materials can discourage employees, particularly those with extensive industry knowledge, from full participation in the learning process.

5) Fear of failure.

The fear of failure can negatively impact an employee's mindset, making them feel unmotivated. This may impair their ability to retain and understand new information.

6) Past unsatisfactory training.

Negative experiences with previous training sessions can create barriers to learning, which further highlights the need for concise, relevant, and effective learning materials.

7) Lack of confidence.

Low confidence can hinder an employee's flexibility and confidence when it comes to learning assignments and exercises.

8) Environmental factors.

Unfavorable environmental conditions, such as extreme humidity, cold temperatures, noisy workplaces, or inadequate facilities, can impede the learning process.

9) Physical and mental health.

Poor physical and mental health can significantly impact an employee's ability to comprehend and acquire essential information, which may affect their learning experience.

Address these barriers and foster a supportive learning environment to ensure more effective and successful learning outcomes for employees.

Compare Clients to Developmental Milestones

Nurses identify, document, and communicate any deviations from normal growth and development in clients. They also assess how anticipated body image changes affect the patient's quality of life and ability to carry out daily activities. The primary expected physical changes encompass puberty, pregnancy, menopause, and aging.

Adapt Management Strategies

Physical treatments are tailored based on the client's age and developmental stage. For example:

1) Administer IM injections in the vastus lateralis muscle for babies.

2) Use pictorial pain assessment tools instead of numerical scales for young children and for older individuals with cognitive impairments.

3) Use touch with young children.

4) Provide patient education to parents or legal guardians.

5) Offer safe and nontoxic toys to avoid aspiration and respiratory obstructions in babies and young children.

Additionally, body image changes can have social and emotional effects. Clients should be supported by the medical team to adjust to these changes, adopt healthy lifestyle choices, set realistic expectations, maintain social relationships, and enhance their self-esteem.

Assist Clients with Expected Life Transitions

Clients need to navigate and adapt to various life changes throughout their lives, such as adolescence, pregnancy, parenthood, and retirement. Life transitions can be difficult for several reasons:

1) Transitions like pandemics or job losses may not have been planned for.

2) Different life transitions can cause both eustress, which motivates growth, and prolonged stress, which may have negative effects on physical and mental well-being.

3) A new routine, even if it is positive, may require some effort to adjust to.

4) Support and guidance from healthcare professionals can help clients cope with life transitions and promote their overall well-being during these periods of change.

Manage Life Transitions

Healthcare workers support patients as they navigate life's changes and transitions. Some ways they can assist include:

1) Provide new parents with newborn care classes to help them handle the challenges of infant care and establish a bond with their baby.

2) Identify community resources that can offer transportation assistance to retired or elderly individuals who must attend medical appointments.

3) Encourage clients to develop compassion.

4) Advise clients to set manageable, targeted goals and tackle them one at a time rather than address everything at once.

5) Support clients in how they monitor their inner self-talk.

6) Guide clients to establish realistic standards and create new habits to facilitate positive transitions.

7) Recommend therapy for clients who experience significant difficulties in communication, work, or mood due to life shifts.

Identify Clients in Need of Immunizations

Active immunity is achieved when the host's immune system generates antibodies in response to infection or vaccination, while passive immunity involves the injection of antibodies produced elsewhere.

Certain groups, such as individuals treated with certain types of corticosteroid treatment or those with compromised immune systems, should take precautions when they receive vaccines, and specific vaccines may be contraindicated. However, most vaccines are safe and recommended for pregnant patients, with exceptions based on their health conditions and advice from healthcare providers.

Vaccinations

1) Hepatitis A: Two doses between 12 and 23 months. Immunity develops 15 days after a single dose.

2) Pneumococcal polysaccharide: Recommended for all adults 65 years and older and individuals aged two years and older with certain medical conditions, who are immunocompromised, or who have a cardiopulmonary illness.

3) Pneumococcal conjugate: Given at two, four, and six months, with a booster dose between 12 and 15 months.

4) Influenza: Recommended annually for medical professionals, nursing home residents, seniors, or patients with cardiopulmonary conditions.

5) BCG: Used in regions with widespread TB but not commonly used in the United States.

6) Varicella: Administered between 12 and 18 months and again between four and six years.

7) MMR (measles, mumps, rubella): Administered once between 12 and 18 months and again between four and six years. It may be given together with DTaP and IPV.

8) IPV (inactivated polio vaccine): Given at two and four months of age, with a booster between 6 and 18 months and four and six years.

9) Haemophilus influenzae B conjugate: Administered at ages two, four, and six months, with another dose between 15 and 18 months.

10) Rotavirus: Given at two, four, and six months.

11) DTaP (diphtheria, tetanus, and pertussis): Initial series of three doses at two, four, and six months, followed by boosters at 18 months and four to six years. Td (tetanus, diphtheria) every 10 years beginning between 11 and 13 years.

12) Hepatitis B: Administered at birth, one month after birth, and six months after delivery. Adults at risk receive two doses spaced one month apart, with a third dose six months after the first.

Vaccine Serums for Passive Immunity

1) Administer hepatitis B immune globulin within seven days after exposure and again 28 days later.

2) Nonimmunized individuals exposed to measles, polio, or chicken pox receive immune serum globulins prophylactically after exposure to any of these diseases.

3) Tetanus immunoglobulin is used if the wound has been open for more than 24 hours or if the patient has not received more than two doses of tetanus toxoid injections before. It is more durable than an antitoxin.

Participate in Health Screening or Health Promotion Programs

Recommendations for screening are based on recognized pathophysiology, such as risk factors for specific illnesses and disorders based on the patient's age, medical history, and family history.

Health Screening Programs

1) Breast cancer screening.

Women over 40 should have a mammogram every one to two years. More frequent screenings may be necessary for women with palpable breast lumps or a personal/family history of breast cancer.

2) Depression screening.

This is conducted based on the client's needs.

3) Colorectal cancer screening.

Though colorectal cancer screening is recommended for both sexes starting at age 50, earlier, more frequent screening may be advised based on pathological risk factors.

4) Chlamydial infection screening.

Sexually active women aged 25 and younger, as well as older women who have risk factors such as new or multiple sex partners, should receive regular chlamydial infection screenings.

Nurses assist, prepare, and advise clients during screening exams. They verify and follow up on test results such as colonoscopies, Pap smears, occult blood stool tests, or mammograms. Results are communicated to the patient's physician and documented in the medical file per institutional norms and procedures.

Screening Risk Programs Associated with Ethnicity

Research is ongoing about how ethnicity affects risk factors. Although correlations between certain races and illnesses may exist, they might not necessarily indicate a causative connection. Genetic anomalies and patterns may pose risks for certain illnesses, but other factors can help prevent them.

Targeted Screening Assessments

In addition to regular and recommended testing, some screenings are targeted at individuals who are at risk for specific ailments or diseases. Specialized tests may be conducted to check for nutritional, auditory, and visual abnormalities in clients at risk in order to rule out potential impairments.

For example:

1) When a parent reports that their toddler is not responding to their name, a targeted screening for auditory acuity may be performed.

2) Nutritional status may be assessed when a baby or young child does not gain weight per established standards.

3) Visual acuity screening may also be conducted on a teenager.

Provide Information for the Prevention of High-risk Behaviors

Registered nurses evaluate their patients' lifestyle habits, such as lack of sleep, unprotected sex, illegal drug usage, alcohol consumption, smoking, poor nutrition, irregular exercise habits, and excessive sun exposure. Individuals can make changes to reduce or avoid risks associated with lifestyle choices.

High-risk Behavior Prevention

Nurses not only help clients identify high-risk behaviors but also provide instruction and guidance on how to modify or stop these dangerous behaviors. For instance, they can:

1) Refer the client to a local smoking cessation program.

2) Educate the client about the link between fatigue, illness, and accidents.

3) Emphasize the importance of calcium and how a deficiency can lead to osteoporosis and other nutritional deficiencies.

4) Promote safe sexual practices to prevent STDs such as HIV.

Nurses offer written and verbal advice to their patients about the management and prevention of high-risk health behaviors based on their individual needs.

Chapter 4: Psychosocial Integrity

Reinforce Education for Caregivers/Family on the Management of Clients with Behavioral Disorders

Caregivers, families, and friends play a vital role as support systems for clients when psychiatric illnesses require behavior management. These supports should provide compassionate care, encourage the patient to adopt healthy habits, and educate the client on how to prevent and defuse problematic behaviors.

<u>Clients with Behavioral Health Concerns</u>

1) Establish a routine to promote behavioral activation.

Behavioral activation is a method used to treat depression in which engagement in enjoyable activities is increased while avoidance and isolation are reduced. Caregivers can help the patient create a depression cycle on paper, plan behaviors, and monitor the patient's emotions before and after engaging in planned activities. Patients often recognize that physical activity contributes to their happiness, which leads to a positive cycle of pleasurable activities, improved social relationships, and an overall enhanced quality of life.

2) Teach deep breathing techniques.

Deep breathing techniques can effectively reduce anxiety, sadness, and general life stress. Caregivers can teach patients a four-count breathing method, which can also be used to treat insomnia before bedtime. For some patients, practices like meditation, prayer, and mindfulness can also be beneficial.

3) Encourage gratitude.

Assist patients to focus on gratitude can be beneficial, starting with recalling minor instances of happiness, such as a good meal, a child's laughter, or a stranger's smile. This practice is particularly helpful for patients with depression and anxiety.

4) Encourage regular check-ins with healthcare providers.

Regular check-ins with a healthcare provider can offer valuable support. This is a safe space where patients can openly discuss their distress and receive nonjudgmental support. The frequency of visits should be based on the healthcare provider's recommendation and the patient's needs.

5) Promote the use of social support.

Social networks, such as friends, family, support groups, and religious organizations, can provide significant support to the patient. Isolated patients may not effectively utilize social resources. Caregivers can help provide relevant contact information or websites.

6) Be present and empathetic.

Show genuine empathy, empower patients by inquiring about their past triumphs over similar challenges, listen without judgment, and use appropriate physical contact and open body language.

7) Respect autonomy.

Respect patients' ability to make choices, even if you disagree with them. Accept their preferences and do not micromanage their decisions.

8) Engage in shared interests.

Participate in activities patients enjoy to foster a sense of connection and support. This will help them steer clear of negative thoughts or emotions. Activities like sports, walks, or music can be beneficial.

9) Create a safe environment.

Remove potential triggers and offer patients a sense of control. This could involve modifications to their environment, like safely storing items that could be used for self-harm, such as knives and sharp objects.

10) Educate yourself on mental health.

Nurses should familiarize themselves with the client's specific condition, symptoms, medications, possible side effects, and how best to provide support.

Incorporate Behavioral Management Techniques

Nurses utilize various techniques and interventions to help clients to develop self-control over their behavior. Reward positive behavior, help them set achievable goals, and establish clear boundaries.

Behavior management techniques include aversion treatment, operant conditioning, contraction, behavior modification, desensitization, and modeling.

1) Aversion treatment is employed when a client exhibits unsuitable behaviors.

2) Operant conditioning rewards desirable behaviors with praise.

3) Contracting requires the creation of a formal, written, and signed agreement that outlines the patient's rights and responsibilities.

4) Behavior modification is a planned and methodical intervention that seeks to alter the patient's behaviors with consistent rewards for good behavior. It discourages undesirable, maladaptive behavior.

5) Desensitization involves intentionally and gradually exposing the patient to stronger stimuli to foster coping mechanisms.

6) Modeling provides the client with opportunities to observe, imitate, and practice appropriate behaviors.

Preventive strategies should be tailored to the client's needs. These include the encouragement of suitable socialization and leisure activities, pet therapy, music therapy, physical activity, the maintenance of regular routines, and the promotion of stress management and relaxation methods.

In cases of aggressive behavior, multidisciplinary therapies may involve medications like olanzapine, ziprasidone, and haloperidol. Additionally, rewards may be offered when clients make efforts to regulate their behavior. Restraint is considered a last resort when other methods have failed, with a focus on eye contact and staying at the same level as the client.

The creation of a stress-free environment is preferable to avoid negative behaviors. Milieu therapy involves planned and methodical modifications to the patient's surroundings while maintaining a therapeutic alliance.

Each instance of inappropriate or risky behavior is addressed and discussed with clients, which facilitates their understanding of how to prevent recurrence. The clients also learn how to prevent future incidents and how to communicate with staff about any issues. The development and maintenance of better self-control are emphasized.

Thorough documentation is essential. Actions taken to address improper and hazardous behavior, duration, location, and potential causes should all be recorded.

Participate in Reminiscence Therapy, Validation Therapy, or Reality Orientation

Reminiscence Therapy

Reminiscence therapy is a form of psychotherapy where patients recall past experiences, which helps them feel better about themselves, boosts self-esteem, and provides comfort, especially for elderly patients. Nurses can use this approach as a part of their care plan to help clients recreate memories from their history. It is essential that nurses listen actively and offer positive responses.

Though talk therapy involves reminiscence, it goes beyond just talk. Here are some techniques:

1) Use scented candles or perfumes to evoke memories, as smells can trigger strong mental and emotional associations.

2) Encourage clients to touch items from their past, like old sweaters, high school sports trophies, or favorite jewelry. Familiar objects can provide comfort.

3) Prepare a client's favorite dishes and discuss their childhood memories related to these delicacies.

4) Watch old family films, look through picture albums and mementos, and discuss journals, letters, and magazine clippings with open-ended questions to jog their memory.

5) Play music from a client's favorite bands or artists they enjoyed in their youth. Music therapy can have various benefits. It can reduce blood pressure, prevent depression, and improve immunity.

Participate in Validation Therapy

Validation therapy is a form of therapeutic communication that helps caregivers connect with individuals who experience moderate to advanced dementia. It emphasizes emotional aspects over factual ones and respects the individual's emotions and views.

The key principles of validation therapy are:

1) Use neutral, factual language when you communicate with patients.

2) Maintain a calm, kind, and loving voice.

3) Avoid arguments with patients, as reasoning may be a challenge for them, which could lead to frustration and anger.

4) Music can be a powerful tool to transport patients to different places and times. Even when they cannot talk, individuals with dementia may still sing songs they remember.

5) Maintain eye contact to make patients feel safe and valued.

6) Use gentle touch if the person appreciates physical contact, but ensure it doesn't invade their personal space.

7) Share your memories with patients, particularly situations they resolved in the past. Although they may not acquire new coping mechanisms, recalling past successful strategies can help them cope with present challenges.

Set aside your emotions and frustrations to listen empathetically and deal with your own feelings later.

Both reminiscence therapy and validation therapy can offer valuable support to individuals with specific cognitive or emotional needs.

Reality Orientation

Reality orientation was inspired by a method used with injured soldiers to encourage them to interact and feel a connection with their environment. It is a method in which the dialogue with the subject constantly makes mention of the environment, which includes the present surroundings, places, and dates.

The tools for reality orientation seek to reinforce the naming of objects and people. This is done through the discussion of recent events, the frequent use of people's names, old photographs and memorabilia, signs on doors, regular references to calendars and clocks, and the discussion of orientation, such as the day, time of day, date, and season.

To help someone who has dementia-related confusion, reality orientation must be combined with compassion and carefully considered. If the process is applied without due consideration of whether it would be suitable for the specific patient, this could result in emotional anguish.

Participate in Client Group Sessions

Nurses encourage patients to participate in group therapy sessions, both as active members and facilitators. Group discussions provide a safe space for individuals to share their experiences, concerns, and thoughts with others. These sessions offer a chance for patients to feel supported. They also provide valuable feedback to the person sharing their thoughts.

Group therapy can take various forms, such as peer support groups for specific illnesses or age-based groups for adults, young adults, teenagers, children, or the elderly. These sessions focus on areas like physical health, mental illness, substance abuse, or stress management.

Groups can be homogenous, made up of individuals of the same gender, or heterogeneous, which includes members of both genders regardless of their psychiatric conditions. Some groups accept new members as others leave, while some remain closed to new participants.

Collect Data about Clients' Psychosocial Functions

Nurses gather information about a client's psychosocial state by observing psychomotor behaviors, mood, appearance, and changes in characteristics. They also assess if there are any potentially dangerous behaviors that need attention.

The patient's appearance, grooming, hygiene, gait, and posture are observed for any noticeable changes.

Mood is assessed through verbal and nonverbal communication, such as signs of being flat, depressed, sad, somber, elated, or happy. Unusual psychomotor movements, sounds, grimaces, or eye contact may indicate the patient's mood.

The client's state of awareness and cognition is also evaluated, which can range from comatose, stupefied, lethargic, and confused to fully awake.

Awake patients can follow directions and respond appropriately. Comatose patients show no response to any stimuli. Lethargic clients respond slowly to forceful stimuli. Drowsy yet alert patients may be roused by verbal or physical cues. Confused patients require cues to respond to directions and questions.

Other states of consciousness include brain death, locked-in syndrome, and persistent vegetative state. Brain death is characterized by the loss of all brainstem reflexes and functions, which includes the cessation of respiratory function, with no response to any stimuli, and the coma being irreversible. Locked-in syndrome patients have limited motor function but retain some cognitive function. The persistent vegetative state is marked by minimal cognitive function and only eye-opening and eye-closing as essential human functions.

The client's ability to abstract, the quality of their speech, and their short-term, intermediate-term, and long-term memory, as well as orientation to time, place, and person, all contribute to the assessment of their cognitive level.

The Mini-Mental State exam is used to evaluate the client's cognition, which involves their ability to follow instructions, communicate effectively, recognize common items, and perform basic arithmetic calculations.

Identify Clients' Use of Effective and Ineffective Coping Mechanisms

Coping mechanisms are strategies used by individuals to deal with stress and unpleasant emotions. They can be classified into adaptive (effective) and maladaptive (ineffective) coping techniques. Adaptive coping involves the identification of the source of stress and positive action taken to address it, while maladaptive coping occurs when the individual avoids or ignores the stressor.

Different Coping Techniques

Examples of adaptive coping strategies include aromatherapy, reading, taking a bath, positive thinking, conversations with a friend, writing, exercise, meditation, and deep breathing. Maladaptive coping strategies are unhelpful in the reduction of stress and include self-isolation, negative thoughts, binge eating, despair, self-harm, the neglect of daily responsibilities, issue avoidance, outbursts of rage, drug use, and excessive alcohol consumption.

Coping Methods

Two commonly used methods of stress management are problem-focused coping and emotion-focused coping.

Problem-Focused Coping: This approach is effective when the client has some control over the stressful situation. It involves taking action to reduce or eliminate the stressor. Examples include how to problem-solve, set boundaries, seek counseling, change jobs, enroll in problem-solving courses, get regular exercise, and consult with a healthcare professional about prescription alternatives.

Emotion-Focused Coping: When the client has little or no control over the cause of stress, emotion-focused coping techniques can help change the emotional response to stress. Examples include a support group, mindfulness practices, focused concentration on the present moment, and deep breathing exercises.

Recognize Stressors that Affect Client Care

The stress response can lead to physiological changes such as hyperglycemia, heightened senses, increased alertness, hypertension, tachycardia, and tachypnea. Though these changes are beneficial in dangerous situations, they are only meant to be short term. Prolonged stress can lead to a range of issues, such as loss of interest in activities, depression, anxiety, unhappiness, rashes, body pain, headaches, stomach discomfort, changes in appetite, and sleep disturbances.

To identify client stresses:

1) Observe the patient's coping mechanisms for daily stress, which include the use of music, religion, hobbies, exercise, support networks, crafts, and communication.

2) Look for unhealthy coping techniques such as smoking or the use of sedatives, alcohol, or illicit substances.

3) Pay attention to nonverbal signs of stress, such as being easily distracted, fidgety, irritable, or withdrawn.

4) Assess patients for personal stresses, such as relationship changes, recent losses, feeling overwhelmed with childcare or work responsibilities, anxiety about medical procedures or treatments, and coping with a new diagnosis.

5) Evaluate patients' perceptions of the circumstances. They may not have a realistic understanding of the stressful situation and might react emotionally. It is essential to educate and support patients in coping.

6) Identify the patients' support network and available resources. Patients may feel less overwhelmed in the face of a difficult situation when they have support from family, caregivers, and community resources.

Assist Clients to Cope/Adapt to Stressful Events and Changes in Health Status

1) Promote rest and exercise to manage stress and its impact on existing medical conditions, such as hypertension, tachycardia, and hyperglycemia. Exercise raises endorphin levels and reduces cortisol levels, which helps to alleviate stress.

2) Offer an objective perspective to help patients recognize behaviors that hinder successful coping and support them so they can make necessary changes.

3) Involve patients in treatment decisions and provide them with options to take an active role in their care and regain a sense of control.

4) Explore past challenges the patients have overcome and discuss how they can apply problem-solving and decision-making skills to their current situation.

5) Provide comprehensive information about procedures, disease processes, and future actions, which empowers patients to feel more in control of their treatment.

6) Use therapeutic communication techniques, such as open-ended questions, reflecting, and active listening.

7) Identify the specific stressors that affect a client. Understand the sources of stress to allow for the application of adaptive coping strategies.

8) Assess clients' current coping mechanisms to determine if they are adaptive or maladaptive and observe how they handle stress.

9) Encourage clients to explore various coping techniques before they settle on those that work best for them.

10) Integrate coping mechanisms into the client's daily routine, such as setting aside time for deep breathing or meditation.

11) Offer assistance in the development of healthy coping mechanisms or the elimination of unhealthy ones, which may involve the recommendation of therapy or counseling.

Collect Data on Clients' Potential for Violence to Self and Others

To prevent violence such as suicide or harm to others, nurses must have a comprehensive understanding of their patients, including risk factors and warning signs associated with such actions. This knowledge enables proper care and supervision of patients at risk for violent behaviors.

Acts of violence can be categorized into violence toward others and violence toward oneself.

Violence Toward Others

Risk factors for violence toward others may include changes in body language and posture, hyperactivity, hallucinations, paranoid delusions, history of violence toward animals, personal or family history of violent acts, neglect, abuse, and substance abuse or addiction.

Violence Against Oneself

Risk factors for violence against oneself may include severe physical illness, prior suicide attempts, interpersonal relationship difficulties, employment problems, personal or family history of violent acts, neglect, abuse, substance abuse or addiction, personal history of psychiatric illness, and history of depression.

Assessment and Data Collection

During a crisis assessment, information about the client is gathered, with a particular focus on the identification of any potential risk for violence.

Signs of Suicide Risk in Clients:

Some signs that indicate suicide risk in clients include improvement in depression, expressed threats of suicide, self-harming behaviors, sleep disturbances, changes in appearance, feelings of shame and guilt, loss of interest, giving away possessions, verbal or written statements about suicide, and saying goodbye.

It is essential to understand that the apparent improvement in a client's mood does not necessarily mean the depression has subsided or that the risk of suicide has diminished. It could also indicate that the client has decided to carry out their suicide plan.

Assist in the Care of Angry or Agitated Clients

1) De-escalation techniques are used to manage potentially angry or violent situations through effective communication and body language. These actions diffuse irritation and anger. Use the patient's name, communicate calmly with visible hands, a relaxed posture and expression, and keep a distance of about two arm's lengths. Other de-escalation tactics the caregiver may use are to show respect, not respond to inappropriate questions, treat others with dignity, outline consequences for behavior, avoid debates, be comfortable with silence, and refrain from the use of medical jargon.

2) Encourage agitated clients to set new priorities and allow them to reevaluate and manage their concerns to gain a better perspective on the situation.

3) Practice mindfulness to help clients gain insight into the world and immediate surroundings, which will reduce anxiety.

4) Biofeedback involves the connection of external electrodes to monitor the patient's bodily responses like breathing, body temperature, pulse rate, and heart rate in reaction to various stimuli. Patients can observe how their internal body

control influences these responses to stress after they engage in different relaxation techniques.

5) Maintain a diary to capture and track thoughts and feelings, which includes events or interactions that trigger specific emotions, to allow for later analysis of patterns or trends.

6) Utilize validation therapy to help patients resolve conflicts and issues by showing that you relate to and empathize with their feelings.

7) Use music therapy as a relaxation technique, either alone or in combination with other methods.

8) Engage in memory therapy. Help clients share personal biographies, memories, and life stories with others to develop a sense of value and self-esteem.

9) Practice meditation and use guided imagery to visualize peaceful scenes and thoughts.

10) Try progressive relaxation, in which patients sequentially contract and release muscle groups in the body.

11) Incorporate deep breathing exercises in which patients take a deep breath, hold it briefly, and exhale gently. They should focus on positive thoughts while they do this.

12) Employ cognitive reframing to teach patients how to intentionally replace negative thoughts and impulses with positive ones.

Plan Care with Consideration of Clients' Spiritual and Cultural Beliefs and/or Gender Identity

Spiritual and Cultural Support

Medical ethics have been influenced by religion, societal change, gender identity, and the attitudes of both healthcare practitioners and patients. Spiritual and cultural support in medical treatment is vital, as diverse religious groups have unique beliefs that apply to healthcare. Religious perspectives encompass pain, grief, and death, and many individuals strongly adhere to their religious traditions.

Healthcare practitioners must recognize the importance of religious beliefs during times of illness and death and must respect these beliefs. Various religions have different funeral rites and beliefs.

1) Catholicism: Embraces Sacrament of the Sick, infant baptisms, fasting, and the eucharist in funeral rites.

2) Jehovah's Witnesses: Discourages the use of illegal substances, tobacco, excessive alcohol, and gambling. Jehovah's Witnesses consider life to be sacred. Thus, suicide and abortion are generally viewed as incompatible with this belief. Premarital and extramarital sex are considered sinful. Although they do not categorically condemn homosexuality, Jehovah's Witnesses expect those who identify as such to remain celibate. They are known for their refusal to accept blood transfusions.

3) Mormonism: Mormon beliefs include Jesus Christ, funerals, communion, baptism, and death forgiveness, with abstinence from alcohol, cigarettes, and caffeine.

4) Islam: Practices include corpses being covered in white fabric and positioned toward Mecca, women taking care of ill family members, prohibition of alcohol, pork, and handwashing.

5) Hinduism: Hinduism has varied beliefs, from atheism to monotheism, with emphasis on personal cleanliness, vegetarianism, and funeral ceremonies.

6) Judaism: Customs include religious circumcision, a kosher diet, and Shiva funeral rites.

When caring for clients, nurses must assess their religious and spiritual practices and beliefs to address any emotional issues related to these aspects. Emotional and psychological symptoms of spiritual or religious sorrow may include despondency, guilt, pain, suffering, hopelessness, loss of purpose, rage, and feelings of abandonment.

Gender Identity

Gender identity also plays a role in medical treatment, as certain illnesses may require distinct diagnoses, treatments, and prescriptions for each sex. People of different genders may have different reactions to vaccines and medications due to a variety of factors, such as hormonal differences, body size, and other physiological variables. Medical professionals must be aware of these variations to ensure safe and effective treatments for their patients.

Provide End-of-Life Care and Education to Clients

Palliative care, also known as end-of-life care, is aimed at the enhancement of quality of life for individuals in their final stages rather than the mere prolongation of life. It focuses on the control and, when possible, reduction of symptoms to offer comfort and support. The type of palliative care a person receives depends on their disease, available care options, and their own or their family's preferences.

Palliative care is available in various places, such as homes, residential care homes, acute hospitals, general practice offices, and specialized community services. It is important to note that palliative care is not limited to the days or hours before death. It can be provided for weeks, months, or even years before the person passes away. Nurses in palliative care settings ensure prompt certification of death, care of the body of the deceased, attention to organ donation requests, and support for the patient's family during the grieving process.

The palliative care team includes general and specialist nurses, physicians, allied health practitioners, counselors/psychologists, hospice personnel, respite employees, grief/bereavement workers, chaplains, complementary therapists, and others.

1) Palliative care is available to individuals who meet these criteria:
2) They have a serious illness that causes them significant distress.
3) They are frail and expected to die within the next 12 months.
4) They have a condition that puts them at risk of death due to a crisis or deterioration.
5) They have an active, progressive illness that is unlikely to be cured, such as cancer (breast, ovarian, pancreatic, leukemia, multiple myeloma, etc.) or diseases that cause organ failure (cardiac disease, pulmonary disease, liver disease, kidney disease, neurological conditions, incurable viral diseases, congenital conditions, and traumatic injury).

Nurses must:

1) Establish a supportive therapeutic relationship where patients and their families can comfortably discuss sensitive and emotional issues.
2) Collaborate with patients and their families to identify and document care-related decisions and provide updates as the patient's condition changes.
3) Educate patients and their families about the illness, prognosis, treatment goals, expected outcomes, and likelihood of mortality, among other things.
4) Provide practical and emotional support to patients' families/caregivers/significant others.

5) Participate in interdisciplinary team meetings to plan and evaluate care.

6) Research and recommend conventional and alternative care options for patients.

7) Deliver direct care, assess its effectiveness, and suggest improvements as needed.

8) Address patients' additional needs and facilitate their fulfillment whenever possible.

9) Collaborate with the multidisciplinary team to support patients' chosen treatment options to the fullest extent possible.

10) Advocate for patients' care to be provided in the location and manner of their preference.

11) Initiate palliative care at the appropriate time for each patient.

12) Ensure that patients who receive palliative care are frequently assessed by a medical practitioner. If the doctor believes death is imminent, the patient and their family should be informed.

Many legal and ethical considerations are relevant to palliative care nursing. These include:

1) Confidentiality.

2) The right to reject care.

3) Capacity and competence.

4) Decision-making through proxy.

5) Euthanasia, also known as assisted suicide.

6) The administration of supplemental nourishment and hydration.

7) Whether to extend or discontinue life-extending procedures.

8) Organ and/or tissue donation.

9) Allow patients to make choices in their best interests, respect their beliefs and ability to articulate their preferences.

10) Beneficence: do good for patients and others.

11) Nonmaleficence: avoid harm to patients or others.

12) Justice: ensure fair and equal treatment for the patient.

Explore Reasons for Clients' Noncompliance with a Treatment Plan

Patient compliance refers to the patient's ability to adhere to the prescribed treatment plan. Noncompliance can lead to health conditions that deteriorate.

Causes of Noncompliance

1) Limited involvement in treatment decisions.

Patients may not have been included in the choice of treatment, which could lead to undesired care and subsequent noncompliance.

2) Lack of knowledge about their illness and how to manage it.

Poor communication with healthcare practitioners can lead to patients who do not understand the consequences if they do not follow the treatment plan.

3) Personal characteristics, such as memory and cognitive difficulties.

Cognitive or behavioral issues may hinder compliance, and some patients may rely on others to help them adhere to the plan.

4) Socioeconomic issues and cost considerations.

Affordability of medications and treatments can impact compliance, along with education level and understanding of the disease.

5) The diagnosis and type of treatment.

A potentially life-threatening diagnosis or a condition without noticeable symptoms may lead to denial and disinterest in treatment. Previous unsuccessful treatments can also affect trust in the current plan, and fear of side effects can hinder compliance with treatment regimens.

Assist in the Care of Clients Who Experience Sensory Alterations

Impaired sensory perception refers to changes in the amount of stimuli, which can lead to altered or reduced reactions in kinesthetic, olfactory, gustatory, tactile, auditory, or visual responses.

Key features of compromised sensory and perceptual changes include altered focus, hallucinations, difficulty with concentration, disorientation, behavioral changes, changed communication patterns, decision-making abilities, sensory precision, clarity, or problem-solving skills.

Care for Clients with Sensory and Perceptual Alterations

1) Identify stimuli that cause symptoms.

Observe how certain stimuli, locations, or times affect the client's sensory and perceptual experiences. Adapt treatment to ensure patient safety.

2) Consider interventions for delirium, dementia, or organic brain syndrome.

- Maintain eye contact and speak at eye level.
- Use closed-ended inquiries.
- Consider dopamine antagonists to treat hallucinations.
- Utilize visual aids and assistive technologies for explanations.
- Reorient the client to time, place, and person.
- Create a calm and distraction-free environment.
- Anticipate and attend to the client's needs.
- Ensure client comfort.

3) Consider interventions for visual impairment.

- Provide the client with information about their local and wider surroundings.
- Offer braille and large-print documents for customers with poor eyesight.
- Check if the client uses corrective lenses, such as eyeglasses or magnifiers.
- Speak to clients with poor vision at eye level and within their functional visual field.

4) Enact interventions for auditory impairment.

- Eliminate unnecessary external sounds and distractions during communication with the client.

- Use written communication instead of vocal communication.
- Offer the client aids like a hearing aid.
- Speak slowly and clearly while sitting at the client's eye level.

5) Evaluate susceptible body areas like the lower extremities, which can help in the treatment of tactile or kinesthetic sensory impairments.

6) To increase the client's desire to eat, provide meals that appeal. This can support the client's ability to cope with gustatory (loss of taste) impairment.

Assist in the Care of Cognitively Impaired Clients

Patients with life-altering diseases who continue to experience neurological abnormalities are diagnosed with cognitive impairment, which affects memory, problem-solving, planning, organization, processing speed, and attention.

Risk Factors

Chronic conditions such as Parkinson's disease, diabetes, stroke, cardiovascular disease, toxic substance exposure, head trauma, family history, a history of lengthy and difficult hospital and ICU admissions, sepsis, ARDS, a history of assisted breathing, chronic delirium episodes, old age, or the existence of pre-existing cognitive problems are all risk factors for cognitive impairment.

Care of Cognitively Impaired Clients

Treat the cause, encourage cognitive rehabilitation sessions, address anxiety or depression linked to cognitive impairment, and provide social support, brain exercises, and physical exercise.

Nurse Management and Areas of Concentration

1) Evaluate patients' functional abilities, which include their psychological, physical, and social circumstances, as well as the severity of their disability.

2) Perform a comprehensive pain assessment that focuses on the identification of verbal and nonverbal clues and recognition of regular and atypical symptoms.

3) Provide close observation of patients with cognitive impairment.

4) Constantly bring patients back to reality to prevent them from having incorrect notions.

5) Use common language to ensure simpler comprehension of instructions and reduce patient misunderstanding.

6) Utilize encouraging comments to boost patients' self-esteem and increase their desire to behave properly.

7) Encourage patients' orientation to reality and everyday activities.

8) Listen intently to patients' worries and maintain a nonjudgmental attitude toward them.

9) Minimize distractions like television and radio when speaking with patients.

10) Encourage family members and close friends to visit and provide necessary support.

Promote Clients' Self-esteem

A person's physical health may be significantly impacted by their sense of self-worth. Negative self-esteem might make it harder for patients to adhere to their doctor's instructions, manage illness, recover after surgery, and recover from accidents.

The nurse is in a unique position to have a significant influence on patients' mental health since she will engage with them more often and for longer periods than maybe any other healthcare provider.

1) Participate in the creation of the patient's care plan.

High self-confidence leads to better outcomes and increases patient satisfaction. Inform patients about their disease and provide them with all the necessary information to aid in decision-making. To ensure the care plan aligns with their values, beliefs, and lifestyle, ask about their preferences. The more collaborative and engaging the care plan, the more empowered patients will feel to adhere to it.

2) Create a natural relationship.

Establish a natural dialogue with patients that goes beyond talk of their disease and therapy to increase self-esteem. Ask about their interests, occupations, pets, and family. Create a rapport with anxious patients or those with needle phobia as a helpful diversionary strategy.

3) Listen actively.

People with low self-esteem often believe that no one is interested in what they have to say. Listen actively, acknowledge patients' remarks, ask relevant questions, avoid distractions, and make eye contact during the conversation. Do not rush through conversation or ignore patients' concerns, as this can damage their trust.

Identify Signs and Symptoms of Substance Abuse, Substance Use Disorder, Withdrawal, and Overdose

Substance abuse involves an overindulgence in addictive substances such as alcohol, prescription medications, or illegal narcotics. Addiction is characterized by the persistent urge to use a drug despite major negative physical or psychological effects, which leads to a lack of control over behavior.

Physiological dependence occurs when a patient stops substance use, and this results in negative bodily consequences, while psychological dependence is the urge to continue drug use to avoid negative emotions or sensations that arise when drug use is halted.

Assessment

Risk factors for drug misuse include peer pressure, psychiatric mental health issues, lack of life success, low pain tolerance, and low self-esteem.

Physical signs and symptoms of substance abuse may include poor attention span, drug-seeking behaviors, academic difficulties, poor job performance, forgetfulness, a low frustration threshold, poor health, cool and moist hands, shakiness, poor hygiene, needle track marks on the extremities, and hyperactivity.

Standardized tests such as the CAGE-AID test, recovery attitude and treatment evaluation, Michigan alcohol screening test, addiction Severity Index, and drug abuse screening test can be used to diagnose substance-related addictions.

Specific Signs and Symptoms of Substance Abuse and Withdrawal

1) Cocaine.

Abuse symptoms include tachycardia, hypertension, high temperature, convulsions, hallucinations, blurred vision, impatience, and increased activity.

Withdrawal symptoms include nightmares, a reduction in psychomotor activity, sadness, or sleeplessness.

2) Amphetamines.

Abuse symptoms include incoherent speech, hallucinations, dilated pupils, paranoia, sleeplessness, poor judgment, lack of mental clarity, weight loss, cravings, and hypervigilance.

Withdrawal symptoms are similar to those of cocaine withdrawal.

3) Benzodiazepines and barbiturates.

Abuse symptoms include nystagmus, poor memory, poor focus, slurred speech, sleepiness, poor coordination, respiratory depression, dizziness, and hypotension.

Withdrawal symptoms include sleeplessness, tremors, anxiety, hallucinations, convulsions, and a high body temperature.

4) Cannabis.

Abuse symptoms include reduced mental function, psychosis, increased hunger, dry mouth, reddish eyes, hypertension, tachycardia, hostility, tremors, poor coordination, and irritability.

Withdrawal symptoms include aggression, sleeplessness, lack of appetite, sadness, fever, tremors, irritability, and anxiety.

5) Sedatives and hypnotics.

Abuse symptoms include slurred speech, lack of coordination, respiratory depression, agitation, convulsions, vomiting, and anxiety.

Withdrawal symptoms include agitation, anxiety, diaphoresis, convulsions, hallucinations, and tremors.

6) Alcohol.

Abuse symptoms include peripheral venous collapse, gastrointestinal hemorrhage, blackouts, gastritis, hepatitis, stomach pains, vomiting, tachycardia, tremors, respiratory arrest, stupor, and a lower state of awareness.

Withdrawal symptoms include delirium, cardiac arrhythmias, anxiety, sleeplessness, tremors, loss of direction, hypertension, and tachycardia.

7) Opioids.

Abuse symptoms include goosebumps, stomach cramps, constricted pupils, tremors, muscular spasms, diaphoresis, short attention span, memory loss, slurred speech, drowsiness, and disorientation.

Withdrawal symptoms include dilated pupils, weakness, muscle spasms, nausea, fever, sleeplessness, and erections.

Provide Emotional Support to Clients

Emotional and physical interventions build trust in the therapeutic patient-nurse interaction, which enables patients to express their emotions freely. The nurse maintains respect, compassion, caring, and therapeutic communication throughout the treatment.

1) Enhance clients' comprehension of any early indicators and danger signals of psychiatric mental health issues.

2) Encourage clients to use relaxation and stress-reduction methods.

3) Provide constructive reinforcement for suitable actions.

4) Encourage clients' participation in both individual and group treatment sessions.

5) Focus on the growth and improvement of clients' coping skills.

6) Encourage the active participation of patients and their families in the treatment plan in a setting that respects patient needs and preferences.

Use Therapeutic Communication Techniques with Clients

1) Only after you have developed a relationship of trust should you address any discrepancies in a patient's past, mental processes, or improper behavior.

2) Use self-disclosure to encourage a trustworthy connection, make the patient feel supported, and provide a foundation for respect, hope, and support.

3) Guide the next stage in the admission and hospitalization process, provide opportunities for clarification, and give a review of the evaluation results.

4) Ask pertinent questions. Start with targeted, rational, close-ended inquiries, followed by open-ended ones.

5) Invite listener engagement and comprehension throughout a dialogue.

6) Bring the discussion's attention to a key issue, cut out tangential or meaningless talk, and center the evaluation on the cause of pain and important historical information.

7) Clarify ambiguous statements and ask the patient to restate perplexing comments.

8) Enlighten the patient about what will happen next and why more testing or observation may be necessary.

9) Use therapeutic silence to encourage patience, thoughtfulness, and consideration of tough choices.

10) Use touch to monitor verbal and nonverbal clues from patients and determine if they are comfortable.

11) Use humor to build rapport, improve physical and mental health, and create a connection that will support the patient emotionally.

12) Give the patient a feeling of control and hope.

13) Speak in a nonjudgmental, impartial manner.

14) Use reflection to promote conversation and attentive listening, and pay close attention to the specifics of what the patient expresses, whether verbally or nonverbally.

Promote a Therapeutic Environment

Both positive and negative aspects of client rehabilitation are influenced by numerous intrinsic client-related components as well as extrinsic factors. Physical recovery from a biological disease may be aided by extrinsic variables such as the patient's family and the community's resources, while comorbidity, like diabetes, an intrinsic element, can hinder it.

Psychological healing may be obstructed by factors like stress, social stigma, lack of access to affordable healthcare, family disruption, and a lack of culturally competent care. However, group meetings for peer and professional support, group therapy, and self-care education can accelerate recovery for patients and their significant others.

A therapeutic milieu, created and maintained by nurses, is an atmosphere that is safe and supportive of therapy. It ensures the environment is free from physical safety risks and any other factors that can endanger patients' mental security and well-being. In a therapeutic setting, efforts are made to remove as many stressors as possible. Components of a therapeutic milieu include client expectations, limits and restrictions, guidelines, and consistency.

For a client at risk of suicide, close and frequent observation and monitoring are essential, which necessitates a room close to the nursing station. Similarly, a client who exhibits violent or disruptive behavior should not share a room with someone who might incite inappropriate, violent, or dangerous actions.

Chapter 5: Basic Care and Comfort

Provide Bowel and Bladder Management Care to Clients

Bowel and bladder management protocols require tailored approaches based on age and individual needs. Nurses identify and address issues like hemorrhoids, fecal impaction, incontinence, diarrhea, constipation, flatulence, and abnormal urine patterns (anuria or polyuria). They assist patients to maintain regular bowel movements and adequate urination.

Monitor Patients

In addition to physical examinations, nurses must establish open communication with patients to demonstrate empathy and ask relevant questions.

Various groups of patients may experience elimination problems. These include cancer patients, the elderly, children with congenital abnormalities, and surgical patients at risk of ileus. Medications like opioids, NSAIDs, antibiotics, and anticoagulants can induce constipation.

Patients at risk for gastrointestinal and urinary dysfunction include those with cancer, neonates, the elderly, individuals with heart, CNS, or renal diseases, bedridden patients, and those with low-fiber or low-fluid diets.

Patients who haven't had a bowel movement in several days should be checked for constipation or intestinal obstruction. Nurses may measure residual urine to assess urinary function. For example, adults usually urinate 30 mL per hour.

It is also necessary to monitor for secondary consequences of elimination issues, such as delirium related to urinary tract infections or positive FOBT (fecal occult blood test) due to ulcers or hemorrhoids.

Management

1) Abdominal massage can improve gastrointestinal tract (GIT) function and ease constipation without the side effects of laxatives.

2) Sitz baths may benefit cancer patients with GIT problems. Preterm babies on enteral feeding may require abdominal massage.

3) Noninvasive measures include abdominal massage, discontinuation of medications that cause gastrointestinal or genitourinary side effects, stool softeners, a high-fiber diet with prunes, and movement.

4) More invasive therapies like enemas, urinary catheters, suppositories, and GIT control may be necessary if initial treatments are ineffective.

5) Ointments like zinc oxide can protect the skin during urinary catheterization for retention. Colostomies and urinary catheter irrigations can aid in excretion.

6) Retention enemas help lubricate the rectum and deliver medication. Cleansing enemas prepare the colon for colonoscopies.

7) If noninvasive methods fail, colostomies and urostomies are possible options, although they require close monitoring for necrosis, dehiscence, B12 deficiency, and infections.

Perform Bladder Irrigation

Bladder Irrigation

Bladder irrigation is a medical procedure commonly used after urological surgeries like transurethral prostate excision. Its purpose is to prevent or dissolve blood clots in the bladder with a sterile liquid that is flushed through. Blood clots can obstruct the catheter, which leads to urine retention, discomfort, kidney injury, or infection. Additionally, bladder irrigation is used to dissolve bladder stones, soothe irritation, treat infections or inflammation, and administer medications directly to the bladder.

There are two types of bladder irrigation: continuous and intermittent. Continuous bladder irrigation takes place over several days. Intermittent bladder irrigation occurs either as needed or at scheduled intervals.

Technique

- For continuous bladder irrigation, the catheter is inserted into the bladder, and two bags of sterile saline solution (and medications, if required) are hung on a pole. The healthcare professional connects both bags to ports on the catheter after the catheter's exterior ports are cleaned. One bag is connected to the pole, and the other is connected to an empty bag on the patient's side and used to collect bodily fluids. The third port secures the catheter's position but is not actively used. Throughout the procedure, the healthcare professional monitors urine production, empties the drainage bag regularly, manages the sterile solution's drip rate, and checks the urine color.

- Initially, the urine may appear dark red and contain debris. Over time, it should change to pink and eventually become clear. When the patient's urine has been clear or pale pink for a day or two, the continuous bladder irrigation is discontinued.

Complications

Possible complications of bladder irrigation include bladder perforation, paraphimosis, UTIs, or catheter obstruction. Skilled care and observation can minimize the risk of these complications.

Catheter Irrigation

Urinary catheters are commonly used for postoperative care, surgical patients, urethral obstructions, incontinence, and difficult urination. Regular catheter flushing or irrigation is essential to maintain cleanliness and functionality. It also helps clear the bladder of debris and prevents mucus buildup.

In general, it is advised to flush the catheter at least once a day. Additional flushes may be necessary if the patient experiences any of these symptoms:

- Catheter bypass (urine leakage around the catheter).
- Swollen abdomen.
- Malodorous or cloudy urine that drains from the catheter.
- Reduced urine flow rate from the catheter.

Technique

- Wash your hands with soap and water. Gather necessary supplies, such as sterile gloves, saline solution, and a syringe with a catheter tip. Fill the syringe with saline solution and put on new gloves, then clean your hands again.
- Position the patient flat on their back with legs spread and knees elevated. Place a pan and absorbent materials between the patient's legs to catch any urine or fluids that leak during the procedure.
- Clean the area around the catheter and drainage tube attachment with an alcohol wipe or medical wipe. Then, disconnect and remove the catheter's drainage tube.
- Use the saline solution to irrigate the catheter and drainage tubing once more. Reattach the drainage tube and observe the urine flow.

Wound Irrigation

Wound irrigation is necessary to reduce the risk of infection and remove exudate and debris. It should be forceful enough to achieve its intended purpose but gentle enough to avoid tissue damage or the spread of bacteria.

Technique

- Wound assessment, site anesthesia, wound perimeter cleaning, and under-pressure solution irrigation are essential components of wound irrigation.
- For irrigation, use an eye cup or a 35 mL syringe with a catheter tip. A 19-gauge catheter and 35 mL syringe produce the required pressure to clear debris and reduce bacterial load. For continuous irrigation, use an 18-gauge catheter and pressure bag with isotonic fluid.
- PPE, such as gloves, face masks, and eye protection, should be worn during wound irrigation. For wound anesthesia, use 1% lidocaine injections around the wound site.
- Normal saline is the preferred irrigation solution due to its similarity to physiological fluids in tonicity. Sterile water is not recommended as it can cause cell lysis due to its hypotonic nature.

Complications

Avoid wound irrigation if the wound bleeds actively, as it may disrupt the development of clots. Incomplete wound irrigation in abscesses may fail to remove debris or purulent discharge from the wound, which can potentially cause sinus formation.

Ear Irrigation

Ear irrigation is a technique used to clean the ears and remove excess earwax, where the ear is gently flushed with liquid. Symptoms of earwax buildup may include ear discomfort, dizziness, and reduced hearing.

Technique

- The patient should sit upright with a cloth on their shoulder to catch any ear discharge.
- Gently pull the ear up and back to facilitate water entry into the ear.

- Insert the syringe into the ear and direct it upward and toward the back of the ear to help the earwax drain out.
- Squeeze the syringe gently to allow water to enter the ear.
- If the patient feels any pressure or discomfort, stop the irrigation.
- Dry the ear with a cloth or a few drops of rubbing alcohol.

Complications

Ear irrigation should not be used for individuals with a history of radiation treatment to the ear, middle ear infections, eardrum surgery, ear damage from sharp objects, or severe otitis externa (inflammation of the ear canal). The procedure carries a risk of eardrum perforation, otitis externa, and middle ear damage.

Eye Irrigation

Eye irrigation is mostly used to remove foreign objects, chemicals, and fluids from the eye. It can also be used to administer medication for corneal and conjunctival conditions. In emergencies, tap water may be used for irrigation.

Technique

- The amount of fluid required for eye irrigation varies based on the type of contamination. Moderate amounts are needed for secretions. Abundant amounts are needed for severe chemical burns. Severe chemical burns may require continuous irrigation with regular saline solution from an IV bottle or bag.
- Equipment includes a sterile basin, eyelid retractor, 60 mL sterile syringe, sterile gauze pads, towels, goggles, gloves, and topical anesthetic with proparacaine hydrochloride.
- Pour 30 to 60 mL of the irrigation fluid into the sterile basin. Apply the sterile ophthalmic irrigation fluid directly from the squeeze bottle container into the eye. Position the patient in a way that allows the stream to enter the inner canthus, wash over the cornea, and exit at the outer canthus.
- For extensive irrigation, set up an IV bag and tubing with no needle and flush the eye for at least 15 minutes. Alkali burns may require hours of continuous irrigation.

- A Morgan lens attached to irrigation tubing can provide continuous lavage and deliver eye medication. Connect the IV tubing and solution bottle to the lens with an adapter. Place the lens beneath the patient's upper eyelid and have them gaze upward to install the device. Then, cover the lens with the lower eyelid and let the patient relax their gaze.

Nasal Irrigation

Nasal irrigation is a technique used for individuals with upper respiratory infections, allergies, or sinus issues. It moistens the nasal airways, improves mucociliary clearance, and removes thick mucus, debris, or germs.

Technique

- Choose from various tools, such as saline, a medical syringe, a bulb syringe, a squeeze bottle, or a neti pot.
- Wash your hands, then mix the solution and pour it into the chosen tool.
- Have the patient tilt their head to the side and bend over the washbasin.
- Insert the syringe tip into the upper nostril and administer the solution with the squeeze bottle or the syringe.
- Repeat the process until the other nostril is clear and the solution flows freely out of it.

Complications

Nasal irrigation can cause a rare but severe infection known as Naegleria fowleri, which infects brain tissue. This amoeba is usually deadly and enters the body through the nose. The infection can only occur if the water used for nasal irrigation is contaminated with Naegleria fowleri. To prevent this, it is important to use sterile water or saline instead of tap water, which may contain harmful contaminants.

Provide for Mobility Needs

Help Patients with Ambulation

- Raise the head of the bed and wait for the patient to adjust. Ensure that there is no dizziness and that their pulse is normal.
- Lower the bed to an appropriate height.

- Assist the patient in a seated position. Place one arm under their back and another under their knees.

- Allow the patient to hang their feet off the bed for a few minutes.

- Help the patient stand, then wait for them to regain their balance.

- During ambulation, support the patient's forearm with your hand and stay close to them for added stability.

Help Patients with Drainage Tubes (Catheters, Chest Tubes, etc.) Ambulate

- Assist the patient out of bed as previously instructed.

- Ensure that drainage containers are kept below the level of the drained bodily cavity.

- Either the nurse or the patient can hold the drainage container during ambulation.

- After ambulation, return to bed and ensure that drainage tubes and containers are properly positioned.

Help Patients via Log Rolling without a Turning Sheet

This technique is utilized when the spinal column must be kept straight, such as after spinal surgery. Log rolling a patient requires two or more people.

- Raise the bed to its highest setting.

- Position one person at the patient's head and shoulders. Position another person at the patient's hips and legs on the opposite side of where the patient will be turned.

- As a team, move the patient toward you.

- Place a cushion between the patient's knees and cross their arms over their chest.

- Walk together to the other side of the bed. Keep the patient's head, spine, and legs straight.

- In a coordinated motion, gently roll the patient toward you. At the same time, maintain their alignment.

- Use cushions for support as needed.
- Increase the height of the side rail for added safety.

Help Weak Patients with Ambulation

- Assist the patient to stand.
- Securely wrap a gait or transfer belt around the patient.
- During ambulation, the nurse should hold the belt from behind to support the patient.
- If the patient is particularly weak, two nurses can provide support, one on each side of the patient.

Range of Motion (ROM) Exercises

Benefits of ROM exercises:

1) They maintain and increase muscle strength.
2) They preserve joint function and prevent deformities.
3) They enhance neuromuscular coordination.
4) They improve tolerance and endurance.

ROM exercises should guide joints through their full range of motion and incorporate all types of movement. These exercises should be performed multiple times a day and must be discontinued if they cause any discomfort.

Types of ROM exercises:

1) Passive exercise: A nurse performs the exercise without the patient's help.
2) Active-assistive exercise: A patient performs the exercise with the nurse's help.
3) Active exercise: A patient performs the exercise independently.
4) Resistive active exercise: A patient works against resistance (manual or mechanical).
5) Isometric or muscle-setting exercise: A patient contracts and releases muscles in a fixed position (e.g., Kegel exercises, quadriceps setting).

Reposition Patients with Specific Health Problems

Hip replacement surgery

Prevent excessive internal and external rotation and adduction. Maintain abduction with a cushion between the patient's legs. Advise the patient not to cross their legs.

Injury to the spinal cord.

Immobilize the patient on a backboard with a natural head position. Use a stiff, padded cervical collar to prevent head movement. Log roll the patient.

Postprocedural myelogram.

Raise the patient's head for oil-based or water-soluble contrast. Lower the patient's head for air contrast.

Puncture of the lumbar region.

Assist the patient into a lateral position with their neck flexed, chin on chest, and knees flexed up to their belly.

Increased ICP.

Raise the head of the bed to 45 degrees (semi-Fowler position) for venous drainage.

Laminectomy.

Keep the patient's back straight and ensure their feet are comfortably placed on the floor.

Craniotomy.

Do not position the patient on the surgery site, especially after bone flap removal. Raise the head of the bed to a semi-Fowler's position for neutral midline drainage of head veins.

Stroke.

Raise the head of the bed to 30 degrees for hemorrhagic strokes to minimize ICP and promote venous drainage. Keep the head of the bed flat for patients with ischemic strokes. Maintain the patient's head in a neutral midline position to aid venous drainage. Avoid excessive neck and hip flexion, which can impact intrathoracic pressure and brain venous outflow.

Angiography.

Immobilize and keep the contrast-injected extremity straight for six to eight hours.

Aneurysm of the cerebral artery.

Maintain bed rest with the head of the bed raised in a semi-Fowler's position to avoid pressure on the aneurysm site.

Detachment of the retina.

Recommend bed rest and a bilateral eye patch to limit eye movement and prevent the spread of detachment. Post-repair activity and posture restrictions are determined by the physician and surgical approach.

Cataract.

Elevate the head of the bed to a semi-Fowler's position and place the patient on their back or nonoperative side to prevent edema at the operation site.

Venous insufficiency, DVT, and leg ulcers.

Leg elevation is often recommended for these conditions.

Peripheral artery disease.

Encourage the patient to hang their legs over the side of the bed or sofa or to walk around if they can. Elevation is not usually recommended because it can reduce blood flow to the already compromised arteries. Do not lift legs higher than heart level, which can excessively slow arterial circulation. Some patients may be advised to slightly lower their legs to enhance blood perfusion.

Pulmonary edema and cardiovascular disease.

Position the patient upright with their legs hanging over the bed edge to reduce venous return and lung congestion.

Catheterization of the heart.

After surgery via the femoral artery, keep the patient in bed for several hours. Raise the head of the bed no more than 30 degrees and keep the leg straight to promote hemostasis.

Extremity vascular arterial grafting.

Maintain bed rest for 24 hours post-surgery to enhance graft patency. Keep the affected extremity straight. Minimize movement and prevent knee and hip flexion.

Amputation.

For the first day after amputation, elevate the foot of the bed to reduce edema. Use cushions to support the stump. Avoid lifting the stump to prevent flexion contractures. Place the patient in a prone position twice a day for half an hour to lengthen muscles and prevent hip flexion contractures.

Minnesota and Sengstaken-Blakemore tubes.

If required, maintain bed elevation to improve lung expansion and limit portal tract blood flow, which allows for efficient balloon esophagogastric tamponade.

Irrigation with rectal enema.

Position the patient in the left Sims' position to enable gravity to move the solution in the natural direction of the colon.

Hypophysectomy.

Raise the head of the bed to avoid increased intracranial pressure.

Mastectomy.

To stimulate lymphatic fluid return after axillary lymph node excision, raise the head of the bed by 30 degrees and place a pillow under the patient's affected arm. Turn the patient gently to the unaffected side and back.

Autograft.

The surgical site is generally immobilized for three to seven days to allow the graft to adhere to the wound bed.

Head and face burns.

Raise the head of the bed to avoid or decrease edema in the trachea, head, or face. Elevate the limbs above heart level to prevent or minimize dependent edema.

Use Measures to Maintain or Improve Clients' Skin Integrity

Maintenance of skin integrity requires proper personal hygiene. Effective communication between patients and healthcare providers is vital. Patients may not want to discuss their personal hygiene needs, so it is essential to create an open and direct dialogue.

Healthcare professionals should always wash their hands before patient interaction to maintain cleanliness. When necessary, they may wear gloves during specific procedures.

Bathing

Bathing not only enhances the patient's sense of cleanliness but also removes dirt, sweat, bacteria, and dead skin cells and improves blood circulation.

Different bathing styles include:

1) Tub bath or shower: This is suitable for patients who can use the restroom independently but may require some assistance with washing. To prevent dryness, use moisturizing soaps or lotions with oil and water.

2) Assisted bath: This is suitable for patients who can wash certain parts of their bodies independently but need some help to wash other body parts and get in and out of the tub or shower. To assist the patient, determine whether they need to use the restroom before bathing, provide a shower chair if necessary, ensure toiletries are easily accessible, remain nearby to offer further assistance, turn on the water, and adjust the temperature for comfort (preferably around 100–105°F). Although gloves are not required during bathing assistance, some patients may prefer their use.

3) Bed bath: This is suitable for patients who are bedridden or unable to wash independently. Bed baths can be performed with a washbasin filled with water or disposable bag baths, which do not require water. Patients often prefer traditional water and soap baths, but bag baths are also effective.

Keep the environment warm, private, and secure. Cover windows, draw the curtains, and lock the doors. Ensure the availability of essential items, such as a laundry hamper, patient amenities, bath towels, disposable aprons, disposable washbasin, nonsterile gloves, clean clothes, and fresh bed linens. Have a bedpan or urinal available, as warm water exposure may trigger the urge to urinate.

With the traditional soap and water method, fill a container three-quarters full with warm water. Ask the patient if they want to clean their face with soap. Remove hearing aids or eyeglasses before the patient's ears, face, and neck are washed. Support their chin with a towel. Then, return the hearing aids or glasses to the patient. Remove the patient's clothing and cover them with a blanket, but leave the cleaning area exposed. Clean the skin from head to toe. Start with one arm and move toward the distal end, then repeat on the other arm. Pay special attention and clean between skin folds.

For the lower half of the patient, repeat the same procedure. For women, use disposable wipes to clean the genitalia from front to back to reduce the risk of urinary tract infections. For men, clean the genital area from the tip of the penis downward. Dispose of used wipes promptly in a plastic trash bag.

Pressure Sores (Decubitus Ulcers)

Pressure sores are also known as decubitus ulcers. These are localized areas where pressure on bony prominences causes skin and subcutaneous tissue necrosis. The pressure compresses small blood vessels, which causes tissue anoxia, ischemia, and, ultimately, necrosis. This can progress to sloughing and ulceration, which may become infected, cause sepsis, and potentially invade deeper structures like fascia, muscle, and bone. Several risk factors contribute to the development of these sores. Risk factors include immobility, incontinence, poor nutrition, poor circulation, decreased physical condition, diabetes, neuropathy, peripheral vascular disease, anemia, or the use of cortisol medication.

Common locations for these ulcers include the ischial tuberosities, trochanters, sacrum, knees, malleoli, heels, and elbows.

Prevention

To prevent pressure sores, maintain clean and dry skin, particularly in areas prone to pressure. Promptly clean skin contaminated with dirt or urine and apply moisturizer to keep the skin supple. Avoid massage directly over bony prominences to minimize the risk of skin breakdown. Regularly change the patient's position at least every two hours or more frequently if necessary. When you reposition the patient in bed, lift rather than slide or pull. Use rotating sheets to reduce friction. Encourage ROM exercises and ambulation to improve circulation and reduce pressure on specific areas. Do not use pressure-inducing tools like braces or donut rings, as they may restrict blood flow.

Provide Care to Immobilized Clients Based on Need

The prevalence of obesity and chronic illnesses continues to increase worldwide, which raises concerns about inactivity. There is a growing emphasis on active lifestyles that can counteract these health issues. Regular physical exercise helps reduce the risk of various chronic illnesses, such as mental health problems, musculoskeletal ailments, different types of cancers, obesity, diabetes, stroke, and coronary heart disease. Encourage regular physical activity to improve a patient's overall health and well-being.

A Nurse's Role in the Management of Immobilized Clients

1) Identify inactive adults.

Nurses can assess activity levels during consultations, health checks, or long-term disease treatment sessions.

2) Offer concise guidance and follow-up.

For individuals who do not meet activity guidelines, nurses should provide encouragement and suggest ways to increase activity levels based on their health status, circumstances, and preferences. Emphasize local options like gyms, sports facilities, fitness programs, and walking groups. Maintain a record of these conversations and provide written recommendations and goals. Follow up during future opportunities.

3) Incorporate short physical activity interventions.

Include short physical activity interventions with chronic conditions (e.g., mental health disorders, type 2 diabetes, stroke, coronary heart disease) and populations at risk of inactivity (e.g., people over 65 or individuals with disabilities).

4) Facilitate quick advice.

Use reading codes to identify evaluation and guidance opportunities. Keep up-to-date information about local amenities.

5) Educate primary care practitioners.

Ensure that primary care practitioners are well versed in physical activity definitions, current guidelines, at-risk groups, physical activity assessments, how to dispel misconceptions about physical activity, and how to offer concise advice to promote behavior change.

6) Follow doctor's orders.

Always read and follow the doctor's prescription, especially after surgeries or treatments. Pay attention to posture and movement recommendations.

7) Practice safe patient movement.

To move a patient, arrange for adequate support and use mechanical aids if necessary. Encourage the patient to assist as much as possible. Maintain proper alignment of the back, neck, pelvis, and feet. Do not twist or bend the knees, and keep the feet wide apart. Position yourself close to the patient, utilize your arms and legs, and use a pull sheet to help move the patient.

8) Use a sliding board.

To transfer a patient onto a stretcher, a sliding board is preferable. Coordinate efforts with the team leader who will carry the most weight. Use an agreed-upon count for a smooth transfer.

9) Position the patient safely.

Place the patient in a safe and appropriate position that considers surgical or medical procedures, recommended therapy, or existing conditions.

Suggested Physical Exercise

Healthcare providers should offer personalized advice on the amount, frequency, duration, and type of physical exercise required to achieve overall health benefits. Although nurses can provide individual advice, it is recommended that everyone participate in physical activity appropriate to their age and capabilities.

The guidelines are as follows:

1) Older individuals.

Aim for at least 150 minutes of moderate-intensity exercise per week, broken down into 10-minute increments. Alternatively, 75 minutes of vigorous-intensity exercise weekly can offer similar benefits. Engage in muscle strength training at least twice a week. Those at risk of falls should engage in balance and coordination training at least twice a week.

2) Early childhood (under the age of five).

Encourage physical activity from infancy. Emphasize water activities and active play. Children who can walk unassisted should be active for at least 180 minutes daily.

3) Children and adolescents (aged five to eighteen).

Aim for a minimum of 60 minutes of moderate to vigorous physical activity every day. Include vigorous-intensity exercise at least three days per week, especially exercise that enhances bone and muscle health.

4) Adults.

Strive for at least 75 minutes of vigorous daily activity. Alternatively, engage in 150 minutes of moderate-intensity exercise per week, with sessions of at least 10 minutes each. A combination of both types of activity is also beneficial.

Complications of Immobility

1) Muscle atrophy.
2) Joint contractures.
3) Osteoporosis.
4) Urinary tract stones due to osteoporosis and dehydration.
5) Orthostatic hypotension caused by a prolonged recumbent posture, which in turn causes decreased vascular tone.
6) Venous thrombosis caused by reduced venous return due to limited leg movement.
7) Hypostatic pneumonia caused by inadequate lung inflation and prolonged immobility, which allows fluid to accumulate in the lungs.
8) Urinary incontinence (inability to urinate in a normal position).
9) Incontinence and constipation due to reduced activity, poor nutrition, and inability to defecate in a regular position.
10) Psychological decline due to isolation and inactivity.
11) Hip external rotation caused by a lack of voluntary muscular control and prolonged supine position.
12) Footdrop (plantar flexion).
13) Pressure sores (decubitus ulcers).
    - Stage I: Characterized by color changes (red, blue, or purple), temperature changes (warm or chilly), and skin stiffness changes.

- Stage II: Involves skin loss. This includes the epidermis and/or a portion of the dermis.
- Stage III: Shows complete skin loss with subcutaneous injury or necrosis.
- Stage IV: Exhibits complete loss of skin with significant destruction, necrosis, or injury to muscle, bone, or supporting structures.

Treatment of Pressure Ulcers:

- Debride slough and eschar with wet-to-dry dressings. Place the gauze dressing when moist and remove when dry.
- Apply a dry-to-moist dressing soaked with sodium chloride to the wound. This will draw out exudate and reduce microorganisms.
- Use commercial dressings and treatments to keep the wound moist, prevent infection, promote healing, and debride the wound as directed.
- Keep a wound assessment record. Include the stage of the pressure ulcer, notes on undermining, pockets, or tracts, tissue condition, and drainage.

Assist Clients with Visual and Hearing Impairments

Visual Impairment

1) When feeding a blind patient, promote self-care through the use of the clock strategy. Describe the location of the food as if the plate is a clock face to help the patient visualize the arrangement.
2) During ambulation, stand slightly in front of the patient and allow the patient to hold the helper's arm for guidance and support.
3) Before interacting with the patient, knock on the door or announce your presence verbally to ensure they are aware of your entrance.

Hearing Impairment

- Do not clean a patient's hearing aid with soap and water. This can damage the device. Instead, use a dry cloth or specific cleaning products designed for hearing aids. Store the hearing aid in a closed container when not in use to prevent dust buildup. Dust can damage the mechanism.

- Check the battery, volume control, on/off switch, and plastic tubing for cracks or loose connections if the hearing aid is not functioning properly.

Effective Communication:

- Speak in a low voice. High-frequency sounds are often lost first for individuals with hearing impairments.
- Do not yell. Communicate clearly and calmly.
- Ensure the patient can see your mouth as you speak. Stand against an unlit background to facilitate lip-reading.
- Raise your arm or hand to get the patient's attention before you speak.

Promote Alternative/Complementary Therapy in Client Care

In the scope of mental health, practitioners incorporate alternative and complementary therapies alongside conventional medical treatments. Among the various complementary therapies, children's play therapy, art therapy, music therapy, and animal-assisted therapy are some of the most common.

Therapeutic Play

Play therapy is a dynamic and effective therapeutic option, especially for children who have experienced trauma. It serves as a means for children to communicate their needs and feelings and help adults better understand their emotions. Often, issues with children can worsen when adults fail to comprehend or respond appropriately to what they are going through.

Art and Music Therapy

For clients who face stress, grief, bereavement, or health difficulties, art and music therapy offer a unique opportunity to express themselves creatively. These therapies address the social, physical, cognitive, psychological, and emotional needs of the client. They are particularly beneficial for those who struggle to convey their emotions verbally. This is because art and music therapy provide a powerful outlet for self-expression.

Animal Therapy

Animal-assisted therapy helps reduce exhaustion, despair, worry, and pain for individuals with various physical and mental health conditions. It has been shown to be particularly helpful for patients with Down syndrome, developmental impairments, schizophrenia, and Alzheimer's.

Provide Nonpharmacological Measures for Pain Relief

There are various nonpharmacological methods available to alleviate pain. These include:

1) Physical therapy: Clients are taught specific exercises to improve strength, mobility, and reduce discomfort.

2) Massage and Ice application: These techniques help with pain and swelling and relax tense muscles.

3) Heat therapy: Clients apply heat to reduce discomfort and relieve muscular spasms.

4) Acupuncture: Fine needles are used to balance the body's energy pathways, which aids in pain relief.

5) Self-hypnosis: Clients can focus their attention on anything other than the pain through self-hypnosis.

6) Biofeedback: Clients learn to manage their breathing and heart rate during pain to achieve a state of calmness.

7) Music therapy: Music can enhance the client's mood and energy levels. Music triggers the production of endorphins, which naturally reduce pain.

8) Guided imagery: Clients visualize a scene in their minds, which diverts attention away from the pain. This alters pain perception and reactions.

9) Yoga and meditation: These practices promote relaxation and well-being and help distract from discomfort.

10) Progressive muscle relaxation: Clients contract and release muscles throughout the body. This process starts from the foot and works upward.

11) Deep breathing: Clients focus on deep, controlled breathing to aid in pain management.

12) Aromatherapy: The use of natural scents from trees and flowers during baths, facials, and massages can relieve stress.

Evaluate Pain with Standardized Scales

Age-appropriate pain scales are utilized by healthcare professionals to quantify and communicate pain levels.

Pain Assessment

Pain assessment involves observation of various signs, such as agitation, groaning, sobbing, vomiting, diaphoresis, clenched teeth, facial rigidity, changes in blood pressure and breathing rate, difficulty opening eyes or talking, and loss of interest in activities or social situations.

Pain Scale

The pain scale often consists of numbers from 0 to 10. Individuals indicate the number that best represents the intensity of their pain. It is important to note that this scale is only used for individuals without cognitive impairments.

- 0 = No discomfort.
- 1 = Very little or hardly any perceptible pain.
- 2 = Mild discomfort or slight irritation.
- 3 = Pain that can be felt but is manageable.
- 4 = Moderate discomfort, so the patient can temporarily ignore it.
- 5 = Moderately severe discomfort, so the patient is unable to ignore it for an extended period but can still function with difficulty.
- 6 = Moderately intense discomfort, so the patient struggles to focus and avoids some regular daily tasks.
- 7 = Severe pain that prevents the patient from performing daily tasks.
- 8 = Extreme pain, so the patient finds all activities challenging.
- 9 = Extreme pain that is difficult to bear, so the patient is unable to converse.
- 10 = The worst possible pain.

Feed Clients with Enteral Tubes

Enteral feeding is the process of providing nourishment through either the mouth or a tube directly inserted into the stomach or small intestine. This method is used for individuals who are unable to consume food orally but still have a functional GIT.

Tube feedings may be necessary when a patient cannot consume enough calories to meet their nutritional needs due to physical limitations or medical conditions like cancer, stroke, or neurological/mobility disabilities.

Types of Enteral Feeding Tubes

1) Gastrostomy tube.

This tube is inserted through the skin of the abdomen and into the stomach.

2) Jejunostomy tube.

This tube is inserted through the skin of the abdomen and into the intestines.

3) Oroenteric tube.

This tube is inserted through the mouth and directed into the stomach or intestines.

4) Nasoenteric tube.

This tube is inserted through the nose and ends in the intestines.

5) Nasogastric tube

This tube is inserted into the nose and ends in the stomach.

6) Orogastric tube

This tube is inserted into the mouth and ends in the stomach.

Complications of Enteral Nutrition

Complications of enteral nutrition may include aspiration if food enters the lungs, diarrhea, skin rashes, nausea, vomiting, infection at the tube or insertion site, and displacement if the tube becomes blocked or dislodged.

Food Delivery Methods

Enteral feeds can be delivered via various methods. Feeding usually starts four hours after tube insertion.

1) Continuous infusion.

Food is administered by gravity or a pump. The head is elevated at a 45-degree angle to prevent aspiration or regurgitation. This method is commonly used for patients confined to bed.

2) Bolus or intermittent drip.

Food is administered over 16 hours at night. A pump delivers two liters of food. This method is popular for enteral feeding at home.

3) Circadian intermittent feeding.

Enteral feedings are administered over eight hours through a pump. This method is used for patients in a semi-recumbent position.

4) Bulb or syringe-based intermittent bolus feeding.

In this method, 400 mL of enteral nutrition is given over 10 minutes, but there is a risk of aspiration, so it is commonly used in ambulatory settings.

Monitor and Provide for the Nutritional Needs of Clients

Enteral Nutrition

Enteral nutrition is recommended for patients who have difficulty swallowing, burns, serious trauma, liver or other organ failure, or severe malnutrition. It is also used when the gastrointestinal system is functional but oral intake does not meet predicted nutritional requirements.

Vegetarians

Types of vegetarian diets:

- Pesco-vegetarian.

Patients consume seafood but not meat or poultry. They may still consume eggs and/or dairy products.

- Vegan.

Patients do not consume any animal products.

- Lacto-vegetarian.

Patients consume dairy products but not eggs, meat, poultry, or shellfish.

- Lacto-ovo vegetarian.

Patients consume eggs and dairy products but avoid meat, poultry, or shellfish.

Ensure that vegetarian patients consume a diverse range of foods to meet their nutritional and energy needs. Educate them about the importance of consuming complementary proteins throughout the day to fulfill their essential amino acid requirements. Vegetarian diets may lack sufficient calories, protein, vitamin B12, zinc, iron, calcium, omega-3 fatty acids, and vitamin D (especially if sunlight exposure is limited). Vegetarians should pay attention to their iron intake and include vitamin C–rich foods in each meal to enhance iron absorption.

Iron-rich Diet

A high-iron diet is prescribed to compensate for iron deficiency that results from insufficient intake or loss. It includes legumes, dried fruit, dark green leafy vegetables, whole-wheat products, egg yolks, meat, and organ meats. This diet is commonly used to treat anemia in patients.

Purine-reduced Diet

The purine-reduced diet limits the intake of purines, which are precursors of uric acid responsible for the formation of stones and crystals. Foods to avoid on this diet include sweetbreads, geese, wild game, meat extracts, gravies, glandular meats, scallops, sardines, mackerel, herring, and anchovies. The diet is used to manage conditions like gout, kidney stones, and high uric acid levels.

Calcium-rich Diet

A diet high in calcium is essential for bone development and bone maintenance throughout adulthood to prevent osteoporosis. It also supports vascular contraction, vasodilation, muscular contraction, and nerve transmission. For lactose-intolerant individuals, non-diary calcium sources should be regularly consumed.

Potassium-modified Diet

A low-potassium diet includes foods like apples, berries, green beans, and bell peppers. It is prescribed for individuals with conditions such as hyperkalemia due to specific medications or medical conditions.

Renal Patients' Nutrition

Individuals with renal conditions, such as acute or chronic renal failure, and those on dialysis require controlled quantities of protein, salt, phosphorus, calcium, potassium, and fluids. Adjustments in fiber, cholesterol, and fat levels may also be necessary based on individual needs. Most dialysis patients need to limit their fluid intake.

Dietary Protein Restriction

For patients on protein-restricted diets, it is important to provide enough protein to maintain nutritional status but avoid the accumulation of waste products from protein metabolism. Approximately 40 to 60 grams of protein is allowed daily. High biological value proteins, which contain all essential amino acids in recommended proportions, are preferred.

Low-protein items, like gelatin, wafers, cookies, and wheat starch-derived bread and pasta, can increase caloric intake and dietary diversity. Carbohydrates in powdered or liquid form may provide additional energy. Although vegetables and fruits contain some protein, they can still be included in extremely low-protein diets. Milk, meat, bread, and starch exchange foods are restricted.

This diet is prescribed to manage renal and hepatic disorders.

Low-sodium Diet

A low-sodium diet can consist of various levels of sodium intake. These include 4 grams per day for a no-added salt diet, 2 to 3 grams per day for moderate restriction, 1 gram per day for severe restriction, or 500 mg per day.

To adhere to this diet, a patient should consume fresh foods instead of processed meals, as the latter tend to contain higher amounts of salt. Examples of high-salt foods to avoid include pretzels, potato chips, soups, fast foods, salad dressings, soy sauce, lunch meats, and packaged, pickled, smoked, instant, frozen, and canned meals.

This diet is recommended for individuals with liver disease, cardiac disease, renal illness, heart failure, and hypertension.

Carbohydrate-controlled Diet

The main components of this diet are carbohydrates, proteins, and fats.

This diet is suitable for patients with type 2 diabetes, hypoglycemia, and hyperglycemia. It is not necessarily suitable for patients with obesity, who may require a calorie-controlled diet.

High-protein, High-calorie Diet

To implement this diet, encourage the consumption of nutrient-dense, high-calorie, and protein-rich foods, such as eggs, pork, fish, poultry, beef, seeds and nuts, peanut butter, whole milk, and milk products. Additionally, include foods rich in calories like honey, avocado, dried fruit, mayonnaise, butter, oil, gravy, milk, and sugar. Encourage snacks between meals, such as milkshakes, quick breakfasts, and nutritional supplements.

This diet is used to manage conditions like malnutrition, muscle-wasting diseases, recovery from surgery or trauma, cancer, wound healing, and burns. It is not generally used as a stand-alone treatment for diseases like respiratory failure, chronic obstructive pulmonary disease, or HIV/AIDS.

Dietary Fat Restriction

A dietary fat restriction diet limits the intake of total fat. This includes saturated, trans, polyunsaturated, and monounsaturated fats. Patients with malabsorption may have difficulty tolerating fiber and lactose, which can cause diarrhea, steatorrhea, and vitamin and mineral deficits. A fecal fat test is used to detect fat malabsorption.

This diet is used to treat symptoms of stomach discomfort, steatorrhea, flatulence, and diarrhea caused by excessive dietary fat intake. It is also used to prevent nutritional losses in individuals with malabsorptive diseases. Additionally, this diet can be beneficial for gastric reflux, gallbladder disease, pancreatitis, and malabsorption issues.

Cardiovascular Diet

In the cardiovascular diet, certain dietary components are restricted, which include total fat (saturated, trans, polyunsaturated, and monounsaturated fats), cholesterol, and salt.

This diet is used to manage conditions such as myocardial infarction, hypertension, hyperlipidemia, and diabetes. It is not specifically used to treat renal failure or nephrotic syndrome.

High-fiber, High-residue Diet

The high-fiber, high-residue diet includes foods that provide 20 to 35 grams of dietary fiber per day. This adds volume and weight to the stool and promotes the quick transit of undigested items through the gut.

Fruits, vegetables, and whole-grain foods are rich in residue. It is essential to gradually increase fiber intake and ensure adequate water consumption to avoid unpleasant side effects like dehydration, diarrhea, bloating, and stomach cramps. Foods that cause gas should be avoided.

This diet is beneficial to treat constipation, irritable bowel syndrome with alternating constipation and diarrhea, and asymptomatic diverticular disease.

Low-residue and Low-fiber diet

This diet is recommended for inflammation, scarring, or reduced gastrointestinal motility that might cause an obstruction. The goal is to provide foods that are less likely to cause obstruction.

Low-residue foods, such as refined pasta, white rice, cooked potatoes without skins, refined cooked cereals, and white bread, are included. Restrict or avoid foods with whole grains, plant fiber, nuts and seeds, and raw vegetables and fruits. Dairy products should be limited to no more than two servings per day.

This diet is used to treat conditions like inflammatory bowel disease, partial intestinal obstructions, gastroenteritis, diarrhea, and other gastrointestinal issues.

Soft Diet

The soft diet is suitable for clients who struggle to eat or swallow, have mouth or gum ulcers, underwent oral surgery, have a broken jaw, underwent plastic surgery of the head or neck, experience dysphagia, or have had a stroke.

Offer food at lower temperatures for patients with mouth sores. Patients with difficulty chewing due to a dry mouth can improve salivary flow by sucking on sour candy. Drinking plenty of water with meals can also help a patient chew and swallow.

All meals and spices are allowed, but it is best to consume liquid, chopped, or pureed foods and conventional foods with a soft consistency. Foods that contain nuts or seeds should be avoided as they may cause discomfort. Whole grains, fried foods, and raw vegetables and fruits should also be avoided.

Mechanically Altered Diet

A mechanically altered diet provides textural changes, such as diced, ground, mashed, or pureed meals. It excludes foods that are salted, smoked, rough, fried, or have abrasive textures. Also avoid raw fruits or vegetables, dried fruits, nuts, and other coarse textures.

This diet is suitable for patients who struggle to chew but can tolerate more texture diversity than a liquid diet provides. It is commonly used for individuals with dental issues, head or neck surgery, or dysphagia.

Complete Liquid Diet

A complete liquid diet consists solely of liquids. It lacks adequate nutritional energy (calories) and various nutrients. It includes clear and opaque liquid foods and foods that are liquid at body temperature. Foods like strained vegetable juices, fruit juices, refined cooked cereals, strained soups, custard, pudding, milk, morning drinks, sherbet, and plain ice cream are considered part of this diet. Often, comprehensive nutritional liquid supplements are employed to meet the dietary demands of patients on a full liquid diet for an extended period.

This may be used as a transitional diet after surgery for patients who were limited to clear liquids. It also may be used for patients who can't chew, swallow, or accept solid meals.

Clear Liquid Diet

The clear liquid diet is low in calories and many nutrients, but it is easily digested and absorbed and leaves only minimal residue in the gastrointestinal system.

The clear liquid diet provides fluids and electrolytes to keep the patient hydrated. It is commonly used as the first meal after full bowel rest, for malnourished individuals, for bowel preparation before surgery or testing, postoperatively, and for patients with fever, vomiting, diarrhea, gastroenteritis, or pancreatitis.

Monitor Clients' Intake/Output

Use an intake and output sheet to keep track of a patient's fluid intake and outflow. Patients who do not consume sufficient fluids throughout the day or who lose too many fluids due to various factors (diuretics, fever, heavy perspiration, burns, bleeding, diarrhea, or vomiting) are at high risk of dehydration.

Patients who receive intravenous fluids, have renal or heart issues, or experience difficulties with fluid balance may develop edema, particularly in the lower extremities. The precise amount of fluid intake and outflow should be noted and tallied each time a patient consumes or loses fluids over the course of 24 hours.

Fluid Output Measurement

Fluid output includes blood, diarrhea, wound drainage, vomitus, and urine. Provide patients with urine collection containers and instruct them to use only these containers for urination. Patients should inform a nurse before they discard the urine. Drainage pouches will contain blood and wound drainage, and vomit should be collected in an emesis bowl. Empty the contents of the patient's bedpan or catheter drainage bag into a graded container. In case of fluid losses that occur outside of containers, such as diarrhea or vomiting that escapes the emesis basin, you may need to estimate the volume.

Fluid Intake Measurement

To measure fluid intake, include all liquid, at-room-temperature meals, enteral fluids, IV fluids, and other beverages consumed by the patient, including water. Add up all the fluid servings for that patient. Use gloves and pour the leftover amounts of each liquid into a graduated vessel. To calculate the total amount of fluids supplied to the patient, add up the liquid in the vessel.

Assist with Activities of Daily Living

Patients may not want to discuss their personal hygiene needs, especially urination. Openly discuss these topics with patients to help put them at ease. Proper hygiene is essential to prevent hospital-acquired infections and complications, especially for patients who have had a stroke. Activities such as routine bathing, assistance with urination, dental hygiene, and hair care help maintain a patient's self-esteem and well-being.

Foot Care

Foot care is important to maintain a pleasant appearance and prevent scratching and infections. Examine the patient's nails, toes, and feet for foot ulcers, extreme pain, thick or brittle nails, and changes in nail texture or color. To take care of the patient's nails, soak them in warm, soapy water for 10 minutes, then place the feet on a towel. Use an orange stick to clean the dirt from beneath the nails and nail clippers to trim them. If the cut edges of the nails are jagged, file them. Apply lotion to the patient's feet.

Hair Care

To ensure the water temperature is pleasant, heat it to around 115°F and test it with an elbow. Place a pitcher of warm water by the patient's side. Position the patient's head at the top of the bed. Put a towel beneath the patient's head and a waterproof bed protector between their shoulder blades. Raise the bed protector's edge to prevent water spillage. Cover the patient's neck with another towel. Place a basin under the patient's head to catch water. Dampen a washcloth with warm water, then gently pour it over the patient's hair. Cover the patient's eyes with a wet washcloth. If necessary, place cotton balls in the patient's ears. Use a cup to gently pour water over the patient's hair.

Massage the patient's scalp with shampoo and rinse thoroughly. Repeat the process with conditioner if needed. Support the patient's head with a dry, clean towel. Replace the patient's head cushion. Dry the patient's hair with a dry towel. Assist the patient to brush and style their hair. Even if a wash is not required daily, regular combing can prevent tangles and distribute oils evenly down the hair shaft. Lightly brush the hair. Start from the ends and work up to the roots. Apply a small amount of petroleum jelly to difficult knots if necessary. Help the patient with their desired hairstyle, then clean and store the combing tools in their proper place.

Dentistry

Ensure the patient does not eat or drink anything if they are NPO (nothing by mouth). Elevate the patient's head and keep their chest dry. If the patient is awake, provide a cup of mouthwash and instruct them to rinse and spit. Use a toothbrush and a dime-sized amount of toothpaste to brush the teeth on all surfaces. Have the patient rinse with more mouthwash and spit as directed.

For unconscious patients, support the head and turn the patient sideways at least 45 degrees. Place an emesis dish under the patient's chin and a cloth beside the patient's head to catch drool. Be cautious when opening the patient's mouth. Do not put your fingers inside. Use a moist mouth swab to clean the patient's tongue and mouth. Moisturize the patient's lips.

Provide Site Care for Clients with Enteral Tubes

Conduct daily skin checks for signs of skin deterioration. Use zinc oxide or petrolatum ointment and wash with soap and water. Teach the patient the correct technique for gastrostomy feeding. Ensure the feeding container is no higher than 18 inches above the stomach, flush with water before and after the meal, and check for any remaining gastric contents. Bolus feeding of 200 to 500 mL usually takes 10 to 15 minutes.

Nasogastric Tube Care

Only tape the tube in place after an X-ray confirms its location in the stomach, usually after 24 hours. Encourage ambulation to facilitate the tube's passage. Position the patient on their back for two hours, then on their right side for two hours, and then on their left side for two hours to encourage gravity and peristalsis. Advance the tube 5–7.5 cm (two to three inches) per hour after it passes the pyloric sphincter.

Postmortem Care

Postmortem care involves care of the patient's body in accordance with the deceased's religious or cultural beliefs. It is essential to respect the family's preferences when you provide postmortem care.

After death, the body undergoes physical changes, such as rigor mortis, livor mortis, algor mortis, and loss of skin elasticity. Administer postmortem care promptly to prevent tissue deterioration. Before any post-death actions, elevate the head of the bed and place a fresh pillow under the patient's head to prevent livor mortis on the face.

In cases of organ donation, keep the patient on life support until vital organs such as the kidneys, pancreas, liver, lungs, or heart are surgically removed. This follows the confirmation of brain death or cessation of the heart, but it depends on the legal and medical context. As part of the organ procurement process, take care of family members during the donation process, tend to the donor's body, and identify potential organ donors.

Assessment

1) Follow specific care instructions or specimen collection guidelines provided by the practitioner.

2) Consult with a spiritual care professional who respects the family's cultural values.

3) Inquire whether the family wishes to participate in body care.

4) Allocate a private space for family and friends to gather and allow them to have time for reflection and mourning.

5) Check the Donate Life Registry to determine whether the patient has given first-person consent for organ donation. Confirm that the request for donation is properly signed and inform the organ procurement team.

6) Ask the doctor or another designated team member to confirm the time of death and inquire whether an autopsy has been requested.

7) Use two forms of identification to ensure the patient's identity.

Preparation

1) If the patient's family requests to view the body, prepare the body and the room with cultural sensitivity. Cover the body with a fresh sheet up to the chin, leave the arms exposed, and remove any unnecessary medical equipment.

2) Allow the family private time to spend with the patient's body. Encourage them to say goodbye according to their religious and cultural customs.

3) Determine which of the patient's belongings should be given to family members and which should remain with the body.

4) Gently brush the patient's hair. Remove any clips or rubber bands.

5) Place a soft pad under the patient's buttocks to manage any discharge of urine and feces as the sphincter muscles relax.

6) Use paper tape or circular gauze bandages to remove soiled dressings and replace them with clean ones.

7) Wash any contaminated body parts. Instruct family members who are involved in cleaning the body to use gloves and gowns for protection from bodily fluids.

8) Unless culturally forbidden, shave male facial hair.

9) If culturally acceptable, gently close the patient's eyes by drawing the eyelids over the pupils.

10) Position the patient's hands on the abdomen.

11) If culturally acceptable, place a cloth under the chin to gently close the patient's mouth.

12) If the patient's dentures are not in place, insert them into the mouth. Place them in a denture cup labeled with the patient's information and ensure they accompany the body to the mortuary if not secured in the mouth.

13) Remove any indwelling medical equipment, such as urinary catheters or endotracheal tubes.

14) Provide the patient's body with privacy, inform any roommates of the situation, and arrange for their relocation to another area.

15) Wrap the patient's body in a shroud provided by the facility. Attach an identification label to the outside of the shroud.

16) Confirm that arrangements have been made for the prompt transportation of the patient's body to the mortuary.

17) Document the entire process in the patient's file.

Provide Measures to Promote Sleep and Rest

Sleep is important for overall physical and mental well-being. It aids in restoration, prevents fatigue, and supports cognitive functions. Sleep hygiene focuses on nonpharmacological techniques to improve sleep quality and duration, which ensures patients can achieve better rest without the need to rely solely on medications. Here are some effective measures:

1) Provide medications to facilitate sleep.

For individuals who experience pain, analgesics can be used before bedtime. Anti-anxiety medications or tranquilizers may help reduce tension and promote relaxation. Hypnotic sedatives can aid a person to fall asleep.

2) Manage emotional stress.

Practice slow, deep breathing techniques for a short period to reduce stress and induce tranquility. Other methods, such as yoga, visualization, and meditation, can also be beneficial.

3) Promote comfort and relaxation.

Ensure that the bed linens are smooth, dry, and clean. The patient should empty their bladder before bedtime, wear loose-fitting nightwear, and maintain personal hygiene to contribute to a sense of comfort and relaxation.

4) Emphasize a sleep-friendly diet.

Avoid large meals, caffeine, and alcohol two to three hours before bedtime. If a bedtime snack is necessary, a glass of milk or light carbohydrates is recommended.

5) Create a comfortable sleep environment.

An ideal sleep environment has appropriate lighting and ventilation, comfortable pillows, a warm bed, and minimal noise. Some individuals may prefer a darker room. Others, such as children or those in unfamiliar surroundings, may benefit from a low light source. Avoid stimulating elements like music, as this can interfere with sleep. In hospital settings, minimize noise disturbances from staff activities to enhance patients' sleep quality.

6) Create a pre-bedtime routine.

Develop a consistent evening routine with calm activities like a warm bath and reading. The bedroom should only be associated with sleep and intimacy, so it is best to remove work-related items like laptops, televisions, and papers because they may disrupt the connection between wakefulness and sleep.

7) Address sleep issues.

For individuals who struggle to fall and stay asleep, it is vital to adhere to a regular sleep schedule. Consistency helps regulate the body's biological rhythm. If sleep does not come easily, it is advisable to get out of bed and engage in calm activities in another room. For example, patients can read or listen to soft music until drowsiness sets in.

Chapter 6: Pharmacological Therapies – Medication Administration Calculations

Perform Calculations for Medication Administration

Three main approaches are used to calculate medication doses: the formula method, ratio and proportion, and dimensional analysis.

Ratio and Proportion Method

To solve a ratio and proportion problem, only multiplication and division are utilized.

Example: If there are 2 mg/mL vials available and a clinician prescribes a 6 mg IV of a drug, the calculation is as follows:

2 mg/mL = 6 mg/x.

Dimensional Analysis Method

Use the same example from above and set up the calculation as follows:

(x mL) = 6 mg/1 x 1 mL/2 mg = 3 mL.

Formula

This straightforward approach involves different units of measurement and conversion factors to find the solution.

For the same example, the formula is as follows:

Dose ordered (6 mg) x Quantity (1 mL)/Have (2 mg) = Amount desired (3 mL).

Reinforce Clients' Education on Medications

It is vital to provide clients and their families with complete information about all the medications they currently take or will take. This education should cover these key points:

1) When to inform their primary care doctor about any side effects, negative reactions, or allergic reactions.

2) Special directions, such as whether to take the prescription before or after meals.

3) Potential drug interactions with other medications, dietary supplements, and over-the-counter drugs.

4) Possible negative effects of the medication, such as warning signs and symptoms to watch out for.

5) The potential side effects and how to recognize their warning signs and symptoms.

6) Medication contraindications that should be strictly followed.

7) Proper dosage and frequency of medication use.

8) The name and intended purpose of the medication.

9) Safe self-administration of medicine, such as techniques for tube feedings, IM injections, insulin, and inhalers.

Evaluate Clients' Response to Medication

Nurses must be well-informed about the interactions, side effects, contraindications, and indications of prescribed medications. If any concerns arise, the nurse should promptly consult the ordering physician or a licensed independent practitioner. Additionally, the nurse must closely monitor the patient for any side effects or negative reactions after medication administration.

Medication Interactions

When you administer IV fluids and pharmaceuticals, it is essential to consider their compatibility. Some medications can be safely injected together in the same syringe if they are compatible. Others cannot. Compatibility can be determined by observing color changes or precipitate formation. However, it may not always be apparent. To ensure safe administration, nurses must refer to a compatibility or incompatibility chart before they combine drugs, medications, and solutions.

Acute Allergic Reaction Symptoms

Allergic reactions to medications can vary from mild to severe. In some cases, they can be life-threatening. Therefore, nurses must thoroughly assess patients for potential pharmaceutical allergies. Patients' medical history should be carefully reviewed, especially if they receive a drug to which they have not been exposed before. All allergies should be documented in the nursing evaluation, drug administration record, and other sections of the patient's medical file per the facility's policies and practices.

Medication Side Effects and Adverse Effects

As part of the patient's medical history, nurses gather and record objective and subjective data on actual or potential side effects, adverse reactions, and allergies to prescribed medications, over-the-counter preparations, and herbal supplements. If a patient experiences a side effect or adverse reaction to a medication or parenteral treatment, nurses must promptly report and document this information. The drug administration should be paused until the prescribing doctor provides further instructions. This may include the continuation of the medication as prescribed or an alternative.

Reduce the Adverse and Side Effects of Parenteral Therapy and Medications

To minimize adverse and side effects, nurses may employ specific interventions. For instance, a patient who experiences nausea and vomiting due to a new medication might be prescribed an antiemetic to alleviate these symptoms. In the case of anaphylactic shock caused by a medication, emergency interventions such as epinephrine and bronchodilators may be administered to save the patient's life. A patient's response to the intervention should be closely monitored.

Rights of Medication Administration

Nurses certified to administer medications to patients must adhere to strict guidelines. They are legally responsible and must interpret patients' records and understand their specific allergic responses to certain medicines. Nurses must ensure precise and timely administration because any errors can cause serious health consequences, which include fatalities.

Medication Preparation

1) Observe patient responses and promptly record them. Administer the medication within 30 minutes of the scheduled time.

2) Inform the patient about potential side effects, expected outcomes, and the purpose of the medication.

3) Administer the correct medication at the right time and dose to the appropriate patient via the correct route.

4) Prior to administration, perform hand hygiene, review the drug label and sequence, and check the expiration date.

Drug Facts

1) The kidneys eliminate most medications from the body.

2) Drug metabolism is influenced by liver health. The liver is where most medications are metabolized.

3) Parenteral medications have a faster onset of action and require lower doses compared to oral medications because they bypass pre-metabolism.

4) Oral medications undergo liver breakdown before they enter the bloodstream. Parenteral medications first reach the liver and then reach systemic circulation.

5) IM medications are absorbed into the muscle before they enter circulation.

Medication Safety Practices

Medication administration and preparation require adherence to the pharmacists' guidance or the manufacturer's recommendations. Errors in medication administration or preparation can jeopardize a patient's health or life.

Hospital pharmacists and dispensing personnel fill prescriptions in a fast-paced environment. Mistakes can occur, especially when urgent medications are required. Nurses must administer medications based on the patient's drug record and understand the purpose of the doctor's prescription. Any changes observed in the patient after medication administration must be documented.

Clinical areas must stock only approved pharmaceuticals and follow standard criteria to order and manage medications. Regular checks of medication stock and expiration dates must be conducted by nursing staff. Up-to-date (nonexpired) and secure storage of pharmaceuticals is the responsibility of nursing staff.

Ensure Medication Safety

1) Conduct a monthly audit of the pharmaceutical supply to dispose of outdated drugs and replace them.

2) Do not store leftover medication for single use in the refrigerator. Do not administer leftover medication to another patient.

3) Discard any injectable stock drugs that were not fully administered to the patient.

4) Dispose of open stock medication bottles or vials after 28 days from the initial use.

5) After a stock medication bottle or vial is opened, record the date, time, and nursing staff initials on the container.

6) Whenever possible, ensure all oral pills are in unit dosage.

7) Order new medications from the pharmacy and return any expired prescriptions to the pharmacy.

8) Keep a log and report any discarded medications in the remarks section.

9) Nursing personnel should verify the expiration dates of all medications by the third week of every month.

10) Always lock up medication stock and keep it out of direct reach of patients.

Reconcile and Maintain Medication Lists or Medication Administration Records

Failure to communicate about a client's prescriptions can cause medication errors. The medication reconciliation process should be performed for all patients, especially during transitions such as admission, discharge, or transfer to another hospital.

The compilation of the medication list includes all current drugs and therapies, such as radioactive pharmaceuticals, diagnostic agents, blood derivatives, immunizations, nutritional supplements, herbal remedies, over-the-counter medications, vitamins, or medications.

Steps for the medication reconciliation process:

1) Inform relevant healthcare professionals about the new prescription list and document it.

2) Use critical thinking and professional judgment.

3) Compare the recently prescribed drugs list with the current medication list and note any discrepancies.

Collect Required Data Before Medication Administration

Before any medication is administered, it is essential to consider the contraindications associated with each drug. These include hepatic illness, renal disease, breastfeeding, pregnancy, allergies, and drug sensitivities.

The nurse must have a comprehensive understanding of the client's current health status, medical history, and any potential drug interactions or allergies.

A thorough assessment of the client's condition (vital signs, relevant test findings, and overall health) should be conducted.

A complete medication order should include the prescribing doctor's signature, the drug name, dose, route, time/ date of administration, and frequency, and the client's full name.

For specific medications like digoxin and antihypertensive drugs, evaluate the client's blood pressure and pulse rate before administration. Similarly, prothrombin time and partial thromboplastin time should be assessed before heparin is administered.

If a nurse identifies a contraindication for a particular patient, they must consult with the prescribing doctor to clarify the medication order.

Administer Medication by Oral Route (Sublingual and Buccal)

Sublingual medications are placed under the tongue. Buccal medications are inserted between the teeth and the inside of the cheek.

To administer these medications:

- Put on gloves.
- Place the medication where it will be most effectively administered (either under the tongue or between the cheek and teeth).
- Instruct the patient not to chew or swallow the medication but to let it dissolve completely.

Administer Medication by Oral Route

Some patients may pocket or retain medications in their cheeks instead of swallowing them immediately. In such cases, give the medication to the patient and remain with them until they have swallowed the medication.

Administer Intravenous Piggyback (Secondary) Medications

1) Connect the secondary IV set (piggyback) to the main intravenous line.
2) Clean the injection port of the main IV line with alcohol before you insert the secondary needle into it.
3) Lower the primary IV with an extension hook to allow the piggyback medication to run at a higher level until it is completed. Once finished, the main IV will automatically resume at the prescribed rate. If simultaneous administration is desired, keep the main and secondary containers at the same height.
4) Remove the secondary set after the entire medication has been infused.
5) Verify the compatibility of the IV solution and any additives with the medication.
6) Monitor for urine output, check for signs of complications at the infusion site (e.g., coldness, pallor, warmth, or redness), and inspect the IV tubing for any kinks or obstructions.

Administer Medication through Various Gastrointestinal Tubes

1) Position the patient at a 30-degree angle in the Fowler's position.

2) Auscultate the epigastric region with a stethoscope after you inject approximately 30 mL of air into the feeding tube. Aspirate the residual content and evaluate the pH to ensure proper tube placement. A pH level higher than six may indicate that the tube is in the respiratory system, not the digestive system.

3) Prepare the medication(s) to be given and attach the syringe without the piston to the end of the NG tube.

4) Allow the medication to flow naturally into the tube after you pour it into the syringe.

5) Flush the tube with 30 mL of water for children or 50 mL for adults after administration to clear and maintain tube patency.

6) Keep the patient in the same position for at least 30 minutes after the medication is administered. If the patient cannot maintain this position, lay them on their right side with their head elevated.

Administer Subcutaneous, Intradermal, or Intramuscular Medications

Intradermal

- Used to inject local anesthetics and conduct skin tests for diseases like histoplasmosis and TB.
- Injection sites: ventral forearm, upper back, and upper chest.
- Use a 25- to 27-gauge, 3/8- to ½-inch needle and apply the medication at a 10- to 15-degree angle into the skin while pulling the skin tight.
- Do not massage the area.

Subcutaneous

Maximum volume: 1.5 mL.

Injection sites: anterior and lateral parts of the upper arm and thigh, upper ventrodorsal gluteal region, scapular region on the back, and the belly, one inch from the umbilicus.

Use a 25- to 27-gauge, 0.5- to 1-inch needle, squeeze the skin, and administer at a 45-degree angle.

Intramuscular (Z Track IM Injection)

- Place the patient on their back and pull the skin to one side.
- Insert the needle into the muscle at a 90-degree angle and wait 10 seconds.
- Use for almost any IM administered ventrolaterally or dorsolaterally, for medications that sting or burn, and for iron injections.
- Injection sites: vastus lateralis muscle for babies, ventrogluteal into the gluteus medius muscle, and dorsogluteal into the gluteus maximus muscle.
- Maximum volumes for the deltoid muscle, children, and older individuals range from 0.5 to 1.0 mL. Adults should inject 4 mL into a big muscle (the gluteus medius).
- Use an 18- to 23-gauge, 1- to 2-inch needle when administering at a 90-degree angle.

Administer Medications by Ear, Eye, Nose, Inhalation, Rectum, Vagina, or Skin Route

Ear

- After ear medication is administered, a small piece of cotton may be placed in the ear canal to prevent drug leakage. It should not be moistened with the medicine itself.
- Advise the patient to rest on their side for 5 to 10 minutes for medication absorption.
- Administer drops, straighten the ear canal, clean the outer ear, and position the patient on the unaffected side.

Eye

- Pull the lower lid down and ask the patient to gaze up.
- Apply pressure to the inner canthus to avoid systemic absorption and a runny nose.
- Inject the medication into the conjunctival sac and place the patient supine with the head rotated toward the affected side.

Vaginal

- Wash the applicator under cold running water.
- Instruct the patient to stay in bed for 15 minutes to allow the suppository to absorb.
- Insert the suppository at least two inches into the vaginal canal.
- Lubricate the suppository and gloved finger if the applicator is not used. If the applicator is used, insert the suppository into the tip of the applicator.
- Check the perineum for odor and discharge before you insert the suppository.

Rectal

- Have the patient void before the suppository is inserted.
- Do not insert the suppository into feces.
- Moisten the suppository and gloved finger with water-soluble lubricant.
- Insert the tapered end beyond the anal sphincter (four inches for adults, two inches for children).
- Instruct the patient to hold the suppository for 15 to 20 minutes and pinch the buttocks until the urge to defecate has passed.

Turbo Inhalers and Metered-dose Inhalers

There are two distinct types of inhalers: turbo inhalers and metered-dose inhalers.

Turbo Inhaler:

1) To open the mouthpiece, pull the sleeve away from it and rotate it counterclockwise.
2) Screw the inhaler back on. Slide the sleeve down to pierce the capsule after you insert the colored portion of the drug into the stem of the mouthpiece.
3) Instruct the client to completely exhale and then take a deep breath in and hold it for a few seconds.
4) The patient may gargle and rinse their mouth afterward until all the medicine has been consumed.

Inhaler with Metered Dose:

1) Shake the bottle and remove the cap.

2) Ask the patient to exhale forcefully. Immediately after the forceful expiration, ask them to tightly wrap their lips over the mouthpiece.

3) As the patient inhales slowly and deeply, press the medicine container against the mouthpiece to release it.

4) Instruct the patient to hold their breath for a few seconds before gently exhaling. This will help to avoid a fungal infection of the mouth. They should then rinse their mouth with water and spit it out.

Topical

1) Open the tube or container. Set the top upside down on a table to avoid contamination of the inside of the cap.

2) Apply the topical treatment to the specified area(s) with a sterile piece of gauze, a cotton-tipped applicator, a tongue depressor, or gloved hands.

3) When you apply the topical treatment to a prescribed body region with hair, use broad, equal strokes that match the direction of hair growth.

Transdermal

Transdermal drugs are given to the client's upper arm or chest, where they are absorbed from the skin's surface. The application location should be hair-free. You may need to shave the area.

Application Process:

1) Clean the area with soap and water. Let it dry.

2) Apply the pre-medicated patch or strip directly to the skin.

3) Spread the medicine across a three-inch region.

4) Cover the location with plastic wrap or a similar semipermeable barrier designed for this purpose.

5) If the patch is not adhesive, tape it in place. Then write the date and time.

Count Controlled Substances and Report Discrepancies

A discrepancy refers to any instance where the amount of medicine present does not match the expected amount. In healthcare institutions, automated dispensing cabinets are commonly used. Blind counts are necessary when a restricted drug bin is accessed. This allows for immediate identification of discrepancies to narrow down the list of potential causes.

Discrepancies in controlled substance counts are seen as a recurring issue that requires resolution. It is no longer acceptable to leave a discrepancy unresolved. Institutions are now required to maintain thorough records of all controlled drugs they use.

Count and Report Discrepancies

Institutions usually require that discrepancies be resolved within a specified time frame based on their restricted drug policy and process. However, the effectiveness and quality of discrepancy resolutions vary across institutions and even within different units of the same organization.

All discrepancies should be noted and addressed properly, with trends closely monitored. Even if the final counts are accurate, a pattern of discrepancies may indicate a problem.

Create Successful Policies

Clinical staff should be properly trained to handle discrepancies. Policies should outline what to do when a resolution is not feasible. The primary goal should be to identify and prevent a recurrence of the problem.

Regular inventory checks are necessary to promptly notice differences in regularly used medications. Discrepancies in rarely used pharmaceuticals may go unnoticed for a long time if a regular inventory is not conducted.

The longer a discrepancy remains unnoticed, the more difficult it becomes to correct. When they design a policy for restricted drug inventory, facilities should consider the frequency of inventory checks. Though a weekly inventory may be sufficient for most cases, facilities that experience widespread discrepancy issues should consider more frequent inventories, at least temporarily.

Calculate and Monitor Intravenous Flow Rate

Ensure IV Flow

Before you administer medication, verify the patency of the vascular access device. To do this, aspirate for blood return and flush it with a 5 mL saline solution.

Calculate Flow Rate

Flow rate can be calculated with smart electronic infusion devices, manual mathematical computation, or a combination of both.

Smart Electronic Infusion Devices:

1) Follow the user manual provided by the manufacturer to program the smart electronic infusion device accurately.

2) Input essential data, such as prescribed dosage, solution concentration, medicine name, and patient weight.

3) Configure the equipment to determine the flow rate electronically.

4) Double-check the flow rate for high-alert drugs with another certified individual to ensure the order and specified infusion rate match.

Manual Mathematical Computation:

1) To calculate the number of drops per minute, use the formula: mL/min x drops/mL = drops/min.

2) Determine the flow rate as follows: (Box 6) mL/hr x 60 min/hr = mL/min.

Check IV Flow:

1) Replace blood and blood product administration sets every four hours when blood or blood components are administered continuously. Otherwise, they should be changed within 24 hours of an infusion's start.

2) Replace specialized administration sets used for propofol delivery every 6 to 12 hours in adults and every 12 hours in children, as per manufacturer's guidelines.

3) Administration sets for parenteral nutrition should be replaced every 24 hours to prevent bacterial development and infection due to fat emulsions.

4) Change administration sets if contamination is suspected. Follow the recommended guidelines to do so. For fluids other than lipids, blood, or blood products, main and secondary continuous administration sets should be changed only once every 96 hours.

5) Examine the vascular access device exit site for signs of phlebitis, extravasation, or infiltration.

6) Adjust the dose as directed if the patient's response is inadequate.

7) Be aware that drugs administered continuously via IV may have adverse side effects, such as urticaria, pruritus, respiratory depression, severe sedation, cardiac arrhythmias, and hemodynamic instability.

Monitor Blood Product Transfusion

Types of Blood Products

1) Factor VIII fractions (cryoprecipitate): Used to treat hemophilia. Contains factors VIII, XIII, and fibrinogen.

2) Platelets: A single unit of platelet transfusion usually increases the recipient's platelet count by approximately 5,000 to 10,000/μL.

3) Fresh frozen plasma: Contains all coagulation factors, with a shelf life of up to 12 months when stored properly in a frozen state. It must be used within 24 hours once thawed.

4) Packed RBCs: Provide twice as much hemoglobin as whole blood of the same volume. Transfusion reactions are potential complications, although they occur less often than with whole blood due to the absence of plasma proteins.

5) Whole blood: Provides all components, but a large amount might cause volume overload. Massive transfusions may result in calcium depletion from citrate, excess potassium and salt, transfusion response, AIDS, and hepatitis, among other complications.

Blood Transfusion Indications

1) Platelets.

Fresh whole blood and a platelet concentration are given.

2) Coagulation factors.

Fresh whole blood, fresh frozen plasma, or cryoprecipitate are used.

3) Proteins.

Albumin, fresh frozen plasma, or the plasma protein fraction is administered.

4) Volume expansion.

Whole blood, plasma, or albumin is used for volume expansion.

5) RBCs.

RBCs are administered to increase oxygen transport.

Care for Blood Recipients

1) Carefully record vital signs, patient's response, quantity infused, start and finish times of the infusion, blood unit number, and blood component.

2) Monitor transfusion reactions:

    - Immunological sensitivity to foreign serum protein or allergic response may occur from the donor or receiver. Symptoms include anaphylaxis, bronchospasm, dyspnea, wheezing, laryngeal edema, or urticaria. Stop the transfusion and administer epinephrine and antihistamine.

    - Incompatibility with Rh or ABO causes a hemolytic response. Symptoms may include renal failure, shock-like symptoms, dyspnea, jaundice, flushing, chills, vomiting, nausea, sternal or lumbar pain, and headaches. Send the blood unit and patient blood to the lab, stop the IV infusion, and start a saline IV.

3) Use an 18- or 19-gauge needle initially. Set the infusion rate to 2 cc/min.

4) Have two nurses double-check the expiry date, patient and blood counts, Rh type, and ABO group.

5) Always use sodium chloride as an intravenous solution. Dextrose solution should never be used as it causes blood cells to clump together.

6) Determine whether there is any history of previous transfusions or transfusion reactions.

Maintain Pain Control Devices

1) Epidural opiates may cause pruritus or itching. To treat pruritus without affecting analgesia, use small doses of naloxone. In some cases, low-dose opioid antagonists may be necessary. Dehydration-related itching can also be treated effectively with diphenhydramine or hydroxyzine, but they may cause greater drowsiness.

2) Vomiting or nausea may require the administration of antiemetics.

3) For the epidural catheter insertion site, change the dressing as directed or if it becomes dirty, moist, or loose. If the catheter site is visible, consult a doctor. Cleanse the surrounding area and watch for signs of infection, which could indicate an epidural abscess.

4) Check the sacrum and heels every two hours for skin integrity to prevent decubitus ulcers and pressure sores.

5) A metallic taste, lips that tingle or ears that ring may indicate local anesthetic toxicity.

6) Assess the extremities every four hours for any sensory or motor loss. It might indicate an epidural abscess, hematoma, or local anesthetic overdose.

7) Monitor the ability to fully empty the bladder and void. This will help identify urine retention and early signs of an epidural abscess or hematoma.

8) Check the epidural catheter site every four hours for signs of infection or site-related issues.

9) Monitor temperature every four hours. Fever could indicate a systemic or epidural infection.

10) Monitor end-tidal carbon dioxide and oxygen saturation. A decline in oxygen saturation is a late sign of opioid oversedation.

11) Ensure the control panel is secured when you use a volumetric infuser or close the PCEA program with a code or key.

12) Check blood pressure every two hours. If hypotension develops, give the patient vasopressor drugs, lie them down flat, and notify the pain relief service, advanced practice nurse, and doctor. Stop the epidural infusion if necessary.

13) Check heart rate every two hours. Bradycardia may signify opioid overdose or sympathetic blocking from a local anesthetic. Tachycardia can indicate shock.

14) Monitor breathing rate for the first 20 minutes after the epidural drug injection to detect respiratory depression.

15) Assess the level of sedation. Changes in the sedation scale may indicate catheter movement into an intrathecal space or an epidural blood artery.

16) Use a pain scale to evaluate the patient's responsiveness to pain relief treatment. Aim to maintain a low pain score both during activity and at rest. The goal of analgesia is to keep pain at a constant and safe level.

Documentation

Documentation should include the effectiveness of pain medications, assessments of their effectiveness, continuous infusion rates and concentrations, settings for PCEA-programmed pumps, unanticipated side effects, measurements of oxygen saturation and vital signs, assessments of sedation scores, degrees of motor and sensory blockade, the type of dressing used, any insertion challenges, pre-procedure checks and timeouts, and informed consent.

Chapter 7: Reduction of Risk Potential

Check and Monitor Clients' Vital Signs

Vital signs are important as objective indicators of essential physiological processes. Their accurate measurement and interpretation are necessary initial steps in the clinical assessment of patients to help identify changes in a patient's condition and ensure appropriate medical interventions.

Blood Pressure

1) Before you measure blood pressure, ensure the patient has not consumed caffeine-containing beverages for at least an hour or smoked nicotine-containing substances for at least 15 minutes.

2) Have the patient empty their bladder before the test, as a full bladder can increase readings by 10 mmHg. Ask them to sit still for at least five minutes before you take their blood pressure.

3) Be aware that talking or active listening may elevate blood pressure readings by 10 mmHg.

4) Ensure the patient's back and feet are properly supported, as unsupported back and feet can contribute 6 mmHg to pressure measurements. Also, make sure their legs are not crossed, as crossed legs can add 2 to 4 mmHg to readings.

5) Support the patient's arm at the level of the heart to prevent an additional 10 mmHg to pressure measurements.

6) To rule out aortic coarctation, measure the patient's blood pressure in each arm and, in younger patients, in the upper and lower limbs.

7) Use the appropriate cuff size to ensure accurate readings. Smaller cuff sizes may result in erroneously high blood pressure readings, and bigger cuff sizes can lead to erroneously low blood pressure readings.

Breathing

1) Breathing patterns.

    - Paradoxical ventilation: The abdomen or chest wall moves outward during expiration and inward during inspiration. This is often seen in chest wall injuries, muscle fatigue, or diaphragm paralysis.

- Orthopnea: Difficult breathing occurs when a patient lies flat, but improvement is seen when the patient sits up or rises. This is commonly observed in congestive heart failure.
- Kussmaul breathing: This is an increased depth of ventilation while maintaining a regular respiratory rate. This is seen in patients with renal failure and diabetic ketoacidosis.
- Cheyne-Stokes respiration: This is an increased ventilation depth followed by pauses in breathing (apnea). This is observed with heavy sedative use, deteriorating congestive heart failure, and elevated intracranial pressure.
- Biot respiration: Intervals of faster and deeper breathing are followed by longer gaps in breathing (apnea), which may indicate elevated intracranial pressure from illnesses like meningitis or space-occupying skull lesions.

2) Breathing depth.

Hyperpnea, characterized by increased depth, occurs with exertion, congestive heart failure, lung infections, and anxious moods. Hyperventilation, on the other hand, involves both an increase in rate and depth of breathing and can be caused by lactic acidosis, diabetic ketoacidosis, exercise, and anxiety. Conversely, hypoventilation with reduced rate and depth may result from metabolic alkalosis, severe sedation, or obesity hypoventilation syndrome.

3) Respiratory rate.

The respiratory rate refers to the number of breaths taken per minute. In most adults, the rate is 12–21 bpm. Tachypnea, with a rate of more than 20 breaths per minute, can occur due to exercise, pregnancy, carbon monoxide poisoning, sepsis, anxiety disorders, aspiration of a foreign body, asthma, pulmonary embolism, or diabetic ketoacidosis. Bradypnea, defined as ventilation of fewer than 12 bpm, may result from the worsening of respiratory illness, respiratory failure, metabolic disturbances, or the use of alcohol, benzodiazepines, or opioids. Apnea, the cessation of lung airflow for up to 15 seconds, can be caused by overdoses of benzodiazepines and narcotics, airway obstructions, or cardiopulmonary arrest.

Pulse

The most frequently used sites to measure peripheral pulses in the lower extremities are the femoral pulse, dorsalis pedis pulse, and posterior tibialis. In the upper extremities, the sites are the brachial pulse, ulnar pulse, and radial pulse.

1) Pulse amplitude.

Low amplitude and rate may indicate poor perfusion conditions and aortic stenosis. Conversely, high amplitude and quick increase may suggest aortic regurgitation, mitral regurgitation, or hypertrophic cardiomyopathy.

2) Pulse symmetry.

Asymmetrical pulses are present in diseases such as Takayasu arteritis, aortic coarctation, and aortic dissection.

3) Pulse volume.

Low volume pulse may indicate insufficient tissue perfusion. This can serve as an indirect systolic blood pressure prediction. For example, radial pulse usually suggests a systolic blood pressure higher than 80 mmHg, a carotid pulse more than 60 mmHg, and a femoral pulse more than 70 mmHg.

4) Pulse rhythm.

Pulse rhythm can be regular, irregular, or abnormally irregular. An abnormally irregular pattern may indicate atrial flutter or atrial fibrillation. Any delay between pulses may indicate aortic coarctation.

5) Pulse rate.

In adults, heart rates usually range between 60 and 100 beats per minute. Rates over 100 beats per minute are referred to as tachycardia, while rates below 60 are considered bradycardia. Sinus arrhythmia involves variations in both pulse rate and breathing, where the pulse rate increases during inspiration and decreases during expiration.

Temperature

The average body temperature ranges from 97.7 to 99.5°F or 36.5 to 37.5°C. The tympanic membrane, oral, rectal, or axillary regions can indicate a patient's temperature. Infrared and electronic thermometers are commonly used for measurement.

Oral temperature is a popular approach, in which the thermometer is placed under the tongue, and the lips form a seal. To take the tympanic temperature, insert the appropriate thermometer into the ear canal. To take the axillary temperature, place the thermometer in the armpit. For a rectal temperature measurement, the thermometer is lubricated and inserted into the anus.

Time of day influences temperature fluctuations second only to the circadian cycle. Women with regular menstrual cycles may experience variations in body temperature known as the circamensal rhythm.

Perform an Electrocardiogram (EKG/ECG)

An EKG is a painless, quick test used to measure the electrical activity of the heart. It is recommended when there is a family history of heart disease or when symptoms of a heart condition are present, such as chest discomfort, fatigue, breathing difficulties, and the presence of a heart murmur or tachycardia.

Types of Electrocardiograms

1) Recording loop.

A loop recorder is inserted under the skin of the patient's chest to detect anomalies that may lead to dizziness or palpitations.

2) Event recorder.

An event recorder is useful for infrequent symptoms, as it captures the heart's electrical activity only when symptoms manifest. Some event recorders require the user to press a button when experiencing symptoms to transmit data to the doctor through their phone. Other event recorders activate automatically when they detect arrhythmia.

3) Holter monitor.

A Holter monitor records the heart's activity over 48 hours or up to two weeks. A log of events is kept by the patient while they wear the monitor. It helps the doctor determine the origin of symptoms. Electrodes are connected to the chest to record data.

4) Stress test.

During a stress test, the patient exercises on a treadmill or stationary bike with continuous monitoring by an EKG. Some cardiac conditions only manifest during physical activity, which makes this test important for diagnosis.

EKG Procedure

1) Ensure the patient removes any metallic items, such as jewelry. If necessary, shave excess chest hair to allow the electrodes to adhere properly.

2) Maintain a comfortable room temperature. Patients should avoid cold water or exercise before the exam.

3) Apply 10 gel-coated soft electrodes to the patient's legs, arms, and chest. Connect them to the EKG equipment.

4) Instruct the patient to remain still, breathe regularly, and remain silent throughout the exam.

5) The EKG device will graph and record the heart's electrical activity.

6) After the test, remove and discard the electrodes.

7) Test results are immediately accessible, so the doctor should review them promptly. In some cases, the doctor may consult a cardiologist. If the findings are abnormal, the doctor will contact the patient to discuss ways to improve heart health. Abnormal EKG results may indicate coronary artery disease, blocked arteries, chamber hypertrophy, chamber dilation, birth defects, insufficient blood flow, enlarged heart, or irregular pulse.

Perform Venipuncture

Venipuncture involves the insertion of a needle into a vein to obtain a blood sample or to support long-term intravenous treatment with fluids or medications.

Venipuncture Procedure

1) Use antiseptic to clean the area. Confirm the reason for drawing blood samples and verify the patient's identity information.

2) Label each tube with the patient's information.

3) Take necessary precautions, such as the use of a clean tourniquet, sterile cotton swabs, sterile needles or cannulas, PPE, and gloves.

4) Locate the antecubital fossa in the inner elbow region of the forearm for blood collection. Apply a tourniquet four inches above the desired location.

5) Instruct the patient to make a fist so the vein bulges with blood. Anchor the vein and pull the skin taut one inch below the venipuncture site. Insert the needle with the bevel side up at an angle of approximately 15 degrees.

6) Collect the blood in the appropriately colored tubes. Tubes with anticoagulants should be fully inverted to mix the blood thoroughly and prevent clotting.

7) Apply gentle pressure to the puncture site after you remove the tourniquet to ensure hemostasis.

8) Dispose of all sharps/needles in designated receptacles.

9) Transport the blood specimen to the laboratory for analysis.

Monitor Blood Glucose

Glucose Tests

1) Venous blood sample.

Venipuncture is used to collect venous blood. The blood is then processed in a commercial-grade facility with quality control procedures.

Benefits:

- Provides more accurate blood glucose measurement compared to capillary blood glucose tests.

Negatives:

- Not suitable for routine specimen collection.
- Involves an unpleasant technique.
- Creates the potential for local tissue injury.

2) Capillary blood glucose

A blood sample is obtained with a fingertip prick. It can also be collected from the palm, forearm, heel, and earlobe, especially while patients are fasting or two hours after a meal.

Benefits:

- Large display on the glucometer.
- Quick testing times.
- Various alternative testing locations.
- Requires a tiny blood sample.
- More comfortable than venipuncture.

Negatives:

- Some manufacturers offer inexpensive glucometers but charge high prices for testing strips and accessories.
- Test strips have short expiration dates.
- Can be expensive overall.
- Results may be affected by the quality of the blood sample, size, humidity, and temperature.
- Results may not be accurate in severely ill patients with hypotension, altered hematocrit, anemia, or hypoglycemia.

Techniques

Use the side of the finger's distal ends on the palm to minimize bone damage. Avoid using the little finger, as the tissue may not be deep enough to protect the bone. Do not use the thumb and index finger as they have more sensitive skin. Do not use the arm if the patient is receiving an intravenous infusion or has recently had a mastectomy on that side of the body. For infants under one year, the lateral or medial plantar surface of the heel is the preferred location.

Steps:

- Remove the glucose testing strip from the container. Do not touch the sensor tip. Place the glucose test strip inside the glucometer, which often turns on automatically.
- Apply a lancet firmly to the area where the sample will be taken. Prime the lancet to no more than 2 mm to reduce the risk of bone breakage.
- Pull back on the lancet's trigger to penetrate the skin.
- To avoid contamination of the blood sample, wipe away the initial drop of blood with sterile gauze, as it could be hemolyzed or contain intracellular fluid. To collect the second drop of blood, touch the tip of the glucose testing strip to it.
- Cover the skin puncture with clean tissue.

Results Interpretation

Further testing to confirm the diagnosis may involve an oral glucose tolerance test. Advise the patient to consume more than 150 grams of carbohydrates daily for three days. The patient should fast for 8 to 16 hours before the test. A fasting blood sample is taken, followed by the consumption of a sweet beverage that contains 75 grams of glucose. Another blood sample is taken two hours after the patient drinks the glucose solution.

1) Diabetes.

A blood glucose level of 200 mg/dL or 11.1 mmol per L two hours after ingesting 75 grams of oral glucose indicates diabetes.

2) Prediabetes.

A blood glucose level between 140–199 mg/dL or 7.8–11.0 mmol two hours after ingesting 75 grams of oral glucose indicates prediabetes.

3) HbA1c.

The HbA1c test measures the proportion of glucose molecules bound to hemoglobin, which generate glycated hemoglobin. The combination that results remains throughout the life span of a red blood cell, usually between 60 and 120 days. HbA1c levels should be between 3.5–6%. An HbA1c test that shows more than 6.5% glycosylated indicates diabetes. Patients with HbA1c values higher than 7.0% require pharmaceutical intervention.

Collect Specimens for Diagnostic Tests (e.g., Blood, Urine, Stool, Sputum)

Urine Sample Collection

1) 24-hour urine sample collection.

Collect a 24-hour urine production sample by having the client discard the first void and then collect all subsequent urine over the next 24 hours. The client should use a commode or bedside urinal. Refrigerate the urine sample to prevent excessive microbial growth.

2) Urine catheter sample collection.

For a regular urinalysis, clamp the catheter drainage tubing with a rubber band below the level of the urine drainage port. Wipe the port with a disinfectant swab for 10 seconds. Draw 25 mL of urine with a syringe and dispense it into the specimen container. For a urine culture, use sterile tools and urine containers to avoid contamination. Take the urine sample to the lab within 20 minutes after you unclamp the catheter to restart proper urine flow.

3) Midstream, clean catch, and random urine sample Collection.

Urine can be collected at any time of the day. Open the clean-catch kit and provide specialized wipes if the patient can clean the perineum themselves. For a clean-catch specimen, clean the perineum and genital area to remove any skin-borne microorganisms that could contaminate the urine sample. This is especially important when a UTI is suspected. Collect the sample in the middle of the urine flow to avoid the first and last urine droplets, which may contain skin germs.

For patients with an uncircumcised penis, retract the foreskin gently. Pull it toward the base of the penis. Use the wipe to cleanse the area from the top down to the base. For patients with phenotypically female genitalia, separate the labia and wipe the area from the top of the vulva downward toward the anus. Keep the labia apart when you collect a midstream specimen for patients with phenotypically female genitalia. Keep the foreskin retracted for those with uncircumcised penises.

Stool Sample Collection

Stool sample collection allows a client's feces to be tested for the presence of parasites, germs, mucus, fat, or blood.

1) Before you collect the stool, ask the individual to empty their bladder. Provide a voiding device if they are unable to use the toilet.
2) Open the specimen container with the inside face up and place the lid on a paper towel.
3) If the client cannot use the toilet, provide a bedpan or bedside commode. If they can use a standard toilet, place a collecting device at the rear of the toilet bowl.
4) If the client can clean themselves, provide tissue paper, a damp cloth, or pre-moistened wipes. If not, assist with perineal care.
5) Observe the stool's overall condition, quantity, color, and smell.
6) Use the tongue depressor attached to the specimen container's lid to collect the feces sample. Add two teaspoons of the sample to the container. Collect samples from any regions that have blood, mucus, or appear watery. Take samples from the center and the two ends of the feces if it is hard.

7) After you carefully close the container, place it back on the paper towel on the restroom counter. Dispose of one glove and grip the transfer bag with the glove-free hand.

8) Transport the sample immediately to the lab. If immediate transfer is not possible, store the sample until it is picked up.

Sputum Sample Collection

Sputum sample collection is an important management tool for pulmonary illness. Usually, specimens are collected through bronchoscopy, tracheal suction, or expectoration. Sputum samples help diagnose respiratory illnesses, such as pneumonia, lung abscess, and bronchitis. An acid-fast sputum smear can be inspected for mycobacterial infection (TB). It is possible to culture sputum to find respiratory germs.

Though tracheal suctioning provides a more accurate diagnostic specimen, it is often not done unless expectoration fails to yield a sample. Expectoration requires postural drainage, chest percussion, hydration, and ultrasonic nebulization.

1) Tracheal suctioning.

Before and after the procedure, provide the patient with oxygen and connect the sputum trap to the suction catheter. Lubricate the catheter with regular saline solution and pass it into the nose without suction. Apply suction for five seconds at a time when you remove the catheter, not as it is being inserted into the trachea. Stop the suction, remove the catheter, and dispose of it properly. Send the specimen to the lab as soon as it is collected. Mark the container with the patient's information, current antimicrobial treatment, initial diagnosis, and the time and date of collection.

2) Expectoration.

Instruct the patient to cough up expectorate into the container. Use chest physiotherapy or nebulization if the cough is ineffective. Before you ship the container to the lab, put on gloves and a mask. Use an aseptic procedure, close the container firmly, and place it in a leakproof bag.

Maintain the Central Venous Catheter

The central venous catheter (CVC) is inserted into the superior vena cava and advanced into the right atrium of the heart through the jugular or subclavian vein. These catheters vary in length of stay and may have up to three lumens.

Indications

CVC is the preferred route of venous access for patients with long-term chronic conditions, those receiving continuous or intermittent treatments like TPN, medications, blood, chemotherapy, or those with insufficient peripheral veins for necessary therapies.

Maintain and Care for the CVC

To maintain and care for the CVC, change the occlusive transparent dressing every seven days or sooner if it becomes moist, dirty, or loosened. Use strict sterile procedures and change dressings at least every 48 hours. Clean the insertion site with a chlorhexidine solution and cover it with an impregnated dressing.

Replace the caps before and after each access, such as when you administer drugs or chemotherapeutic agents. Flush the line with heparin solution to keep the CVC open. Replace the injection cap on each lumen every seven days. Both the nurse and patient should wear masks when the CVC device is accessed and cared for.

Do not perform blood pressure measurements or collect laboratory specimens on the side of the central venous access device.

Complications of the CVC

Complications of CVC placement may include infection, emboli, thrombosis, hemothorax, pneumothorax, and unintentional heart perforation.

Monitor Diagnostic or Laboratory Test Results

Arterial Blood Gases Test

Blood gas analysis interprets metabolic, circulatory, and respiratory issues through the analysis of $PaCO_2$ (ventilation status) and PaO_2 (oxygenation status).

ABG Components

- SaO_2 is the calculated arterial oxygen saturation with a range of 95–100%.
- Base excess or deficit is the calculated relative base excess or deficit in arterial blood with a range from -4 to +2.
- HCO_3 is the estimated bicarbonate concentration in arterial blood with a range of 21–26.

- PaCO2 is the measurement of carbon dioxide partial pressure in arterial blood with a range of 35–45.
- PaO2 is the partial pressure of oxygen in arterial blood and should range between 75–100.
- pH is the measured acid-base balance of blood with a range of 7.35 to 7.45.

Interpretation of the ABG Results

First, observe the pH level to determine if alkalosis (pH > 7.45) or acidosis (pH < 7.35) is present. For a normal pH, consider the cutoff point as 7.40 (e.g., pH = 7.42 is alkalosis, and pH = 7.37 is acidosis). Next, analyze the respiratory (PaCO2) and metabolic (HCO3) components of the ABG data. Respiratory alkalosis is indicated by pH > 7.4 and PaCO2 > 40. Respiratory acidosis is indicated by pH < 7.4 and PaCO2 > 40. Check for a value (HCO3 or PaCO2) that is inconsistent with the pH to see if it indicates compensation for the original acidosis or alkalosis.

Example 1:

On room air, the ABG has these values: pH = 7.43, PaCO2 = 31, PaO2 = 137, HCO3 = 22, base deficit = 1.5, and SaO2 = 93%.

- The pH is within a healthy range, which indicates no alkalosis or acidosis.
- The HCO3 is normal but on the lower end, and the PaCO2 is decreased, which suggests respiratory alkalosis.
- PaCO2 is consistent with pH, which confirms respiratory alkalosis without any compensation, as HCO3 is within the usual range.
- The PaO2 is within the normal range, which indicates no aberrant oxygenation.

Example 2:

On room air, the ABG values are pH = 7.38, PaCO2 = 52, PaO2 = 59, HCO3 = 31, and SaO2 = 90%.

- The pH falls within the normal range, which indicates acidosis as it is below 7.40.
- Both the PaCO2 and HCO3 are elevated, which points to metabolic alkalosis and respiratory acidosis, respectively.

- PaCO2 is consistent with pH, which confirms respiratory acidosis without compensation. The raised HCO3 suggests metabolic alkalosis, which indicates non-acute primary disease, as compensation takes days to occur.
- PaO2 is reduced, which indicates a problem with oxygenation. The severity and necessary interventions, if any, will depend on the patient's history and physical examination.

ABG's Clinical Relevance

In ER and ICU settings, oxygenation is assessed in patients with severe ARDS, acute respiratory failure, or sepsis. Calculating the alveolar-arterial oxygen gradient can help identify the source of hypoxemia. This can determine if the issue is related to impeded diffusion, a shunt, a V/Q mismatch, or hypoventilation.

To accurately gauge oxygenation status, the percentage of cardiac output going into pulmonary units not involved in gas exchange or the intrapulmonary shunt fraction is calculated. The shunt percentage is usually calculated with 1.0 delivered FiO2. The oxygenation index, which includes the degree of ventilatory assistance required to maintain oxygenation levels, is considered a stronger indication of lung damage than the P/F ratio. To calculate it, multiply the ventilator's reading of the Paw (mean airway pressure) by the fraction of FiO2 divided by PaO2. The oxygenation index is used as a management tool to determine the need for interventions such as EMO, surfactant administration, or inhalation of nitric oxide.

PaCO2 measures both cellular and pulmonary CO2 production. It is a sensitive indicator of ventilatory failure, especially when additional oxygen is administered. The physiological dead space, calculated as the difference between mixed expired PCO2 and PaCO2 divided by PaCO2, is a useful measurement of total lung function.

Metabolic acidosis may develop in patients with renal or gastrointestinal HCO3 loss, medication or toxin intake, renal failure, septic shock, or diabetic ketoacidosis. Metabolic alkalosis may result from factors such as hypokalemia, diuretic use, hypovolemia, protracted vomiting, electrolyte imbalances, or renal illness.

Blood Urea Nitrogen Test

This test determines the waste product created during protein digestion, which is then filtered by the kidneys and excreted in the urine.

Normal BUN Levels

- Adult males: 8–24 mg/dL.
- Adult females: 6–21 mg/dL.
- Children between 1 and 17 years: 7–20 mg/dL.

Abnormal BUN Values Interpretation

Elevated BUN levels, along with high creatinine levels, may indicate renal failure. Other factors, such as gastrointestinal bleeding, heart attacks, stress, aging, burns, dehydration, a high-protein diet, and certain drugs, can also raise BUN levels. BUN levels below normal may be seen in cases of liver disease, overhydration, a petite frame, or a low-protein diet.

Cholesterol Tests

Atherosclerotic cardiovascular disease is a major cause of cardiovascular disorders. Cholesterol levels, such as triglycerides, VLDL, LDL, or HDL, are essential to assess heart disease risk.

Test Instructions

Not every patient is required to fast before a cholesterol test.

- Fasting lipid profiles are necessary to diagnose hypertriglyceridemia and pancreatitis, estimate residual risk in treated individuals, and screen and monitor hyperlipidemia in patients with genetic hyperlipidemia or a family history of early ASCVD.
- Non-fasting blood lipid profiles are appropriate to diagnose metabolic syndrome or conduct the initial risk assessment of a primary prevention patient who is not undergoing treatment.

Normal Cholesterol Levels

- HDL cholesterol: ≥1 mmol/L (40 mg/dL).
- Lipoprotein: ≥0.50 g/L (50 mg/dL).
- Non-HDL cholesterol: ≤3.8 mmol/L (145 mg/dL).
- Apolipoprotein A1: ≥1.25 g/L (125 mg/dL).

- IDL + VLDL: ≤0.8 mmol/L (30 mg/dL).
- LDL cholesterol: ≤3.1 mmol/L (115 mg/dL).
- Total cholesterol: ≤5 mmol/L (191 mg/dL).
- Triglycerides: ≤1.7 mmol/L (150 mg/dL).
- Apolipoprotein B: ≤1.0 g/L (100 mg/dL).

Complete Blood Count (CBC)

A CBC alone is not conclusive for diagnosis. Additional tests are required to determine the presence of diseases.

1) Platelets.

Platelets regulate bleeding and help blot clot. Changes in platelet counts may indicate significant medical conditions and increase the risk of excessive bleeding. A normal platelet count is 150,000–450,000 per milliliter.

2) White blood cells.

White blood cells are essential to fight infection. Abnormal changes in their quantity or composition may indicate malignancy, inflammation, or infection. A normal WBC count range is 3,500–10,500 cells/mcL.

The various types of WBCs include neutrophils, eosinophils, basophils, monocytes, and lymphocytes. The percentage ranges are 0.5% to 1% basophils, 2% to 8% monocytes, 1% to 4% eosinophils, 20% to 40% lymphocytes, and 55% to 70% neutrophils.

3) Red blood cells.

Normal hemoglobin levels are 135–175 g/L for men and 120–155 g/L for women. The normal range of RBC count is approximately 4.32–5.72 million per milliliter for men and 3.90–5.03 million per milliliter for women. Normal hematocrit levels are 34.9–44.5% for women and 38.8–50% for males.

Additional RBC indices include:

- Mean corpuscular volume (MCV) indicates RBC size.
- Mean corpuscular hemoglobin (MCH) indicates the amount of hemoglobin in each RBC.

- Mean corpuscular hemoglobin concentration (MCHC) indicates the concentration of hemoglobin in a certain volume of blood.
- Red cell distribution width (RDW) measures red blood cell size variation.
- Reticulocyte count examines the quantity of freshly formed red blood cells.

Creatinine Test

Test Indications

- Monitor the performance of a donated kidney.
- Detect medication side effects that might impact kidney function.
- Assess the progress of renal disease therapy.
- Evaluate kidney function in patients with diabetes, hypertension, or other conditions that increase the risk of renal disease.

Results Interpretation

1) GFR (glomerular filtration rate).

GFR is determined via serum creatinine levels along with consideration of age and sex. A GFR of less than 60 indicates renal disease.

2) Albumin-to-creatinine ratio.

This ratio assesses the amount of albumin in urine relative to creatinine. Results below 25 mg/g for adult women and below 17 mg/g for adult males indicate healthy kidney function. An above-average result may suggest renal disease, diabetic nephropathy, or diabetic kidney disease.

3) Creatinine clearance.

Creatinine clearance measures the kidneys' ability to remove creatinine from the blood and excrete it in urine. It is determined through the analysis of creatinine concentration in a 24-hour urine sample and a simultaneous serum sample. Values outside the expected range for a specific age group may indicate compromised renal function or conditions that affect the kidneys' blood supply. The usual range is between 77 and 160.

4) Serum creatinine level.

Elevated serum creatinine levels may indicate impaired renal function. For serum creatinine, normal ranges are usually 0.74 to 1.35 for adult men and 0.59 to 1.04 for adult women.

PT, PTT, and INR Tests

These tests assess blood coagulation and can detect bleeding disorders. They are also useful to predict a patient's response to anticoagulant medication and help to assess blood's ability to clot before surgery.

However, they serve different purposes:

- The PTT test examines the intrinsic coagulation pathway within a blood vessel.
- The PT test, also known as the PT/INR test, measures the function of the extrinsic coagulation pathway, which is activated when damage occurs to the tissue surrounding blood vessels.

Prothrombin Time (PT)

PT measures how long it takes for a blood clot to form based on the production by the liver of a protein called prothrombin. Prothrombin, or clotting factor 2, is one of 13 molecules involved in coagulation.

Normal and Abnormal Values

- For patients who do not take anticoagulants, the PT reference range is between 11 and 13.5 seconds.
- Elevated blood clotting times above the reference range indicate slower blood clotting and may be seen in conditions such as sickle cell disease, Von Willebrand disease, hemophilia, liver disease, anticoagulant use, or vitamin K deficiency.
- When the value falls below the reference range, blood clotting is faster than normal, which could be due to conditions like pulmonary embolism, deep vein thrombosis, medications that contain estrogen, or excessive vitamin K intake.
- Although the PT test doesn't require fasting, meals rich in vitamin K, such as soybeans, dark green vegetables, green tea, pork, or beef liver, may influence the results.

International Normalized Ratio (INR)

INR readings are essential to prevent blood clots in patients who take warfarin. The standard PT/INR range for individuals on warfarin is two to three seconds. Low INR readings indicate a higher risk of life-threatening blood clots. High INR readings indicate the possibility of life-threatening hemorrhage.

Partial Thromboplastin Time (PTT)

PTT assesses the intrinsic and common pathways of coagulation. This involves the conversion of prothrombin (factor II) into thrombin (activated factor II), catalyzed by several other clotting factors. Factor XI (also known as antihemophilic factor C) is one of the components of the intrinsic pathway, not thromboplastin.

The PTT reference range is between 25 and 33 seconds. A higher PTT value indicates slower than normal blood clotting and may be seen in conditions such as leukemia, antiphospholipid syndrome, lupus, Von Willebrand disease, hemophilia, liver disease, excessive heparin use, or vitamin K deficiency. A lower PTT value may be caused by metastasized ovarian, colon, or pancreatic cancer. It may also be caused by an advanced whole-body infection that consumes clotting factors too quickly, which leads to faster blood clotting.

Unlike warfarin, which is taken orally, heparin is administered intravenously to patients at risk of blood clots or after surgery. Warfarin interferes with vitamin K activity, while heparin interferes with thromboplastin action. The surgeon determines the amount of heparin required for each patient's surgery.

Identify Signs or Symptoms of Potential Prenatal Complications

Examination and Investigations

- Check the patient's blood type, CBC, and rhesus D status.
- Calculate the woman's body mass index with her height and weight measurements.
- Screen for fetal anomaly, thalassemia, sickle cell disease, and infectious diseases, such as hepatitis B, syphilis, and HIV.
- Conduct an ultrasound scan between 11 + 2 weeks and 14 + 1 weeks to test for Patau's syndrome, Edward's syndrome and Down syndrome to identify multiple pregnancies and establish gestational age.

- Perform an ultrasound scan between 18 + 0 weeks and 20 + 6 weeks to locate the placenta and check for fetal malformations.

- Offer rhesus-negative women a blood type and antibody test, CBC, and start anti-D prophylaxis at 28 weeks.

- Measure symphysis fundal height for singleton pregnancies after 24 + 0 weeks and plot it on a growth chart. The urgency of an ultrasound scan may depend on concomitant clinical signs, such as decreased fetal movements or elevated maternal blood pressure.

- Suggest abdominal palpation at every consultation after 36 + 0 weeks to help women expecting a singleton to detect potential breech presentation. Offer an ultrasound scan to confirm the presentation if a breech is suspected. Discuss various options and their advantages, disadvantages, and ramifications. This includes elective cesarean delivery, breech vaginal delivery, and external cephalic version (ECV), which involves turning the infant from a breech to a head-down position.

Nausea and Diarrhea

- Reassure expecting mothers that mild to severe morning sickness and vomiting are common during pregnancy and usually resolve by 16 to 20 weeks.

- Encourage pregnant women with mild to moderate nausea and vomiting to try nonpharmacological alternatives, like ginger.

- Offer antiemetic medication to expectant mothers who decide to take medication for their nausea and vomiting.

- Consider intravenous fluids, preferably as an outpatient procedure, and explore acupressure as a complementary therapy.

Heartburn

- Provide advice on dietary and lifestyle adjustments.

- Try an antacid or alginate for a few days to alleviate symptoms.

Vaginal Discharge

Vaginal discharge accompanied by symptoms like itching, discomfort, unpleasant odor, or pain requires attention. If there's uncertainty about the cause of symptomatic vaginal discharge in pregnant women, consider a vaginal swab. Treat vaginal candidiasis with vaginal imidazole. Use oral or vaginal antibiotics to address bacterial vaginosis.

Unexplained Vaginal Bleeding

For rhesus D-negative women at risk of isoimmunization with vaginal bleeding after 13 weeks of pregnancy, administer anti-D immunoglobulin. After 13 weeks, refer pregnant women to secondary care for review. Factors such as the extent of bleeding, risk of premature birth, and potential placental abruption should be considered when you decide whether to hospitalize pregnant women with unexplained vaginal bleeding beyond 13 weeks. If the placental location is unknown, offer an ultrasound. Contemplate corticosteroids for fetal lung maturation in cases of elevated preterm delivery risk within 48 hours with consideration of gestational age.

Preeclampsia Signs

Preeclampsia signs include suddenly swollen feet, hands, or face, vomiting, severe pain below the rib cage, blurred or flashing vision, and intense headaches. Use strip reagent automated reading equipment to check for proteinuria. If dipstick screening indicates positive proteinuria (1+ or more), measure the protein: creatinine ratio or albumin: creatinine ratio. Avoid using the first-morning void and refrain from regular 24-hour urine collections to measure proteinuria. If the protein: creatinine ratio is above 30 and the preeclampsia diagnosis remains uncertain, consider repeating the test with a fresh sample alongside clinical assessment. If the result using albumin: creatinine ratio is 8 or higher and there are doubts about the preeclampsia diagnosis, consider repeating the test.

Gestational Diabetes Mellitus

To assess the risk of gestational diabetes, consider these factors: disproportionately diabetic, first-degree relative with diabetes, history of pregnancy-related diabetes, previous macrosomic infant who weighed 4.5 kg or more, and BMI above 30 kg/m2. If a woman shows glycosuria of 1+ or higher on 2 or more occasions or 2+ or above on one occasion during regular prenatal care, further testing should be done to rule out gestational diabetes. For women at risk, perform the 75-g two-hour OGTT to check for gestational diabetes. Suspect gestational diabetes if the FPG (fasting plasma glucose) level is 5.1 mmol/L or higher or the two-hour plasma glucose level during a 75-g OGTT is 8.5 mmol/L or higher.

Focused Data Collection Based on Clients' Condition (e.g., Neurological Checks, Circulatory Checks)

Neurological Data Collection

1) Pupillary response evaluation.

Evaluate pupil response as part of the neurological assessment. Normal pupils are spherical and range in size from 2 to 6 mm bilaterally. Anisocoria, where one pupil is slightly smaller than the other, is a common variation. To test pupil sensitivity, shine a light beam into the eye's outer canthus. A healthy reaction is a quick and similar response. Any alteration in pupil size or responsiveness may indicate serious neurologic damage.

2) Motor function assessment.

Examine both sides of the patient's body for motor function. Note any asymmetry, as unilateral atrophy can indicate weakness. To test the patient's upper and lower extremities, have them resist your attempts to move their arms while they hold them parallel to the floor or bed. Additionally, ask them to make a fist with their fingers and release when instructed. Difficulty in releasing the fist may suggest brain damage.

3) Cranial nerves.

Assess various cranial nerves for proper function:

- Olfactory nerve: To test the sense of smell, ask the patient to identify familiar scents, like cinnamon and coffee.
- Optic nerve: Measure visual acuity with a Snellen chart and the Rosenbaum near-vision card.
- Oculomotor, trochlear, and abducens Nerves: Evaluate these nerves together through the cover-uncover test, six cardinal gaze positions, and corneal light reflex test. Assess pupil symmetry, shape, size, and responses to light.
- Trigeminal nerve: To evaluate sensory function, touch the patient's jaw, face, and forehead with a wisp of cotton. To test the pain threshold, use the point of a safety pin on the same areas. To evaluate motor function, ask the patient to clench their teeth and assess the masseter and temporal muscles for equal strength.

- Facial nerve: To test sensory function, place items with different flavors on the anterior tongue. To assess motor function, observe facial expressions and eye closure.
- Acoustic nerve: To assess hearing, perform the Rinne and Weber tests.
- Vagus and glossopharyngeal nerves: Check the gag reflex and observe the uvula's midline location and upward movement of the soft palate.
- Spinal accessory nerve: Test the strength of the sternocleidomastoid and upper trapezius muscles.
- Hypoglossal nerve: To assess tongue symmetry and strength, have the patient press their tongue against their face while you apply resistance.

By conducting these neurological checks, healthcare professionals can obtain essential information about a patient's neurologic status.

4) Memory.

To assess remote memory, which involves recalling past events like a wedding date or a child's birth date, you may need verification from a second party. To evaluate short-term memory, ask the patient to narrate a recent event. To test their immediate recall, give them three unrelated words, such as pencil, grape, and car, and have them repeat the words back to you. Then ask them to recall the words after five minutes.

5) Orientation.

During orientation, ask specific questions about the patient's name, location, and the date. Keep in mind that hospitalized patients might know the month but not the day of the week or the exact date.

6) Consciousness level.

To determine the patient's level of consciousness, address them by name at a regular volume. If there is no response, repeat their name louder. Gently shake the patient if necessary. If they still don't respond, consider unpleasant stimulation like supraorbital pressure, sternal rubbing, or trapezius contraction. If a patient only responds to painful stimuli on one side of their body, evaluate the nonreactive side to understand their level of responsiveness.

The Glasgow Coma Scale has a maximum score of 15 and a minimum score of 3. A patient with a score of 8 or less is considered unconscious.

Motor response:

- 1: No motor response.
- 2: Extension to pain.
- 3: Flexion to pain.
- 4: Withdraws from pain.
- 5: Localizes pain.
- 6: Obeys commands.

Verbal response:

- 1: No verbal response.
- 2: Incomprehensible sounds.
- 3: Inappropriate words.
- 4: Confused speech.
- 5: Fluent and oriented.

Eye response:

- 1: No eye-opening.
- 2: Opens to pain.
- 3: Opens to command.
- 4: Opens spontaneously.

Cardiovascular Data Collection

Cardiovascular symptoms include poor peripheral circulation, faintness, an irregular heartbeat or rhythm, shortness of breath, abrupt and unexplained weight gain, peripheral edema, and chest discomfort.

Examination

1) Precordium examination.

Check for any scars, abnormalities, or unusual pulsations that may be caused by the heart's underlying chambers and major vessels.

2) Jugular distension.

Observe for jugular distension. This occurs when there is increased pressure in the superior vena cava, which causes a bulge in the jugular vein. It should not be present when the head of the bed is upright or at a 30- to 45-degree angle.

3) Skin color.

To evaluate perfusion, check for pallor or cyanosis on the fingers, lips, and face. Cyanosis in the nail beds, lips, and skin indicates reduced oxygenation and perfusion. Pallor of the mucous membranes or skin may suggest reduced red blood cell production, oxygenation, or blood flow. In dark skin tones, check for pallor on the inner side of the lip, conjunctiva, or palms.

4) Extremities examination.

- For DVT, assess the calves for pain, warmth, color, and size variations. Look for unilateral acute onset of strong muscular pain that worsens with foot dorsiflexion, calf edema, soreness, redness, and warmth.
- Examine the lower extremities (legs, feet, and toes) bilaterally. Note feeling, movement, temperature, and color. Look for superficially dilated veins, peripheral edema, capillary refill, and skin ulcers.
- Observe the hands, arms, and fingers bilaterally. Note any feeling, movement, warmth, or color. Bilateral inconsistencies may indicate an injury or underlying ailment. To measure capillary refill time, squeeze the nail bed until it blanches and time the color return. A capillary refill time of more than two seconds may be a concern.

5) Thrills or heaves.

A sensation of an upward surge beneath the breastbone and on the front chest wall to the left of the sternum, referred to as a lift or heave, may indicate right ventricular hypertrophy. A thrill refers to a palpable tremor felt on the precordial skin or over an area of disturbance, such as an arteriovenous fistula or graft.

6) Edema.

Palpate the affected region to check for pitting by pressing on the skin over a bone such as the tibia. Use a scale from 1–4 to assess the indentation and the time needed to return to the initial position. Edema with a rating of 1+ implies a quick rebound. 4+ denotes a severe depression with a recovery period of more than 20 seconds.

7) Pulses.

Examine the dorsalis pedis, carotid, posterior tibialis, brachial, and radial pulses, as well as their rhythm. Rate bilaterally. If Doppler ultrasonography is available, use it to determine if the finding is new or long-standing before deciding whether a pulse is absent or present.

8) Heart sounds.

Auscultation is performed at various locations: mitral, tricuspid, Erb's point, pulmonary, and aortic zones.

- The mitral region (apical or left ventricular region) is located at the mid-clavicular line at the intercostal space number five.
- The tricuspid (or parasternal) region is found at the fourth intercostal space to the left of the sternum.
- Erb's point is situated at the third intercostal space to the sternum's left, just below the aortic region.
- The pulmonary region is located at the second intercostal space to the sternum's left.
- The aortic region is found at the second intercostal space to the sternum's right.

Auscultation usually starts in the aortic region. Note that the S2 will be audibly louder than the S1 when you listen over the region of the aortic and pulmonic valves. For the mitral region, ask female patients to elevate their breasts to place the stethoscope on the chest wall. Count the apex pulse over 60 seconds. The normal range for an adult is a regular beat with a rate between 65–110.

Other Heart Sounds

- A pleural friction rub, caused by inflammation in the pericardium, is most easily discernible when the patient is in an upright position, leans forward, and holds their breath.

- To hear S4 and S3 sounds, if present, ask the patient to lie on their left side while you listen over the apex.
- A ventricular gallop or S3 occurs when the ventricles fill up due to fluid overload or cardiac failure. This follows the S2.
- An atrial gallop or S4 comes just before the S1 and may indicate coronary artery disease or decreased ventricular compliance.
- A mid-systolic click related to mitral valve prolapse may be audible at the sternal border at the lower left part of the apex.
- Murmurs, which result from turbulent blood movement, may be detected in various areas, such as the aortic, tricuspid, and pulmonary. This may indicate valve defects or other conditions.

Check for Urinary Retention (e.g., Bladder Scan, Ultrasound, Palpation)

Urinary retention is diagnosed through a comprehensive approach that includes medical history, physical examination, and specific tests to assess the urinary system.

Medical History

Inquire about bowel habits, eating and drinking routines, current medications (both over-the-counter and prescription), history of pregnancy and delivery (for females), prostate issues (for males), past and present health conditions, and any lower urinary system symptoms.

Examination

Conduct a thorough examination. This includes a lower abdominal palpation to check for any abnormalities or discomfort, a neurological assessment to evaluate nerve function, a rectal examination to assess the prostate (in males), and a pelvic examination to examine the pelvic organs (in females).

Imaging Exams

Utilize imaging tests such as MRI to visualize the spine and urinary system, voiding cystourethrogram to observe the flow of urine from the bladder through the urethra, and ultrasound to obtain detailed images of the urinary tract.

Laboratory Tests

Perform blood tests to assess renal function and identify any underlying issues related to kidney function.

Urinalysis

Conduct urinalysis to diagnose conditions such as diabetes, renal problems, and UTIs.

Cystoscopy

Use a cystoscope (a long, thin device) to inspect the urethra and bladder for structural abnormalities, signs of infection, inflammation, or potential presence of cancer.

Urodynamic Evaluation

Conduct a urodynamic evaluation to understand how the bladder, urethra, and sphincters store and release urine effectively. This evaluation includes several tests:

1) Electromyography to analyze the muscle response of the bladder and sphincters to nerve signals.

2) Cystometry to measure the bladder's capacity, pressure buildup, and the sensation of the urge to urinate.

3) Video urodynamics to record images and measurements as the bladder fills and empties.

4) Pressure-flow study to assess the bladder pressure and urine flow rate.

5) Uroflowmetry to measure the volume and rate of urine flow during voiding.

Postvoid Residual Urine Assessment

Postvoid residual urine can be assessed with either a catheter or ultrasound technology to determine the amount of urine that remains in the bladder after urination.

Application and Verification of Compression Stockings and/or Sequential Compression Devices (SCD)

In patients at risk for DVT, such as those with cardiac conditions or recovering from major surgery, anti-embolic stockings and SCDs are utilized as preventive measures.

Anti-embolic Stockings

These stockings come in various pressure levels and can cover the foot to the calf or thigh. Ensure that the prescribed stockings fit appropriately, neither too loose nor too tight, to facilitate blood return to the heart and minimize the risk of clots. Openings over or under the toes allow medical staff to assess blood circulation, skin color, and temperature in the lower leg.

Sequential Compression Devices

SCDs consist of multi-compartment plastic sleeves that are placed over the client's legs and connected to an air pump via a tube. The air pump inflates each compartment from the bottom to the top and then deflates them in a cyclic pattern. This process helps push the blood from the legs back toward the heart.

Procedure to Apply SCDs

1) Ensure the bed's wheels are locked in place before you adjust it to a suitable height.

2) For SCDs, unfold the sleeves after you remove them from the plastic cover. Position one sleeve under the client's leg. Align the back of the knee with the knee opening and the ankle with the ankle opening. Wrap the sleeve snugly over the leg and repeat the process on the other leg. When you connect the tube to the air pump and turn it on, a green light will usually indicate a successful connection.

3) For anti-embolic stockings, place the client in a supine position and expose one leg. Turn the stocking inside out from the heel up while you hold it with both hands. Properly position the heel pocket over the client's heel before you slide the stocking over the toes, foot, and heel. Repeat the same process for the other leg and pull the stocking up to the desired position.

Check the Appropriate Use

1) Inspect the client's feet and toes for soreness, swelling, tingling, sensation, movement, temperature, and color.

2) Remove the boots every eight hours for about 30 minutes. Clients are allowed to take the boots off at night, but they should be put back on before getting out of bed the next day to prevent leg swelling from standing or sitting.

3) Avoid the boots if there are ulcers, sores, dermatitis, skin breakdown, or lower leg edema.

4) Ensure that the legs are dry before you apply the boots.

Identify Clients' Risks and Implement Interventions

Identifying Clients' Risk

The complexity of healthcare environments is recognized as a factor that can lead to human error. For example, identical packaging may cause mix-ups in medication administration in hospitals. Such errors can be attributed to various factors, such as lack of patient involvement in care, insufficient medication administration verification, ineffective provider communication, and the absence of standardized practices for medication storage.

It is important to acknowledge that human error is inevitable in high-stress circumstances. The key to improvement requires the creation of error-proof environments with well-designed systems, procedures, and practices to protect individuals from errors. This requires a strong safety culture in which workers share significant safety beliefs, values, and attitudes.

Millions of people suffer injuries or even death each year due to unsafe and subpar medical treatment. Various medical procedures and healthcare-related risks pose significant challenges to patient safety and add to the burden of harm caused by inadequate care. Patient safety incidents encompass conditions such as DVT, sepsis, radiation errors, unsafe transfusion practices, diagnostic mistakes, unsafe injection practices, surgical errors, healthcare-associated infections, and medication errors.

Client Risk Interventions

Successful implementation of patient safety measures requires qualified healthcare professionals, data-driven safety improvements, strong leadership, and clear policies.

It is essential to recognize how patient safety impacts the efficiency and costs of healthcare systems in relation to patient harm.

Monitor Continuous or Intermittent Suction of Nasogastric Tubes

1) Properly restock supplies and maintain equipment per agency policy and manufacturer's instructions.

2) Record and measure NG irrigations and drainage on the intake and output chart. Follow the timetable and agency policy. Create a graphic with client comments and a drainage description. Monitor NG tube output every eight hours, which

includes water intake from irrigation. If drainage is heavy, collection containers may need to be emptied more frequently. Accurately document the client's reaction to NG drainage.

3) Check the NG tube and suction the device at least once every two hours. If the client's condition or drainage changes, conduct more frequent inspections and report to the doctor.

4) Observe for bowel noises, assess the client's abdomen for distension, and check for discomfort, fullness sensation, or vomiting, as these may indicate improper NG suction or tube blockage.

5) Verify the NG tube's position to ensure it has not moved into the trachea due to manipulation or movement.

6) Examine the suction equipment to confirm proper drainage movement through the tubing, appropriate suction level (high, medium, or low), and continuous or intermittent suctioning.

7) Inspect the drainage from the NG tube for odor, consistency, color, and quantity. Stomach drainage may have a pale yellow to green color due to bile presence. In cases of bloody drainage, Hematest should be performed to confirm blood presence after stomach surgery. Coffee-ground-like discharge could be indicative of bleeding.

8) Validate doctor's orders for irrigation method, suction type, and NG tube placement.

Use Precautions to Prevent Injury and/or Complications Associated with a Procedure or Diagnosis

Nurses must:

1) Take preventive measures to mitigate the effects of immobility, such as DVT, urinary stasis, and contractures.

2) Practice thorough hand hygiene and use PPE when necessary.

3) Conduct specific tests and evaluations to identify clients at risk for skin breakdown or falls.

4) Implement isolation and cough hygiene measures.

5) Keep suctioning equipment and supplies readily available at the bedside for patients at risk of aspiration.

6) Initiate and maintain seizure precautions for clients with a history of seizure disorders.

7) Enforce NPO status before surgery to prevent aspiration.

8) Monitor clients with newly placed casts on extremity fractures to prevent denting, as this may lead to circulatory and neurological damage. Advise clients not to apply pressure on the cast until it is fully dry.

9) Position patients who receive continuous tube feedings in a semi-Fowler's position at a minimum of 30 degrees to prevent aspiration.

10) Implement necessary safety measures related to patient positions.

11) Adhere to sterilization and infection control protocols.

Evaluate Client Oxygen (O2) Saturation

Oxygen saturation measures the amount of oxygen in the blood. Oxygen saturation below 95% may warrant further investigation or intervention. This depends on the patient's specific clinical situation. It is not always considered a medical emergency. Always refer to clinical guidelines or the attending healthcare professional's directions.

Measurement Methods

Two methods are used to determine oxygen saturation: pulse oximetry and ABG.

- ABG: Measures oxygen and carbon dioxide levels in the blood to assess hemoglobin's oxygen and carbon dioxide exchange.

- Pulse oximetry: This measures the percentage of oxygen saturation in arterial blood. A probe is attached to the client's finger, nose, or earlobe to read wavelengths reflected from the blood using a sensor. Results are provided within seconds.

Causes of Hypoxia

Hypoxia, a decrease in blood oxygen saturation, may result from conditions such as exposure to cyanide or carbon monoxide, altitude sickness due to low oxygen in the air (e.g., flying at high altitudes), congenital heart defects, pulmonary embolism, certain heart conditions, anemia, pneumothorax, asthma, COPD, or respiratory infections.

Assist with Client Care Before and After Surgical Procedure

Preoperative Preparation

The preoperative phase starts when the decision for surgery is made and ends when the patient is transported to the operating room.

Nurse responsibilities include:

1) Pre-admission tests.

Perform or instruct the patient on preoperative shower and bowel preparation, assess the need for postoperative transportation and care, and initiate the first preoperative examination.

2) Waiting area.

Provide psychological support, administer medication if needed, establish an intravenous line, verify and mark the surgical site, review records, and assess the patient's condition, baseline pain, and nutritional status.

3) Entry into the surgical center.

Develop a care plan, outline perioperative phases and expectations, ensure the patient has signed the surgical consent form, explain potential risks and possible outcomes, assess the likelihood of postoperative issues, and complete the preoperative evaluation.

Postoperative Preparation

The postoperative period starts when the patient is brought to the recovery area and concludes with a follow-up assessment at a clinic or home.

Nursing duties include:

1) Intraoperative information.

Report the patient's level of consciousness before surgery, physical restrictions, any events during surgery, medications or analgesics administered, blood transfusions, insertion of drains or catheters, patient's reaction to surgery and anesthesia, type of anesthetic used, and type of surgery performed.

2) Assessment and recovery.

Determine if the patient is ready for transfer to an in-hospital unit or home discharge, administer blood, fluids, or medications as directed, ensure patient safety (prevent injury, maintain circulation and airway), and assess the patient's pain level.

3) Transfer to the surgical ward.

Plan patient discharge, assess mental state, assist in recovery and preparation for home, and monitor physical and mental reactions to surgery.

4) Home care.

Provide follow-up care through office or clinic visits or phone calls. Assess patient's response to surgery and anesthesia, as well as impact on body image and function.

Reinforce Clients' Education about Procedures and Treatments

1) The patient should understand the purpose of the evaluation.
2) The evaluation should be adaptable and tailored to individual needs.
3) The patient's dignity, independence, and interests should take priority, and active engagement is essential.
4) Patients may bring a companion with them.
5) Use appropriate terminology and phrasing.
6) Consider the patient's diversity, beliefs, values, culture, and circumstances.
7) Analyze the patient's gender, sexuality, race, disability, and religion with sensitivity.
8) Be attentive and respectful of the patient's background and history.
9) Consider the needs of the entire family. This includes the patient and caregivers.
10) Consider cost-effectiveness.

Monitor Clients' Responses to Procedures and Treatments

Nurses assess the effectiveness of all care, treatments, and procedures, as well as whether the client's expectations for the results have been met. They also evaluate the client's response to all prescribed medications, including drug interactions, adverse reactions, side effects, and therapeutic outcomes. Drug interactions occur when a drug interacts with another substance, which alters the effects of one or more medications. Anaphylactic reactions to medications indicate severe adverse effects that can be fatal. Side effects are unintended effects of a drug that do not reflect its anticipated therapeutic effects. They can vary in significance and sometimes cause patient discomfort. Objective and subjective information gathered during ongoing reassessments, client comments, and diagnostic test results compared to baseline data are used in this evaluation.

Insert, Maintain, and Remove Urinary Catheters

Urinary Catheter Insertion

1) Urinary catheter insertion requires aseptic conditions and proper equipment.

2) Clean the genital region with soap and water if soiled. Place the client supine with knees bent and hips contracted.

3) Practice hand hygiene, prepare the tools, and pour sterile normal saline into the tray.

4) For males, gently lift the penis, pull back the foreskin if uncircumcised, and hold it with a sterile gauze swab. Insert the catheter and direct the penis down when reaching the first sphincter.

5) For females, separate the labia, clean the urethral opening and labial folds with swabs held in forceps, and discard the swabs.

6) Lubricate the catheter before insertion and gently inflate the balloon with sterile water to the specified volume. If the patient experiences pain, ensure the catheter is in the bladder. Deflate the balloon before you remove the catheter.

7) Attach the catheter to the drainage system. Ensure it is secured and the drainage bag is below the level of the bladder.

Maintain the Urinary Catheter

1) Ensure the urine flow is unobstructed, use a securement device, perform perineal care daily, keep the drainage bag below the bladder, review the need for the catheter daily, and use the smallest diameter catheter possible.

2) Perform regular bathing and clean the insertion site daily with warm, soapy water, especially if secretions accumulate. Boys with uncircumcised foreskins should gently return the foreskin to its normal position after washing.

3) Investigate any abnormal signs in urine, such as blood, unpleasant odor, or cloudiness.

Urinary Catheter Removal

1) Assemble removal tools, wash your hands, put on gloves, and deflate the balloon fully before you gently remove the catheter.

2) Check the catheter's integrity after removal and report if any issues are found.

3) Ensure the patient urinates within six hours after catheter removal. If not, use a bladder scanner to measure urine volume. If more than 450 ml, encourage urination and drain urine with a straight catheter. If the patient still cannot urinate after another six hours and the scan shows more than 500 ml of urine in the bladder, contact the physician for further instructions.

Insert, Maintain, and Remove Nasogastric Tubes

Insertion

1) Measure and note the length of the NG tube from the tip of the nose to the tip of the xiphoid process before passing it.

2) Have the patient lean forward and sip water through a straw while you insert the lubricated tube into the nasopharynx. Drinking water helps close the epiglottis and prevent the tube from entering the trachea.

3) Unconscious patients may require X-rays to confirm proper placement. Aspirate gastrointestinal fluids and assess the pH to check for placement. A pH of less than 5.5 usually indicates proper placement in the stomach.

4) Clamp the tube or connect it to the suction device if needed after you secure the NG tube to the nose with tape and attach the tubing to the client's hospital gown with a safety pin.

5) Check for gastric residuals before each bolus feeding and every four to six hours during continuous feedings.

Maintain a Nasogastric Tube

To maintain an NG tube, monitor the tube's patency and the patient's mouth and nose daily. Each instance of NG drainage is counted and recorded, such as its volume, color, and other details. If the tube is used for meals or medication administration, it should be irrigated both before and after each instance.

Nasogastric Tube Removal

To remove the NG tube, first, remove the safety pin and the locking tape anchor from the nose. Then, disconnect the suction tubing and ask the client to take a deep breath as you gently draw out the tube.

Maintain and Remove Peripheral Intravenous Catheters

Maintain the Peripheral IV Catheter

1) Longer peripherally inserted central catheters (PICCs) may remain in place for several weeks or months. Shorter peripheral catheters can usually be left in place for 72 to 96 hours or as per facility policy.

2) The appropriate gauge of intravenous catheter is selected based on the patient's specific needs. Smaller gauges, such as 24-gauge, are often used for children and the elderly. Larger gauges, such as 16-gauge, are used for significant trauma patients and rapid transfusion needs. An 18- or 20-gauge is often suitable for most adults for general and emergency use. For short-term peripheral access lasting less than 24 hours, a butterfly may be used. An angiocatheter is utilized for peripheral intravenous treatment that lasts longer than 24 hours.

3) Veins in the nondominant hand's distal area are chosen for catheter insertion. Veins near dialysis access devices, areas of paralysis, mastectomy, or phlebitis are avoided. The use of upper extremity veins is preferred to prevent lower extremity phlebitis and emboli.

4) The nurse monitors and maintains the intravenous line to ensure that it is patent and the flow rate is as directed. Dressings are replaced as needed, or at least every 72 hours for gauze dressings and every seven days for transparent dressings. Any signs of infiltration, extravasation, infection, hematoma, fluid overload, or embolism are carefully observed at the intravenous site.

Removal of the Peripheral IV Catheter

The removal of the peripheral IV catheter requires aseptic procedures. Proper documentation of the removal is necessary for continuous patient care, audit, and data collection on rates of phlebitis and infiltration.

Pressure should be applied to establish hemostasis before you gently remove the device in a steady motion. Careless removal may result in a painful hematoma and potential infection. The integrity of the cannula should be checked to ensure the entire device has been removed. After you verify that bleeding has stopped, the area must be covered with a sterile dressing.

Assist with the Performance of a Diagnostic or Invasive Procedure

Registered nurses play a role in both noninvasive and invasive components of diagnostic examinations. They assist patients and other healthcare professionals during diagnostic testing. This may involve the administration of medications, positioning of patients, and, if needed, transport of patients to and from the test.

These basic guidelines and practices apply to all client diagnostic tests:

1) Dispose of all materials and tools used in the diagnostic procedure.

2) Properly label all specimens collected at the patient's bedside, such as the time and date of collection, the patient's full name, and instructions for preservation and transportation to the laboratory.

3) Observe general safety measures and wash your hands before and after each specimen collection or bedside diagnostic test.

4) Confirm the client's consent for the requested diagnostic test.

5) Provide the client with information about the test preparation, the protocol to be followed, and the purpose and explanation of the diagnostic test.

6) Monitor patients during diagnostic testing. Assess any necessary monitors (such as heart monitors or ventilators) as well as the patient's physical condition and vital signs.

7) Review test results. Promptly notify the patient's doctor of abnormal or critical findings that require immediate action and document the results in the patient's medical record.

Chapter 8: Physiological Adaptation

Recognize and Report Basic Abnormalities on a Cardiac Monitor Strip

Normal Rhythm

In a normal sinus rhythm, both atrial and ventricular rhythms are regular. QRS complexes have a constant duration of 0.06–0.12 seconds, and the heart rate ranges from 60 to 100 beats per minute. The PR interval lasts between 0.12 and 0.20 seconds, and each QRS complex is preceded by a round P wave.

Sinus Bradycardia

Sinus bradycardia differs from normal sinus rhythm in that the heart rate is less than 60 beats per minute. Contributing factors may include an inferior wall myocardial infarction, hypothermia, hypoglycemia, elevated intracranial pressure, drugs such as beta blockers and digitalis, and hypothyroidism. Warning signs include breathlessness, intolerance to exertion, syncope, weakness, clammy and chilly skin, and chest discomfort.

Sinus Tachycardia

Sinus tachycardia differs from normal sinus rhythm in that the heart rate exceeds 100 beats per minute. Causes may include excessive use of coffee, alcohol, and nicotine or preexisting cardiac disease, pain, stress, hyperpyrexia, hypertension, and hyperthyroidism. Symptoms may include syncope, palpitations, breathlessness, and chest discomfort.

Atrial Rhythm Disorders

Atrial arrhythmias occur when the sinoatrial node, the heart's natural pacemaker, fails to provide the necessary impulses for the heart's regular functioning.

Types of atrial arrhythmias include:

1) Supraventricular tachycardia.

In this arrhythmia, atrial and ventricular heart rates are 150–250 beats per minute. QRS complexes last 0.06–0.12 seconds, the PR interval may not be visible, and the P wave may be hidden by the QRS complex. Causes may include atherosclerosis, hypoxia, stress, and hypokalemia. Symptoms include dyspnea, fatigue, diaphoresis, syncope, palpitations, and polyuria.

2) PACs (premature atrial contractions).

PACs occur when the P wave is premature and followed by a compensatory pause. The PR interval lasts 0.12–0.20 seconds, the P wave is upright and occurs before each QRS complex, and the cardiac rhythm is irregular. However, the heart rate is normal. Causes may include stress, digitalis, electrolyte abnormalities, ischemia, and hypertension. Symptoms may include missed beats and palpitations.

3) Atrial fibrillation.

Atrial fibrillation is characterized by a QRS complex duration of 0.06–0.12 seconds and a uniform shape. It is distinguished by the absence of the PR interval, the presence of F waves instead of P waves, an irregular and variable ventricular rate rhythm, and a high atrial rate of 350–400 beats per minute. Contributing factors may include pulmonary embolism, hyperthyroidism, coronary artery disease, rheumatic heart disease, pericarditis, mitral valve malfunction, heart failure, and hypertension. Symptoms include fainting, disorientation, fluttering, dyspnea, and palpitations.

4) Atrial flutter.

Atrial flutter is characterized by a regular atrial rhythm, a fast atrial rate of 250–400 beats per minute, an irregular ventricular rhythm, and a fluctuating ventricular rate. The QRS complexes last 0.06–0.12 seconds, have a uniform shape, an imperceptible PR interval, a saw-tooth-like flutter wave, and abnormal P waves. Contributing factors may include ischemia, cardiomyopathy, a mitral valve abnormality, and COPD. Symptoms include angina pain, palpitations, dyspnea, and weakness.

Ventricular Rhythm Disorders

Ventricular arrhythmias are cardiac irregularities that lack any atrial activity or P waves and have an unusually wide QRS complex that lasts longer than the usual 0.12 seconds. They occur when the AV junction and the sinoatrial node fail to send their electrical impulses, so the ventricles take over the function of the heart's pacemaker.

Some ventricular arrhythmias include:

1) Torsades de Pointes.

Torsades de Pointes is characterized by the QRS complex bending both downward and upward, a prolonged QT interval, and an irregular or regular rhythm with a heart rate ranging from 150 to 250 beats per minute. Causes include hypomagnesemia, hypokalemia, and phenothiazine usage.

2) Asystole.

Asystole presents as a flat curve with no heart rate, P waves, PR interval, or QRS complex. Causes include myocardial infarction, pulmonary embolism, cardiac tamponade, and artificial pacemaker failure.

3) Ventricular fibrillation.

Ventricular fibrillation can be fine or coarse and lacks identifiable rhythm or rate of contraction. Without prompt medical attention, it can lead to death due to the absence of cardiac output. Causes include hypothermia, electrolyte imbalances, severe injury, myocardial infarction, drug overdoses, and untreated ventricular tachycardia.

4) Ventricular tachycardia.

Ventricular tachycardia occurs when the atria are not receiving any impulses. Urgent medical attention is essential to prevent progression to ventricular fibrillation and cardiac arrest. The ventricular rhythm is regular, the atrial rhythm is undetectable, and the heart rate is 101–250 beats per minute. Causes include myocardial infarction, digitalis, and heart failure. Symptoms may include no pulse, hypotension, dyspnea, palpitations, angina-like chest discomfort, and hemodynamic deterioration.

5) Agonal rhythm.

Agonal rhythm is a specific form of idioventricular rhythm with a heart rate of under 20 beats per minute. The rhythm is generally regular at a slow pace. Signs include loss of consciousness, no detectable blood pressure or pulse, and causes such as trauma or myocardial infarction.

6) Idioventricular rhythm.

Idioventricular rhythm is characterized by a T wave deflection, steady rhythm, and ventricular rate of 20 to 40 beats per minute. Causes include myocardial infarction, cardiomyopathy, hyperkalemia, and digitalis. Symptoms may include weakness, hypotension, and chilly, mottled skin.

7) Idioventricular arrhythmia that accelerates.

This arrhythmia occurs when both the AV and SA nodes do not function correctly. The heart rate ranges from 40 to 100 beats per minute, and the rhythm is often regular. Causes include hyperkalemia, cardiomyopathy, digitalis, and myocardial infarction. Symptoms may include weakness, hypotension, and cold, mottled, pale skin.

Provide Care for Clients' Drainage Devices (e.g., Wound Drain, Chest Tube)

Chest Tube Care

Chest tube insertion aims to remove fluid or air from the pleural space (the area that surrounds the lungs).

Nursing care includes:

1) Apply topical anesthetic to the insertion site for pain reduction.
2) Help the doctor identify the tube insertion location (slightly below the pectoralis muscle between the fourth and fifth ribs) and clean the area with chlorhexidine.
3) Elevate the afflicted side's arm over the head and tilt the patient's bed at the head up by 60 degrees.
4) Utilize sterile gloves and aseptic techniques.
5) Monitor the patient's vital signs.
6) Set up a drainage system once the chest tube is secured firmly with a suture or adhesive tape.
7) Apply a dressing to the site when the doctor has removed the chest tube. It may or may not be necessary to suture the insertion site based on the doctor's judgment.
8) Inform the physician, check the patient's vital signs, and prepare for a CXR if the chest tube system unintentionally disconnects. Do not clamp the chest tube without a specific order from a physician, as this could lead to a tension pneumothorax.
9) Clean the incision and take blood cultures if the insertion site is infected.
10) Check the drain chamber for significant blood loss, apply pressure to the area, cover it with an occlusive bandage, and verify coagulation findings if there is bleeding at the insertion site.

Wound Drain Care

Wound drains are tubes placed near surgical incisions in postoperative patients to drain fluids, blood, or pus.

Nursing care includes:

1) Secure the drain and inform the treatment team if its position changes.

2) Notify the treatment team and retape the surgical drain dressing if there is a leak at the drain site.

3) Ensure the drain is positioned below the insertion point.

4) Perform frequent pain assessments and administer analgesics as needed.

5) Monitor the patient for sepsis symptoms. If infection is suspected, swab the insertion site or consult the medical team about the need to test samples from any oozing.

6) Record the type and quantity of fluid in the drain bottle.

7) Check the drain's patency and insertion site before and after the patient is moved and at the start of each shift. Maintain suction to avoid infections, increased discomfort, or hematoma from a blocked drain tube.

Help Restore Normal Body Temperature

Hyperthermia occurs when the body produces or absorbs more heat than it can dissipate. This results in a core body temperature usually above 100.4°F (38°C). Causes include hyperthyroidism, certain drugs, such as anticholinergics and diuretics, hypothalamic injury, intense physical activity, and infection. Management involves cooling measures such as the application of cool wet cloths to the skin or the use of cooling blankets to bring the client's temperature down to normal. It is important to ensure adequate hydration and address any underlying issues.

Hypothermia occurs when the body loses heat faster than it can produce heat, which leads to a core body temperature below 95°F (35°C). Causes include diabetes, hypothyroidism, aging, trauma, and exposure to severe cold environments. To warm the person, cover them with blankets, provide warm oral fluids or intravenous fluids in severe cases, and address the underlying cause.

Provide Care for Clients with a Tracheostomy

A tracheostomy involves the placement of an indwelling tube through a neck incision to facilitate airflow or remove secretions from the trachea. Tracheostomy care is initially required every two hours for suctioning and cleaning. As the inflammatory reaction subsides, once-daily care is sufficient.

Evaluation

1) Assess the appearance of the incision.

2) Check the tracheostomy dressing or ties for any drainage.

3) Observe the substances produced at the tracheostomy site.

4) Monitor the client's respiratory condition.

Nursing Care

1) If tracheal secretions need suctioning, place the patient in a semi-sitting position to promote lung expansion and suction the entire length of the tracheostomy tube to clear secretions and ensure an open airway.

2) Pour normal saline and soaking solution into containers from the tracheostomy kit or sterile basins.

3) Remove the inner cannula from the double cannula tube and soak it in a solution recommended by the healthcare provider or facility protocol to remove any crusted secretions before you reinsert it.

4) Clean the lumen and the entire inner cannula with a brush cleaner soaked with saline. Gently tap the inside edge of the cannula to remove excess saline.

5) Reinsert the inner cannula.

6) Clean the incision site and the tube flange with gauze dressings saturated with normal saline.

Provide Care to Clients with an Ostomy (e.g., Colostomy, Ileostomy, Urostomy)

Ostomy Care for Bowel and Enteral Diversion

Nurses provide care and instructions to clients with bowel diversion ostomies and enteral ostomies. They educate clients about ostomy management. This includes matters such as how to communicate with their doctor, how to handle adverse effects, ostomy care, and the intended use of the ostomy.

To care for enteral tube feedings, nurses administer feedings, monitor intake and output, ensure correct tube placement, maintain tube patency, and manage the surgical entry site. They also assess residual measurements and watch for any complications.

To care for urinary diversion ostomies (urostomies), nurses monitor urine output, maintain skin integrity around the stoma, prevent infection, and educate the patient. Additional monitoring is necessary for complications such as renal calculi, UTIs, stomal infections, stenosis, or stoma retraction.

Steps

- If required, perform irrigation on the proximal loop.
- Encourage daily hydration intake of at least 2500 mL.
- Educate the client to avoid foods like cabbage, broccoli, and baked beans, which produce gas.
- Expect serosanguinous stomal discharge for the first few days after surgery.
- Cleanse the perineal wound four times daily in a warm sitz bath and use a T-binder after an abdominal-perineal resection.
- Observe the characteristics of the first stool and signs of peristalsis returning.
- Administer vitamin K to control postoperative bleeding.
- Ensure that stool preparations include enemas for stool cleansing and antibiotics (neomycin) for three to five days to reduce bacterial growth.
- Advise that the client only consume clear liquids the day before surgery, followed by three to five days of low-residue eating.

Provide Care to Clients on Ventilators

Mechanical ventilation supports alveolar function during inspiration and prevents alveolar collapse during expiration. It reduces the client's respiratory effort, expands lung capacity, improves gas exchange, and enhances oxygenation. Nurses must carefully observe the therapeutic benefits of mechanical ventilation on respiratory function and blood gases while being aware of associated risks.

Issues with Mechanical Ventilation

1) Hospital-acquired ventilator infections.

Vigilance for infection symptoms and respiratory issues, adherence to infection control protocols, sterile suctioning, and frequent handwashing are essential for management.

2) Hyperventilation.

Conditions like fever, sepsis, pain, anxiety, improper ventilator settings, or certain medications may cause hyperventilation in mechanically ventilated patients. Nurses must monitor carbon dioxide level, tidal volume, and minute volume.

3) Hypoventilation.

Unplanned extubation or disconnection from the mechanical ventilator can lead to hypoventilation. Management includes the use of safety alarms, rapid response to low pressure, and cautious handling of tubing and airways during patient movement, such as relocation or bed transfers.

4) Nitrogen depletion.

Atelectasis can result in nitrogen depletion as nitrogen is expelled from the patient's body tissues and lungs. This may occur if the client receives more than 80% oxygen.

5) Oxygen toxicity.

High oxygen concentrations can be toxic. Monitor ABG levels and maintain PaO2 between 50 and 60.

6) Cardiovascular complications.

Reduced venous return, cardiac output, and myocardial blood flow are potential complications. Management may involve adjusted ventilator settings, maintenance of optimal fluid balance, and adequate systemic perfusion.

7) Alveolar overdistension.

High ventilating pressures and tidal volume can cause alveolar overdistension and atelectrauma. This may lead to complications such as barotrauma, such as pneumothorax, pneumomediastinum, and subcutaneous emphysema. Management options include extracorporeal membrane oxygenation, high-frequency jet ventilation, high-frequency oscillatory ventilation, and reduced tidal volume and PEEP.

Provide Care for Clients Who Receive Peritoneal Dialysis or Hemodialysis

Dialysis aims to remove excess fluid, treat acidosis, maintain healthy electrolyte levels, and clear the blood of waste products resulting from protein metabolism.

Peritoneal Dialysis

Peritoneal dialysis is a medical procedure that uses the body's peritoneum as a natural filter. The peritoneum is a membrane in the abdomen that acts as a semi-permeable barrier. During peritoneal dialysis, a special fluid called dialysate is introduced into the abdominal cavity. Waste products and excess fluids pass from the blood vessels in the abdomen, through the peritoneum, into the dialysate, which is then drained away.

Nurses must:

- Monitor intake and output.
- Drain by gravity.
- Allow the solution to sit for 30–45 minutes.
- Initiate inflow for 10–20 minutes.
- Warm the dialysate solution to body temperature.
- Ask the patient to urinate before the treatment.
- Monitor vital signs before and after the procedure.
- Weigh the patient.

Risks associated with peritoneal dialysis are:

- Protein loss: Most serum proteins pass through the peritoneal membrane and are lost in dialysate fluid.
- Peritonitis and breathing problems may occur due to an engorged abdomen.

Hemodialysis

Hemodialysis involves blood shunted from the patient's circulatory system through a dialyzer and then returned to circulation.

Access points:

1. Venipuncture-accessed arteriovenous fistula. It may take three to four months to mature before it is suitable for use, but can last for many years.
2. Arteriovenous graft. It may take three weeks to be ready for use and can last for many years.

3. Catheterization of the femoral and subclavian veins. This provides quick access for emergency hemodialysis but is not recommended for long-term usage.

After dialysis, nurses should observe for peripheral paresthesia, leg cramps, confusion, elevated blood pressure, nausea, vomiting, and hypovolemic shock that could result from rapid fluid removal.

During hemodialysis, nurses must monitor patients for headaches and nausea, avoid the use of sedatives, antihypertensives, and vasodilators, and weigh the patient frequently.

For femoral or subclavian cannulation, nurses should observe for bleeding from the catheter, hematoma development, and palpate peripheral pulses in the extremity with the cannula.

For arteriovenous fistula and arteriovenous graft care, nurses should report pain, drainage, skin discoloration, or bleeding, avoid tight clothing over the site, avoid IM or IV injections, avoid taking blood pressure on the affected arm, auscultate for a bruit and palpate for a thrill to confirm patency.

Perform Wound Care and/or Dressing Change

Wound care involves dressing and cleansing the wound. The wound area is cleaned from the cleanest section to the most contaminated parts with sterile normal saline or antiseptic solutions. Each time the incision is gently cleaned, a new piece of gauze is applied with care so as not to disturb the granulating tissue.

Nurses evaluate the color, quantity, and characteristics of the exudate, along with the wound's location, size, and color.

Wound healing falls into three categories: tertiary, secondary, and primary intention healing. Pressure ulcers are treated based on the type of debridement needed (autolytic, enzymatic, mechanical, or surgical) and their color (black, yellow, or red).

Lavage Pulse

Pulsed lavage uses a high-pressure and pulsatile lavage device with saline to remove exudate and irrigate wounds. Nurses should use appropriate PPE to prevent occupational-related infections. Pulsed pressure lavage that is increased too much can lead to wound disruption.

Hydrotherapy

Hydrotherapy involves a whirlpool, sometimes with an antibacterial solution, with water heated to approximately 37°C. It is recommended for significant wounds, unhealable necrosis, and severe, serious burns. However, due to shared usage, there is a risk of pathogen contamination in these whirlpools.

Monitor Wound Infection Symptoms

Infections can manifest with systemic symptoms such as fever, chills, and fatigue. Symptoms specific to a wound infection may include redness, pain, swelling, or pus-like discharge at the wound site. Local symptoms may include swelling, heat, redness, and pain at the wound site. Nurses closely observe for these infection-related symptoms and diagnostic laboratory findings such as elevated CPR, ESR, and WBCs.

Assist Clients with Pacemakers

Pacemakers are electronic devices that provide regulated electrical stimulation to the heart muscle for rhythm modulation.

Nursing Care Objectives

1) Provide psychological support to address emotional issues.

2) Educate patients and their families about potential problems, activity limitations, and pacemaker operation.

3) Ensure an infection-free insertion site.

4) Encourage good hygiene, proper wound care, frequent site checks, and daily dressing changes for wound healing and skin integrity.

5) Monitor for pacemaker issues like lead dislodgment, infection, allergic reactions, malfunction, interactions, and thrombosis.

6) Regularly monitor ECG or telemetry to assess pacemaker settings, rhythm, and heart rate.

7) Avoid the pacemaker battery area during cardiac arrest and defibrillation. It may be necessary to reprogram the device if revival occurs.

8) To improve cardiac tissue perfusion, limit movement near the insertion site and monitor for symptoms like dyspnea, neck vein pulsations, palpitations, chest discomfort, edema, fatigue, or syncope.

9) Enhance mobility within prescribed parameters through regular exercise and deep breathing. Immobilize extremities near the pacemaker insertion site with devices like arm boards or slings.

Remove Wound Sutures or Staples

To remove surgical sutures or staples:

- Clean and disinfect the surgical incision with a topical antiseptic.
- Use sterile forceps to lift each knot and employ sterile scissors to cut the suture.
- After you remove all sutures, cleanse the surgical site with antiseptic again.
- Apply strips over the incision to promote further healing and closure.
- Remove staples with a surgical staple remover. Prior to this procedure, ensure the correct identification of the patient with two distinct identifiers.

Assist with Client Wound Drainage Device Removal

Steps for Wound Drainage Device Removal

1) First, assess analgesic needs and consider procedural sedation if necessary. Arrange pain management and nonpharmacological measures to minimize discomfort and distress during the process. Administer analgesics 30 minutes before the procedure for full effect.
2) Clean the area around the wound and remove sutures using aseptic procedures.
3) Gently rotate and apply smooth, quick traction to remove the drain.
4) Apply an occlusive dressing and tie off any sutures.
5) Before you remove pigtail drains, uncoil them to prevent tissue injury or pain.
6) If needed for culturing, cut the tube's tip.
7) Record the drain's removal and its condition in the progress notes.

Inability to Remove the Wound Drainage Device

If resistance occurs after mild rotation and gentle pull, do not continue. Alert the medical team and surgeon. Do not pull the drain tube with undue force to prevent internal tissue injury or fractured drain tubes.

Intervene to Improve Clients' Respiratory Status (e.g., Breathing Treatment, Suctioning, Repositioning)

Breathing Treatment

1) For short-term high oxygen needs, use high concentrations (up to 100% FiO2). These can be delivered through a non-rebreather mask or invasive mechanical ventilation such as an endotracheal tube or tracheostomy. The actual liter flow will depend on the delivery device and the patient's condition.

2) Moderate amounts (3 to 5 L/min through a nasal cannula) are recommended for conditions that hinder oxygen circulation, such as pulmonary embolism or congestive heart failure.

3) For prolonged oxygen administration, use low concentrations (1 to 2 L/min through a nasal cannula).

Breathing Treatment Methods

1) Venturi mask.

This accurately delivers 24% to 50% oxygen concentrations. Remove and wash the mask every two to three hours.

2) Nonrebreathing mask.

This provides 90% to 100% oxygen with a one-way valve and reservoir bag.

3) Standard mask.

This provides 40% to 65% oxygen at 6 to 12 L/min flow rates.

4) Nasal cannula.

This delivers 24% to 40% oxygen at 1 to 4 L/min flow rates. Insert prongs one centimeter into each nostril.

Suction

- Use a sterile catheter to remove secretions from the airway during tracheobronchial suctioning.

- Avoid suction use during catheter insertion.

- Hyperventilate the patient on 100% oxygen before and after suctioning.
- Disconnect the ventilator before suctioning.
- Place the patient in an upright position during suctioning.
- Rotate the catheter while intermittently suctioning for 10 seconds.
- Place your thumb over the catheter's opening to create suction.
- Reconnect the ventilator.

Position

1) Thoracentesis.

Place the patient in a seated position, leaned forward on a table, and have them support their weight with their arms. This position opens the spaces between the ribs and allows for easier access to the pleural space.

2) Bronchoscopy.

Put the patient in a semi-Fowler's position to prevent choking or aspiration due to reduced swallowing abilities.

3) Radical neck dissection.

Place the patient in a semi-Fowler's or Fowler's position to keep the airway patent and reduce edema.

4) COPD.

Position the patient with their arms over multiple cushions, leaned forward and seated, to facilitate better breathing.

Educate Clients About their Care and Condition

Clients have the legal and ethical right to accept or refuse treatments and procedures based on their comprehension of the process, alternatives, risks, advantages, problems, the procedure's purpose, and the person executing it. In cases where the client lacks mental capacity or understanding, is unconscious, or is a minor, education is provided to their spouse, parent, legal durable power of attorney, healthcare proxy, or guardian. All treatments and operations require the client's permission. The nurse must ensure the patient or legal representative signs the permission form in their presence, freely and without outside pressure.

Identify Signs and Symptoms Related to Acute or Chronic Illness

Nurses must be knowledgeable about both acute and chronic illnesses, such as symptoms and indicators of each disease, pathophysiology, diagnostic tests, risk factors, modifiable risk factors for improved health, self-care techniques, drug information, potential alternatives, and follow-up care frequency. Clients may also receive assistance from various community services.

Provide Care for Clients with Fluid and Electrolyte Imbalances

Fluid Imbalances

Hypovolemia refers to a lack of body fluids. Hypervolemia indicates excessive fluid in the blood, particularly blood plasma.

Hypervolemia can be caused by hypernatremia, cardiac failure, renal failure, liver failure, or excessive fluid supplementation. Symptoms include bounding and rapid heartbeat, tachycardia, peripheral edema, dilated jugular veins, ascites, crackling and rales of the lungs, dyspnea, and hypertension. Treatment options include diuretics, salt, and hydration limits.

Hypovolemia can result from diarrhea, vomiting, severe dehydration, or hemorrhage. Treatment options include blood and blood products, plasma expanders, and IV fluids like lactated Ringer's.

Electrolyte Imbalances

1) Phosphate.

The normal range for serum phosphate is 0.81–1.45 mmol/L. Hyperphosphatemia (phosphate level above 1.45 mmol/L) can be caused by conditions such as rhabdomyolysis, systemic infections, diabetic ketoacidosis, and severe renal illness. It may lead to symptoms such as atherosclerosis, myocardial infarctions, poor circulation, bone wasting, and cramping. Treatment involves phosphate binders and restricting phosphate-containing foods. Hypophosphatemia (phosphate level below 0.81 mmol/L) can be caused by conditions like osteomalacia, hepatic failure, leukemia, and severe malnutrition. Symptoms include confusion, agitation, and cardiac dysrhythmias. Treatment includes high-phosphorus diets and oral or intravenous phosphate supplements, not potassium phosphate, unless there is a concurrent potassium deficiency.

2) Magnesium.

Normal blood magnesium levels range from 1.7 to 2.2 mg/dL. Hypermagnesemia (magnesium level above 2.2 mg/dL) can result from long-term use of magnesium-containing laxatives and certain medical conditions. Symptoms include hypotension, depression, muscle weakness, and respiratory paralysis. Treatment options include IV dextrose, insulin, calcium, and renal dialysis. Hypomagnesemia (magnesium level below 1.7 mg/dL) can be caused by conditions like alcoholism, severe burns, and uncontrolled diabetes. Symptoms include cramps, spasms, convulsions, and muscle weakness. Treatment involves fluid and IV magnesium.

3) Calcium.

Normal calcium levels are between 8.5–10.6 mg/dL. Hypercalcemia (calcium level above 10.6 mg/dL) can be caused by conditions like tuberculosis and hyperparathyroidism. Symptoms include constipation, exhaustion, and skeletal pain. Treatment options include IV fluids, diuretics, and bisphosphonates. Hypocalcemia (calcium level below 8.5 mg/dL) can be caused by various medications and medical conditions. Symptoms include arrhythmias, seizures, and muscle pains. Treatment includes vitamin D and calcium supplements.

4) Potassium.

The normal range for potassium is 3.7–5.2 mEq/L. Hyperkalemia (potassium level above 5.2 mEq/L) is associated with renal illness and can cause cardiac dysrhythmias and muscle weakness. Treatment options include renal dialysis and potassium-lowering medicines. Hypokalemia (potassium level below 3.7 mEq/L) can result from fluid losses due to various factors. Symptoms include constipation, palpitations, and muscle weakness. Treatment involves the administration of potassium supplements. The underlying problem must also be addressed.

5) Sodium.

Normal sodium levels range from 135 to 145 mEq/L. Hypernatremia (sodium level above 145 mEq/L) can be caused by conditions such as Cushing's syndrome and dehydration. Symptoms include confusion and thirst. Treatment includes salt restrictions and care for underlying issues. Hyponatremia (sodium level below 135 mEq/L) can result from conditions such as severe diarrhea and renal failure. Symptoms include fatigue and seizures. Treatment options include fluid restrictions and hormone replacement therapy if necessary.

Respond and Intervene in a Situation that Threatens Life (e.g., Cardiopulmonary Resuscitation)

Cardiopulmonary Resuscitation

Cardiopulmonary arrest involves a significant disruption of the heart's electrical impulses and results in sudden cardiac function loss, cessation of breathing, and loss of consciousness. Initial treatments for sudden cardiac arrest include CPR and defibrillation to address conditions such as asystole and ventricular tachycardia.

Airway obstructions may be partial or total. Nurses can observe the patient's cough and respiratory sounds. The absence of coughing indicates a complete blockage. If necessary, intubation can be performed. Visible foreign objects can be removed, but caution should be exercised to avoid pushing them deeper into the airway. Encourage the patient to cough as well.

Observe the patient's chest and upper abdomen movement, listen for breath sounds, and check if the chest rises and falls to determine spontaneous breathing.

Nurses are trained in basic life support, which includes the performance of chest compressions during CPR. Defibrillation involves an electric shock delivered to the heart. Automated external defibrillators are user-friendly and do not require extensive knowledge of cardiac rhythms.

Recognize and Report Changes in Client Condition

After you evaluate the client's condition, identify and monitor any changes and take appropriate action. This may involve autonomous nursing tasks, further assessments to inform your judgment and reports to the physician as necessary.

Nursing evaluations encompass risk factors that may predispose clients to specific conditions. For example, immobile clients are at higher risk of complications related to immobility. Those with neurological deficits are more prone to falls. Sensory impairment increases the risk of accidents and medical errors, and poor nutrition may lead to cardiac disease and delayed wound healing.

In addition to a comprehensive head-to-toe evaluation and health history, specialized assessments are performed as needed. Clients with respiratory disorders undergo evaluations of their ABG and breath sounds, while those with cardiac issues receive focused assessments of heart sounds and ECG readings.

Test 1: Questions

(1) Which foods may be the cause of diarrhea, fever, and abdominal pain in a diverticulitis patient?

(A) Whole-grain cereal.

(B) Baked fish.

(C) Steamed carrots.

(D) Mashed potatoes.

(2) What is the appropriate approach for a patient with atopic dermatitis?

(A) Decrease the daily fluid intake.

(B) Moisten the skin daily.

(C) Use antipyretics.

(D) Infection prevention.

(3) A 75-year-old female told her family not to put her on a mechanical ventilator if she needed resuscitation. Which of these statements is true about her request?

(A) It is a consent for death.

(B) It is an advance directive.

(C) It is hospice care.

(D) It is palliative care.

(4) Which of these statements is true about combining Phenergan and Demerol as analgesics?

(A) This causes an excitatory effect.

(B) This causes an antagonist effect.

(C) This causes a synergistic effect.

(D) This causes an agonist effect.

(5) What is the role of the nasogastric tube after laryngectomy?

(A) Oral mucosa healing promotion.

(B) Suture line contamination prevention.

(C) Stomach decompression by suction.

(D) Dysphagia and swelling prevention.

(6) Which of these statements is true about the contagious varicella stage?

(A) It occurs from the rash onset until crusted lesions develop.

(B) It occurs from the rash onset until its disappearance.

(C) It occurs during crusting and vesicular lesions.

(D) It occurs from the rash onset until crusted vesicles develop.

(7) What can a patient advocate provide?

(A) Legal guidance.

(B) Insurance guidance.

(C) Medical guidance.

(D) All of the above.

(8) Which of these statements is true about a nephrotic syndrome patient who takes Cytoxan?

(A) The nurse should keep the inflamed joints warm.

(B) The nurse should use water and soap to bathe the patient.

(C) The nurse should give the patient a diet low in protein.

(D) The nurse should advise the patient to increase hydration.

(9) What is a side effect of clomiphene use?

(A) Painful intercourse.

(B) Vaginal bleeding.

(C) Multiple births.

(D) Infertility.

(10) What is the role of IV cimetidine in a severe burn patient?

(A) Prevent Curling's ulcers.

(B) Improve renal function.

(C) Improve electrolyte balance.

(D) Prevent infection.

(11) What can promote a patient's self-advocacy?

(A) Do not allow the patient to choose a healthcare provider.

(B) Stay present throughout significant events.

(C) Do not allow the patient to ask questions.

(D) Do not give the patient any updates on his medical condition.

(12) What is not true about care plan decision-making?

(A) Patients' choices should be respected even if a patient is not competent.

(B) Patients' choices should be respected if a patient is competent.

(C) The healthcare practitioner is responsible for informing the patient about his condition.

(D) In a medical emergency, consent can be presumed unless it is evident that the patient would reject the intervention.

(13) What is the systematic nursing care problem-solving approach?

(A) The nursing method.

(B) The Nurses Practice Act.

(C) The nursing process.

(D) The nursing care plan.

(14) Which nursing plan should be followed for a patient with severe back pain who is taking codeine sulfate?

(A) Check for hypertension.

(B) Check for peripheral pulses.

(C) Check for bowel activity.

(D) Check for fluid balance.

(15) Which side effects of carbamazepine, which is used to treat trigeminal neuralgia, may occur?

(A) WBC count = 2500/mm3.

(B) BUN level = 12 mg/dL.

(C) Sodium level = 139 mEq/L.

(D) Uric acid level = 3.5 mg/dL.

(16) What is a sign of aspirin intoxication?

(A) Photosensitivity.

(B) Constipation.

(C) Diarrhea.

(D) Tinnitus.

(17) What is true about a patient prescribed birth control pills and phenytoin for seizure control?

(A) There is an increase in thrombophlebitis risk.

(B) The birth control pill's effectiveness is decreased with phenytoin.

(C) It can be stopped if it causes a gastrointestinal effect.

(D) The patient should avoid pregnancy when prescribed phenytoin.

(18) What is not among the benefits of an interprofessional team?

(A) It promotes safe, quality care.

(B) It decreases the risk of negative outcomes.

(C) It increases positive outcomes.

(D) It decreases healthcare employee retention and job satisfaction.

(19) What is a type of conflict?

(A) Task-based.

(B) Value-based.

(C) Interpersonal-based.

(D) All of the above.

(20) What is an important step of ear irrigation?

(A) Face the irrigated ear upward by turning the head.

(B) Use the irrigation solution in a steady, slow stream to the eardrum.

(C) Keep the irrigated side in an upward position after irrigation.

(D) The solution should be warmed before irrigation.

(21) How do you do a visual acuity test with a Snellen chart?

(A) Check if the patient can read the smallest line while standing at 40 feet.

(B) Check if the patient can read the largest line while standing at 40 feet.

(C) Assess both eyes simultaneously before assessing the left and right eye individually.

(D) Assess both eyes simultaneously after assessing the left and right eye individually.

(22) When a nurse finds that the parenteral nutrition bag of a patient is empty, which solution is considered appropriate until a new parenteral nutrition is delivered to the nursing unit?

(A) 0.9% sodium chloride in 5% dextrose.

(B) Ringer's lactate in 5% dextrose.

(C) 10% dextrose.

(D) 5% dextrose.

(23) Four patients are under the supervision of a nurse. Which of the patients should the nurse evaluate first?

(A) A patient who got nasal oxygen and experienced respiratory issues during the prior shift.

(B) A postoperative patient who is ready to be released.

(C) A patient who must change into new clothes every day.

(D) A patient with a chest X-ray appointment.

(24) What is an effective instructional strategy during staff in-services?

(A) Feedback.

(B) Interaction.

(C) Case-based learning.

(D) All of the above.

(25) A patient who takes furosemide and digoxin came for a regular check-up. Which laboratory results should concern the nurse?

(A) Serum Mg of 1.7 mEq/L.

(B) BUN of 15 mg/dL.

(C) Serum K+ of 2.8 mEq/L.

(D) Serum digoxin of 1.3 ng/mL.

(26) What PPE should be worn during silica particle exposure in a silicosis patient?

(A) Eye protection.

(B) Gloves.

(C) Gown.

(D) Mask.

(27) What medical supportive equipment should be prepared when IV naloxone hydrochloride is administered to an opioid overdose patient?

(A) Central line insertion tray.

(B) Resuscitation equipment.

(C) Paracentesis tray.

(D) Nasogastric tube.

(28) After abdominal surgery, a nurse prescribed oral acetaminophen and IM meperidine for a patient's severe pain. The patient said that she still has severe pain. What is the appropriate action?

(A) Help the patient start a relaxation exercise to relieve the pain.

(B) Use a pain scale to assess the patient's pain level.

(C) Increase the patient's dose of meperidine.

(D) Increase the patient's dose of acetaminophen.

(29) What is the importance of a transparent dressing to cover a stage I pressure ulcer?

(A) The dressing promotes healing by letting the light through.

(B) The dressing makes the patient more comfortable.

(C) The dressing promotes healing by retaining moisture.

(D) The dressing protects the skin from injury.

(30) What is the role of data-driven clinical decision-making?

(A) To diagnose disease.

(B) To identify disease symptoms.

(C) To merge a range of tested diseases.

(D) All of the above.

(31) Which laboratory tests can indicate a therapeutic effect of epoetin alfa?

(A) WBC count = 8000 cells/mm3.

(B) BUN level = 12 mg/dL.

(C) Platelets count = 380,000 cells/mm3.

(D) Hematocrit level = 33%.

(32) Which condition is contraindicated for tacrolimus drug prescription?

(A) Coronary artery disease.

(B) Diabetes insipidus.

(C) Ulcerative colitis.

(D) Pancreatitis.

(33) What is not one of the Five Rights of Delegation?

(A) Proper person.

(B) Situation.

(C) Task.

(D) Education.

(34) Which foods can increase the LES pressure in a GERD patient?

(A) Nonfat milk.

(B) Fatty foods.

(C) Chocolate.

(D) Coffee.

(35) What is the appropriate hemorrhoidectomy postoperative action?

(A) Place the patient in the Fowler's position to decrease bleeding and rectal area pressure.

(B) Put a dressing over an ice pack.

(C) Advise the patient to eat a low-fiber diet.

(D) Decrease the patient's fluid intake to prevent urine retention.

(36) Why does information technology need management?

(A) It helps in decision-making.

(B) It provides a solid nurse-patient relationship.

(C) It improves healthcare quality.

(D) It damages the patient's confidentiality.

(37) A patient has specific privacy needs in the corporeal-physical domain. Nurses know that they should:

(A) Knock on the patient's door.

(B) Not introduce the patient to others in the ward.

(C) Ask permission for university students to be present during diagnostic and therapeutic procedures.

(D) Not touch the patient's body when unnecessary.

(38) When you call a patient at a predetermined date to check on the patient's progress, this is known as:

(A) Follow-up.

(B) Assessment.

(C) Diagnosis.

(D) Nursing care planning.

(39) When a nurse plans a patient's discharge, they will:

(A) Provide self-care at home before discharge instructions.

(B) Obtain a written medical order.

(C) Assist the client to leave the hospital.

(D) All of the above.

(40) What does a nursing report include?

(A) A patient's medical history.

(B) The reason for hospital admission.

(C) The medication time of the last dose and dosage amount.

(D) All of the above.

(41) Which medication can cause bleeding gums and bruises?

(A) Ibuprofen.

(B) Atenolol.

(C) Estrogen.

(D) Metformin.

(42) What aims to inspire a person to realize their fullest potential?

(A) Self-actualization.

(B) Self-esteem.

(C) Love.

(D) Safety.

(43) What is the best position to place a patient for rectal examination to detect inflamed hemorrhoids?

(A) Lithotomy.

(B) Sims'.

(C) Knee-chest.

(D) Dorsal recumbent.

(44) What PPE should be worn while a patient's bleeding is treated?

(A) There's no need for precautionary equipment.

(B) Gown and mask.

(C) Goggles, mask, gloves, and gown.

(D) Gloves only.

(45) What is the commitment to do no injury to another person called?

(A) Nonmaleficence.

(B) Paternalism.

(C) Autonomy.

(D) Justice.

(46) What is of concern during nursing care?

(A) Clear amber urine in the urinary catheter.

(B) The patient can offer assistance during his bath.

(C) A red area on the hip that does not disappear after massage.

(D) A red area on the back that disappears after massage.

(47) What is the most essential precaution for infection spread prevention?

(A) Use gloves.

(B) Wear a gown.

(C) Wash your hands.

(D) Isolate infected patients.

(48) A patient will have electroconvulsive therapy after involuntary hospitalization. What is true about informed consent?

(A) The patient should assign informed consent.

(B) The patient's family should assign informed consent.

(C) There is no need to assign informed consent.

(D) The doctor should assign informed consent.

(49) What indicates the need for a mammogram?

(A) A 50-year-old asymptomatic female.

(B) A breastfeeding female.

(C) A female with breast sports trauma.

(D) A 25-year-old female complaining of premenstrual breast pain.

(50) What is the correct administration technique for a metered-dose inhaler of two puffs of beclomethasone dipropionate and two puffs of salmeterol?

(A) A single alternative puff of each drug starting with beclomethasone.

(B) A single alternative puff of each drug starting with salmeterol.

(C) Start with two puffs of salmeterol, then two puffs of beclomethasone.

(D) Start with two puffs of beclomethasone, then two puffs of salmeterol.

(51) What are some side effects of ethambutol?

(A) Inability to distinguish red from green.

(B) Body secretions that are discolored and orange-red.

(C) Gastrointestinal side effects.

(D) Hearing impairment.

(52) What is true about isoniazid?

(A) Vitamin supplements should be avoided during therapy.

(B) Swiss cheese should be consumed in a high quantity.

(C) If yellow skin or eyes happen, it should be reported to the doctor.

(D) Alcohol should be consumed in large quantities.

(53) What should be considered during an MRI?

(A) The patient takes digoxin.

(B) The patient wears a hearing aid.

(C) The patient has a pacemaker.

(D) The patient has an iodine allergy.

(54) A female patient diagnosed with hypomagnesemia presents with confusion, hypotension, Trousseau's and Chvostek's positive signs, facial tics, and cramps. She takes furosemide, potassium, aspirin, and Digitalis. Which tests could be done on her?

(A) EEG.

(B) ABG.

(C) Potassium and calcium levels, which will be low.

(D) Potassium and calcium levels, which will be high.

(55) A patient who received an IV streptokinase continuous infusion suddenly complains of itching and becomes anxious. What is the correct action?

(A) Start a continuous infusion of diphenhydramine.

(B) Ask the patient to sit up in bed and decrease the infusion rate to half.

(C) Inform the doctor and stop the infusion.

(D) Give the patient protamine sulfate and oxygen.

(56) Which medications should a nurse ask about before a throat culture?

(A) Antibiotic.

(B) Acetaminophen.

(C) Throat lozenge.

(D) Aspirin.

(57) What is the diagnosis of a 35-year-old female who presents for a breast biopsy and cries at the appointment because her mother died from ovarian cancer?

(A) Spiritual distress.

(B) Ineffective coping.

(C) Anxiety.

(D) Fear.

(58) How should the nurse prepare a dead body for transportation to the mortuary?

(A) The arms should be folded against the chest, and the head should be down.

(B) Bathe the body after the dentures are removed.

(C) Put the identification tags on after the body is bathed.

(D) There is no specific preparation indicated.

(59) Which PPE should be worn during ambulation of a mycoplasma pneumonia patient?

(A) Gown and gloves.

(B) An N95 respirator.

(C) A surgical mask.

(D) A face shield.

(60) What is used to analyze how effectively different healthcare system components operate together?

(A) Balance metrics.

(B) Outcome metrics.

(C) In-process metrics.

(D) Structural metrics.

(61) What indicates a patent hemodialysis fistula?

(A) The left-hand fingernail bed's capillary refill is less than two seconds.

(B) Fistula auscultation shows absent bruit.

(C) Left wrist radial pulse is present.

(D) Fistula palpation shows a thrill.

(62) What should be considered in the preprinted physician orders?

(A) Orders are well-organized, accurate, and thorough.

(B) The type and layout, such as appropriate room for handwritten inputs, white space, point size, and font.

(C) Clear and consistent recommendations for drug safety and instructions.

(D) All of the above.

(63) What is a heparin antidote?

(A) Vitamin K.

(B) Aminocaproic acid.

(C) Potassium chloride.

(D) Protamine sulfate.

(64) What are some complications of hydrochlorothiazide?

(A) Penicillin allergy, hypoglycemia, and hyperkalemia.

(B) Sulfa allergy, hyperglycemia, and hypokalemia.

(C) Osteoporosis.

(D) Hyperkalemia and hypouricemia.

(65) A pregnant female craves white clay dirt. Which study corroborates her pica?

(A) WBC count = 13,000.

(B) Hemoglobin = 8.

(C) Glucose = 120.

(D) Hematocrit = 39%.

(66) What is the correct action a nurse should take if a patient reports irregular contractions but is expected to experience Braxton-Hicks contractions?

(A) The patient is in the pre-labor phase, and the maternity unit should be informed.

(B) Tell the patient those contractions are normal throughout pregnancy.

(C) Tell the patient she should maintain bed rest for the rest of the pregnancy.

(D) Inform the doctor.

(67) When a nurse started an NG tube feeding, she found a residual 170 mL. What is the appropriate action she should take?

(A) Continue to administer the feeding and remove the residue.

(B) Administer the feeding after she elevates the head of the bed 45 degrees.

(C) Continue the feeding and return the residue to the NG tube.

(D) Stop feeding.

(68) What is the best position for a severe burn patient who will have an autograft from the lower limb?

(A) Cover the limb with the blanket.

(B) Put the limb in a flat position.

(C) Immobilize and elevate the limb.

(D) Put the patient in a prone position.

(69) What is the best position for a DVT patient?

(A) Put the affected limb in a dependent position.

(B) Elevate the affected limb.

(C) Put the affected limb in a flat position.

(D) The patient can choose any position he desires.

(70) Based on the self-limitations of nursing practice, what element do interpersonal interactions impact?

(A) Conscious attention.

(B) Professional sensibility.

(C) Personal attention.

(D) Contextual attention.

(71) What is deliberate contact with another person's body without their permission known as?

(A) Assault.

(B) Battery.

(C) Defamation.

(D) Fraud.

(72) What is an example of disciplinary actions that could cause an RN's license to be suspended?

(A) The creation of a false record for a customer.

(B) Abuse of a patient either physically or verbally.

(C) A violation of patient confidentiality.

(D) All of the above.

(73) What is the most often used quality improvement methodology?

(A) Lean.

(B) Six Sigma.

(C) Plan-do-study-act.

(D) None of the above.

(74) What are some contraindications of atropine eye drops?

(A) Glaucoma.

(B) Diabetes.

(C) Hypothyroidism.

(D) Bradycardia.

(75) What is a preterm labor risk factor?

(A) 22-year-old primigravida of average height and weight.

(B) Hemoglobin of 12.5.

(C) History of cardiac disease.

(D) 32-year-old primigravida.

(76) What should the nursing care plan for thrombocytopenia in a chemotherapy patient include?

(A) Lower limb exercises.

(B) No injections.

(C) Decreased fluid intake.

(D) Position the patient semi-upright.

(77) What does Level 1 evidence-based ranking include?

(A) Case studies.

(B) Case-control studies.

(C) Cohort studies.

(D) Meta-analysis.

(78) Which immunity types will develop after an immunoglobulin injection?

(A) Artificial passive immunity.

(B) Natural passive immunity.

(C) Artificial active immunity.

(D) Natural active immunity.

(79) What can be given to a patient on a clear liquid diet?

(A) Apple juice.

(B) Sherbet.

(C) Fruited gelatin.

(D) Milkshake.

(80) What should be assessed after a prolonged stay in a lithotomy position for perineal prostatectomy?

(A) Bladder.

(B) Arm movements, sensation, and radial pulse.

(C) Bowel sounds.

(D) Lower extremity pain, paresthesia, and pulses.

(81) What patient allergies should be assessed upon first contact?

(A) Food allergy.

(B) Medication allergy.

(C) Contrast media allergy.

(D) All of the above.

(82) A postoperative colostomy patient started to pass malodorous flatus from the stoma. What should the nurse assume?

(A) The patient's preoperative bowel preparation was inadequate.

(B) The NG tube should not be removed.

(C) It is an early sign of bowel ischemia.

(D) It is an expected, normal finding.

(83) What do stool characteristics of Crohn's disease include?

(A) Oozing stool.

(B) Diarrhea that alternates with constipation.

(C) Chronic constipation.

(D) Diarrhea.

(84) What precautions are unnecessary for a postoperative Bill Roth II procedure patient?

(A) Deep breathing exercises and coughing.

(B) NG tube irrigation.

(C) Early ambulation.

(D) Leg exercises.

(85) A 32-year-old male cholecystectomy patient has 700 mL drainage of green color in the T-tube. What is the appropriate step the nurse should take?

(A) Locate the patient's surgical documentation.

(B) Inform the doctor.

(C) Irrigate the T-tube.

(D) Clamp the T-tube.

(86) Which type of hepatitis virus can be transmitted through contaminated food?

(A) Hepatitis D.

(B) Hepatitis C.

(C) Hepatitis B.

(D) Hepatitis A.

(87) If a nurse finds flames and smoke in a patient's room, what should she do?

(A) Discharge all the unit's residents.

(B) Close the room door.

(C) Remove the patient from the room.

(D) Fight the fire.

(88) What is a respiratory acidosis sign in lung disease patients?

(A) Paresthesia, dizziness, and bradypnea.

(B) Confusion, restlessness, and headache.

(C) Respiratory depth and rate decrease.

(D) Hyperactivity and bradycardia.

(89) What does a nursing care plan for a traction patient include?

(A) Keep the head of the bed at an angle of 90 degrees.

(B) Verify the pulleys are where the knots are.

(C) Keep the weights off the floor.

(D) Place the weights on a firm surface.

(90) During care for an infant with colostomy due to an imperforate anus, the nurse finds an edematous and red stoma. What is the appropriate next step?

(A) Elevate the buttocks.

(B) Apply ice immediately.

(C) Find the patient's documentation.

(D) Inform the doctor.

(91) What is the position of the left arm of a female patient who has undergone a left radical mastectomy?

(A) Left atrium dependent.

(B) At left atrium level.

(C) On a cushion and elevated.

(D) Elevated above shoulder level.

(92) For someone with hypothyroidism who is prescribed levothyroxine and warfarin, what is the appropriate action?

(A) Decrease the levothyroxine dose.

(B) Increase the levothyroxine dose.

(C) Decrease the warfarin dose.

(D) Increase the warfarin dose.

(93) What do CNS complications of cimetidine include?

(A) Hallucinations.

(B) Confusion.

(C) Dizziness.

(D) Tremors.

(94) To determine infliximab effectiveness, what should a nurse do?

(A) After the complete transfusion, do a gastric fluid Hema test.

(B) Before and after transfusion, measure hepatic enzymes.

(C) Assess the bowel movement's consistency and frequency.

(D) After the complete transfusion, do a leukocyte count test.

(95) What are common symptoms of a duodenal ulcer?

(A) Right arm pain.

(B) Food intake relieves the pain.

(C) Vomiting and nausea.

(D) Weight loss.

(96) What are some early signs of dumping syndrome?

(A) Abdominal pain and cramping.

(B) Chest pain and double vision.

(C) Indigestion and bradycardia.

(D) Pallor and sweating.

(97) Which symptom can indicate a peptic ulcer perforation?

(A) Board-like, rigid abdomen.

(B) Vomiting and nausea.

(C) Leg numbness.

(D) Bradycardia.

(98) A feverish patient is using a cooling blanket. What is the next step in this patient's medical management?

(A) Place a blanket and sheet over the patient.

(B) Cover the groin area with ice.

(C) Turn the patient every two hours.

(D) Put a padded blade on the tongue.

(99) What is the role of the semi-sitting position in a post-abdominal surgery patient?

(A) Respiratory distress prevention.

(B) Incision tension reduction.

(C) Circulation promotion.

(D) Venous return stasis prevention.

(100) Which laboratory tests should be done before a liver biopsy?

(A) Serum creatinine level.

(B) CBC.

(C) Prothrombin time.

(D) Serum electrolytes.

(101) What should a nursing care plan for a myasthenia gravis patient include?

(A) Make sure the patient is active in the afternoon.

(B) Bathe the patient multiple times daily.

(C) Monitor the patient's swallowing and gag reflexes before he eats.

(D) Bathe the patient each evening.

(102) Which statement is true about multiple sclerosis?

(A) A cane can be used to help the patient balance.

(B) The patient should avoid contact with relatives.

(C) Symptoms will disappear after three months of treatment.

(D) It is characterized by a slow recovery.

(103) A 22-year-old female patient presents with a grand mal seizure. What is the first management step?

(A) Inform the doctor.

(B) Move the patient's head to the left side.

(C) Use a restraint.

(D) Use a tongue blade with padding.

(104) To assess cranial nerve XI, what should be done?

(A) Use the Snellen chart.

(B) Request the patient do a shoulder shrug.

(C) Use a flashlight to examine the patient's pupils.

(D) Ask the patient to recognize the aroma of cloves.

(105) What is the most difficult management instruction for a COPD patient?

(A) Get pneumonia and flu vaccinations.

(B) Drink plenty of fluids daily.

(C) Use pursed-lip breathing.

(D) Stop smoking.

(106) A 14-year-old boy presents with a positive mono spot test, lymph node enlargement, sore throat, and fatigue. What is the next step in his medical management?

(A) Isolate and stay home until the blisters fade.

(B) Don't engage in extracurricular activities.

(C) Ensure good nutrition and bed rest.

(D) Take antibiotics for five days.

(107) What is an indication of a low therapeutic level of iron prescribed to an iron-deficient anemia toddler?

(A) Ecchymosis of the legs.

(B) Daily naps.

(C) Light brown stool.

(D) Yellow skin.

(108) What are some varicose vein risk factors?

(A) Use of a computer at work.

(B) A weight of 59 kg and a height of 160 cm.

(C) A person who runs and exercises daily.

(D) Multiple previous pregnancies.

(109) What are some signs of right-side heart failure?

(A) Constipation.

(B) Renal failure

(C) Facial edema.

(D) Neck vein distension.

(110) A patient develops an acute decrease in urine output, which averages 18 mL/hr for three hours. After he receives 550 mL of IV fluids, the urine output becomes 23 mL/hr, and laboratory tests show a serum creatinine level of 3.1 mg/dL and BUN of 56 mg/dL. What is the diagnosis?

(A) UTI.

(B) Glomerulonephritis.

(C) Acute renal failure.

(D) Hypovolemia.

(111) A male patient diagnosed with myocardial infarction develops pink-tinged frothy sputum, tachypnea, and tachycardia. What will be found during chest auscultation?

(A) Diminished air entry.

(B) Scattered rhonchi.

(C) Crackles.

(D) Stridor.

(112) A 46-year-old diabetic male presents with chest pain. He is scheduled for cardiac catheterization surgery. Which antidiabetic drug should be stopped for 48 hours before and after the operation?

(A) Metformin.

(B) Repaglinide.

(C) Glipizide.

(D) Regular insulin.

(113) What laboratory test should be done before anti-tuberculosis drugs are prescribed?

(A) Urinalysis and CBC.

(B) Hematocrit and CBC.

(C) ALT and AST.

(D) Serum BUN and creatinine.

(114) A leukemic patient presents with stomatitis. What is the appropriate patient management?

(A) Use a cotton swab to clean his mouth.

(B) Use an overbed cradle-to-mouth swab.

(C) Use mouthwash to clean his mouth.

(D) To clean the patient's teeth, use dental floss.

(115) Which statement is incorrect for a sickle cell anemia child?

(A) Dairy should be avoided.

(B) Paracetamol can be used as an analgesic.

(C) Increase consumption of juice.

(D) High elevation will not affect the patient.

(116) What is an implication of smoking for a patient with peripheral leg vascular disease?

(A) It causes severe stress.

(B) It causes heart strain and hypertension.

(C) It causes a decrease in the blood supply to the legs by vasoconstriction.

(D) It is contraindicated in blood disorders.

(117) During the assessment of a patient admitted for cardiac catheterization, the patient says she has a shrimp allergy. Which statement is true?

(A) The side effects of a shrimp allergy should be discussed with the patient.

(B) The nurse should tell the hospital's kitchen to avoid shrimp in the patient's meals.

(C) The nurse should take a history of any other allergies.

(D) The nurse should inform the doctor.

(118) What is the appropriate management for a patient with a pulse deficit?

(A) Monitor the pulse at home.

(B) Inform the doctor.

(C) Schedule the patient for a weekly re-evaluation.

(D) This is a normal presentation.

(119) What is included in KUB?

(A) Enema administration.

(B) Catheterization.

(C) Procedure explanation.

(D) NPO.

(120) What is a symptom of alcohol withdrawal?

(A) Pallor.

(B) Tremors.

(C) Dizziness.

(D) Hypotension.

(121) What is the nursing care priority for a recently delivered baby?

(A) Get an Apgar score.

(B) Get the baby's footprints and give it an identification bracelet.

(C) Wrap the baby in a warm blanket.

(D) Use a bulb syringe for airway suction.

(122) A nurse finds that a Kaposi's cutaneous sarcoma patient has draining skin lesions. What PPE should the nurse use?

(A) Gloves to bathe the patient and gloves and a gown for linen changes.

(B) A mask, gloves, and gown.

(C) Gloves and a gown.

(D) Gloves only.

(123) Which vitamin deficiency can be associated with chronic gastritis?

(A) Vitamin E.

(B) Vitamin C.

(C) Vitamin B12.

(D) Vitamin A.

(124) What is a sign of hepatitis A infection?

(A) Upper left quadrant pain.

(B) Weight gain.

(C) Dark stools.

(D) Malaise.

(125) What is a reason for prednisone administration in an ulcerative colitis patient?

(A) Bowel bacteria reduction.

(B) GIT acid neutralization.

(C) Peristaltic activity reduction.

(D) Bowel inflammation suppression.

(126) Which patient should have immediate surgery?

(A) A patient with an irreducible inguinal hernia.

(B) A patient with acute appendicitis.

(C) A patient with mild vaginal bleeding for one week.

(D) A patient with cholecystitis.

(127) What is the diagnosis for a chronic limitation airflow patient who presents with a barrel chest?

(A) Bronchitis and bronchial asthma.

(B) Chronic obstructive bronchitis.

(C) Bronchial asthma.

(D) Emphysema.

(128) What are some signs of flail chest?

(A) Dyspnea.

(B) Paradoxical chest movements.

(C) Hypotension.

(D) Cyanosis.

(129) Which of these statements is not true about cholestyramine drugs?

(A) It is important to eat a high-fiber diet with them.

(B) Patients should only take the medication with water.

(C) Patients take the medication to decrease cholesterol.

(D) Vitamin supplements should be continued.

(130) What must be checked before a blood transfusion begins?

(A) Patient identification number.

(B) Blood type and group.

(C) Presence of clots.

(D) Blood product expiration date.

(131) What indicates that a patient will benefit most from a platelet transfusion?

(A) Decreased blood oozing from gums and puncture sites.

(B) Normal temperature.

(C) Increased hemoglobin level.

(D) Increased hematocrit level.

(132) What should the nurse ask a patient before a blood transfusion?

(A) If he knows the risks and complications of transfusion.

(B) If he has had a transfusion and developed shock before.

(C) The reason why he needs a transfusion.

(D) If he has a history of transfusions.

(133) What is the appropriate action when the exposed tubing of a continuous IV infusion falls and hits the top of the medication cart?

(A) Disinfect it with an alcohol swab.

(B) Disinfect it with betadine.

(C) No action is necessary.

(D) Obtain new IV tubing.

(134) After 45 minutes of a 1-liter bag transfusion of 0.9% sodium chloride in 5% dextrose, the patient complains of chills, dyspnea, and a bad headache. 350 mL remains in the bag. What is the appropriate action?

(A) Remove the IV catheter.

(B) Sit the patient up in bed.

(C) Slow the IV infusion rate.

(D) Call the physician.

(135) What should be assessed to avoid hyperglycemia complications of parenteral nutrition?

(A) Increased urine output, thirst, and weakness.

(B) Abdominal pain, chills, and sweating.

(C) Oliguria, vomiting, and nausea.

(D) Thirst, weak pulse, and fever.

(136) A patient with hyperbilirubinemia is receiving phototherapy. What should the nurse ensure?

(A) Ensure the infant's eyes are covered.

(B) Ensure the patient's heart rate is measured.

(C) Ensure the mother is not allowed to touch the infant because of the risk of infection.

(D) Ensure the baby is kept NPO.

(137) What is the dietary recommendation for a patient who takes furosemide?

(A) Watermelon.

(B) Radishes and cucumbers.

(C) Apple.

(D) Apple juice and eggs.

(138) A kidney transplant patient develops a tender kidney, hypertension, and a fever of 38.5 six days after transplantation. On X-ray, there is an enlargement of the transplanted kidney. What is the diagnosis?

(A) Kidney obstruction.

(B) Chronic rejection.

(C) Kidney infection.

(D) Acute rejection.

(139) What is an important final test to evaluate a renal disorder?

(A) Decreased WBC count.

(B) Decreased RBC.

(C) Elevated serum creatinine level.

(D) Decreased hemoglobin level.

(140) What is a sign of benign prostatic hyperplasia?

(A) Decreased urinary stream force.

(B) Urge incontinence.

(C) Urinary retention.

(D) Nocturia.

(141) What should be assessed in an acute congestive heart failure patient who is given bumetanide IV?

(A) Potassium serum level.

(B) Blood pressure.

(C) Urine output.

(D) Weight loss.

(142) Which PPE should a nurse wear while caring for a colostomy patient with methicillin-resistant Staphylococcus aureus infection?

(A) Face shield, goggles, gown, and gloves.

(B) Shoe protectors, gowns, and gloves.

(C) Goggles and gloves.

(D) Gown and gloves.

(143) How often should a nurse check the skin integrity of a restrained patient?

(A) Every 30 minutes.

(B) Every 5 hours.

(C) Every 7 hours.

(D) Every 12 hours.

(144) Which daily serum laboratory studies should be checked in a patient who received a unit of granulocytes?

(A) WBC.

(B) Hemoglobin.

(C) Erythrocytes.

(D) Hematocrit.

(145) A patient recently diagnosed with impaired renal function and myocardial infarction is admitted to the cardiac unit and experiences coughing and tachypnea after administration of IV fluids at 100 mL/hr. What is the possible cause?

(A) Circulatory overload.

(B) Systemic infection.

(C) Air embolism.

(D) Hematoma.

Test 1: Answers and Explanations

(1) (A) Whole-grain cereal.

Diverticulitis symptoms are often observed in patients who consume nuts, whole grains, raw vegetables, celery, or popcorn. Other answer choices are inappropriate since they are permitted in a diverticulitis patient's diet.

(2) (D) Infection prevention.

Individuals with atopic dermatitis must avoid scratching as it can lead to skin infection. Additionally, options A and B can further dry out the skin, which exacerbates the symptoms of atopic dermatitis. It is important to note that fever is not directly related to atopic dermatitis.

(3) (B) It is an advance directive.

It is important to discuss and prepare for medical decisions in case patients become critically ill or unable to communicate their preferences.

(4) (C) This causes a synergistic effect.

When two drugs are used together, their impact is stronger than when used individually. The combination of these medications has a depressant effect instead of a stimulating one. An antagonist effect occurs when the drugs' actions conflict with each other. On the other hand, agonist effects mimic the effects of natural substances found in the body.

(5) (B) Suture line contamination prevention.

The NG tube is mostly used to enable feeding without suture line contamination. There is no need for suction since the laryngectomy did not affect the oral mucosa.

(6) (A) It occurs from the rash onset until crusted lesions develop.

Varicella's contagious phase lasts from when the rash appears until all lesions disappear. Other answer selections are erroneous because they provide an incorrect estimate of when the infection began.

(7) (D) All of the above.

Patient advocacy is an essential part of healthcare. It protects patients' rights to receive proper care, preserves their dignity, promotes equality, and ensures they can make their own healthcare decisions.

(8) (D) The nurse should advise the patient to increase hydration.

The patient using Cytoxan should drink more fluids daily to prevent hemorrhagic cystitis.

(9) (C) Multiple births.

Clomiphene, a fertility medication that enhances ovulation, can lead to multiple births. It does not cause vaginal bleeding or uncomfortable erections.

(10) (A) Prevent Curling's ulcers.

Patients with burn injuries usually develop Curling's (stress) ulcers. Cimetidine is a histamine blocker that lowers stomach acid and aids in preventing ulcer growth.

(11) (B) Stay present throughout significant events.

There are various approaches to empower patients to become their own advocates. Some approaches are to ask for clear communication, select a medical team, prepare a medical summary, aid patients to access services both within and outside the hospital, educate patients, and be physically available to them.

(12) (A) Patients' choices should be respected even if a patient is not competent.

This is not true. The nurse must assess each patient's decision-making ability and obtain and revoke consent as needed based on patient data.

(13) (D) The nursing care plan.

When a patient's needs are assessed, a nursing care plan is created to address any identified present or future challenges. Communication can be informal, but documentation is always necessary and can take various forms, such as digital, handwritten, or preprinted care plans.

(14) (C) Check for bowel activity.

When giving codeine sulfate, healthcare professionals must monitor vital signs, assess pain relief, evaluate respiratory function, track bowel movements, detect urinary retention, and encourage hydration.

(15) (A) WBC count = 2500/mm3.

Dysrhythmia, thrombophlebitis, cardiovascular disorders, and blood dyscrasias such as leukopenia, thrombocytopenia, agranulocytosis, and aplastic anemia are side effects of carbamazepine.

(16) (D) Tinnitus.

A person who consumes more than 4 grams of acetylsalicylic acid daily may experience salicylism, a mild form of intoxication. The most common symptom of this is tinnitus. Additionally, salicylate can cause hyperventilation as it activates the respiratory center. It may also lead to fever because it interferes with the body's metabolic processes, which link heat production and oxygen usage.

(17) (B) The birth control pill's effectiveness is decreased with phenytoin.

Because phenytoin speeds up estrogen metabolism, it may reduce the efficacy of certain birth control pills.

(18) (D) It decreases healthcare employee retention and job satisfaction.

Interprofessional teamwork has many benefits. It decreases errors, promotes quality care, decreases fragmentation and duplication of care, increases healthcare provider retention and job satisfaction, decreases the risk of negative outcomes, and increases positive outcomes.

(19) (D) All of the above.

There are multiple causes for conflicts, such as interpersonal relationships, differences in values, and task-based disagreements.

(20) (D) The solution should be warmed before irrigation.

If the temperature of the irrigation solution differs from the temperature of the patient's body, it can be uncomfortable or painful. To facilitate earwax removal and resolution, the patient should tilt their head so the irrigated ear faces downward. After the irrigation, the patient should lie on the affected side to allow the fluid to drain completely. It's important to ensure that the top wall of the ear canal, rather than the eardrum, receives a steady, gradual flow of solution.

(21) (D) Assess both eyes simultaneously after assessing the left and right eyes individually.

The left eye is tested first with the right eye covered, and then the reverse is done with the right eye. Then both eyes are examined simultaneously. The patient stands 20 feet away from the chart while visual acuity is tested both with and without corrective glasses.

(22) (C) 10% dextrose.

The solution with the greatest glucose concentration should be hung until the new PN solution is ready since the patient is in danger of hypoglycemia.

(23) (A) A patient who got nasal oxygen and experienced respiratory issues during the prior shift.

The airway is always given priority. Thus, the nurse will respond to the patient who has been having trouble breathing first. The demands of the patients mentioned in other answer options would be categorized as intermediate priority.

(24) (D) All of the above.

Effective instructional strategies include feedback (give the student information about performance), interaction (between the provider and the learner), clinical simulations, and case-based learning (use fictitious or real-life clinical scenarios).

(25) (C) Serum K+ of 2.8 mEq/L.

The normal range for serum potassium (K+) is between 3.5 and 5.5. If a patient's serum K+ is low, they may be at risk for digoxin toxicity. The patient in question is on furosemide, a diuretic that can deplete potassium levels. The ideal range for BUN is 12–20. Normal serum magnesium levels should be between 1.3 and 2.1 Mg. The ideal range for digoxin serum levels is between 0.8–2.0 ng/mL.

(26) (D) Mask.

Excessive and chronic inhalation of silica crystalline particles leads to silicosis. The patient should wear a mask to prevent inhalation of this material, which might lead to restrictive lung disease after years of exposure.

(27) (B) Resuscitation equipment.

If a patient experiences an opioid overdose, the nurse who administers naloxone should have access to resuscitation equipment, such as vasopressors, mechanical ventilators, and oxygen.

(28) (B) Use a pain scale to assess the patient's pain level.

Nurses must acquire sufficient information to make the best decision since they have the liberty to determine which drug and delivery method will be most effective. In this instance, it's important to identify the site and intensity of the pain in order to select the best painkiller.

(29) (C) The dressing promotes healing by retaining moisture.

Moist skin will heal faster.

(30) (D) All of the above.

A data-driven clinical decision is often used to handle difficult tasks, such as chronologically merging a range of tested diseases, symptoms, and diagnoses. The goal is to provide recommendations and options that prioritize the patient's well-being.

(31) (D) Hematocrit level = 33%.

The anemia brought on by chronic renal failure may be treated with epoetin alfa. A therapeutic effect is seen when the hematocrit is between 31% and 34%.

(32) (D) Pancreatitis.

Tacrolimus should be cautiously administered in individuals with immunosuppression, impaired pancreatic function, or hepatic or renal impairment. Also, patients with a history of cyclosporine or this medication-related hypersensitivity should not use tacrolimus.

(33) (D) Education.

The Five Rights of Delegation should be followed when assigning tasks. They are proper person, situation, task, monitoring and assessment, and communication.

(34) (A) Nonfat milk.

Nonfat milk is one of the foods that will reduce reflux and improve the symptoms of GERD by raising lower esophageal sphincter pressure. Other options reduce LES pressure, which worsens reflux symptoms.

(35) (B) Put a dressing over an ice pack.

Following a hemorrhoidectomy, nursing care is focused on managing discomfort and preventing bleeding. An ice pack can lessen the bleeding and improve comfort.

(36) (D) It damages the patient's confidentiality.

Confidentiality in the healthcare system refers to the privacy of the patient's personal information. Medical information should be disposed of, transmitted, and/or saved with specific security procedures and tools.

(37) (B) Not introduce the patient to others in the ward.

It is important to respect a patient's personal space. It's necessary to ask for permission if other people, such as university students, are present during diagnostic or therapeutic procedures. Additionally, do not introduce the patient to others in the ward. It's also important to knock on the patient's door and to avoid bodily contact unless it's medically necessary.

(38) (A) Follow-up.

Nurses should follow up with a patient to check on progress.

(39) (D) All of the above.

To ensure a smooth discharge process, multiple steps must be considered. Request that the room be cleaned, summarize the client's condition prior to discharge, assist the client in leaving, notify the business office, and issue discharge instructions. It is also important to obtain written medical orders, meet eligibility requirements for home healthcare, discuss home care self-care topics with the patient, establish patient goals, and assess healthcare needs.

(40) (D) All of the above.

Nursing reports cover vital information about a patient, such as recent changes in symptoms or conditions, pain management approaches, level of consciousness, allergies, dietary restrictions, medication dosage and time of last dose, reason for hospital admission, and medical history.

(41) (A) Ibuprofen.

Bleeding is an adverse effect of ibuprofen. Antihypertensive atenolol can result in hypotension or a sluggish heartbeat. A negative impact of estrogen is clotting. For Type 2 DM, metformin is prescribed.

(42) (A) Self-actualization.

Self-actualization aims to inspire people to realize their fullest potential and range of abilities. Self-esteem is the need to be appreciated and acknowledged as a valuable individual. Love is the individual's intrinsic need for affection, a sense of community, and acceptance from others.

(43) (B) Sims'.

The Sims' position is ideal for examination and patient comfort since it relaxes the patient's rectal muscles. Even though the knee-chest position may be employed for a rectal examination, a patient with acute inflammation may find it quite painful. An examination of the heart, axillae, breast, lungs, and anterior thorax requires the patient to be in the dorsal recumbent position.

(44) (C) Goggles, mask, gloves, and gown.

When there is a chance that bodily fluids will spill or spray, common precautions include goggles, masks, gloves, and gowns.

(45) (A) Nonmaleficence.

Nonmaleficence is the commitment to do no injury to another person.

(46) (C) A red area on the hip that does not disappear after massage.

A region that remains red after massage suggests that the skin may deteriorate and require urgent care. If the patient is rotated often, a red spot that vanishes with massage is a pressure area that shouldn't deteriorate.

(47) (C) Wash your hands.

Regular handwashing is the best strategy to stop the transmission of illness. It is more effective than gloves or gowns. It's helpful to isolate infectious patients. However, most patients are admitted before a test is administered, and isolation may not begin until the tests are completed.

(48) (A) The patient should assign informed consent.

Involuntarily admitted patients retain their right to informed consent and are regarded as legally competent until a court of law determines their incapacity. The informed consent should be assigned by the patient.

(49) (A) A 50-year-old asymptomatic female.

Women over 50 are advised to have a mammogram every year. Mammograms are unnecessary for women who exclusively breastfeed or who have sports injuries. Before menstruation, sore breasts are common.

(50) (C) Start with two puffs of salmeterol, then two puffs of beclomethasone.

A glucocorticoid is beclomethasone dipropionate, while salmeterol is a bronchodilator. When both medications are given simultaneously, bronchodilators are always given first. This enables the bronchodilator to open the airways, increasing the glucocorticoid's effectiveness.

(51) (A) Inability to distinguish red from green.

Optic neuritis, which is brought on by ethambutol, reduces visual acuity and a patient's capacity to distinguish between red and green. Hearing impairment occurs because of streptomycin antitubercular treatment. Rifampin causes secretions to become orange-red.

(52) (C) If yellow skin or eyes happen, it should be reported to the doctor.

It is important for patients who take isoniazid to avoid foods that contain tyramine, such as Swiss cheese, as they can trigger reactions such as headaches, tachycardia, sweating, flushing, itching, and skin redness. Alcohol should also be avoided, and any symptoms of hepatitis, such as yellow skin or eyes, should be reported to a doctor. Pyridoxine (vitamin B6) may help prevent peripheral neuritis.

(53) (C) The patient has a pacemaker.

Patients with pacemakers cannot get MRIs. Digoxin and iodine do not prevent MRIs. A hearing aid can be removed before an MRI is performed.

(54) (C) Potassium and calcium levels, which will be low.

Low serum calcium and potassium levels are associated with hypomagnesemia. The patient's hypocalcemia is manifested by hyperreflexia, as shown by Trousseau and Chvostek positive symptoms, facial tics, and muscular cramps, as well as the patient's low blood potassium levels since the patient takes furosemide, a diuretic that depletes potassium.

(55) (C) Inform the doctor and stop the infusion.

Streptokinase caused the patient's anaphylactic response. The infusion should be stopped, the doctor should be informed, and the patient should receive epinephrine, corticosteroids, and antihistamines.

(56) (A) Antibiotic.

To find any potential germs, a throat culture must be performed. Antibiotics prevent microbial development.

(57) (D) Fear.

Fear is an emotional state that arises from a specific cause. In this case, the patient can express sadness because of her mother's death due to ovarian cancer. Conversely, anxiety is a feeling of discomfort triggered by a vague sense of danger. A patient who experiences spiritual anguish has had their belief system disrupted.

(58) (C) Put the identification tags on after the body is bathed.

After it is bathed, the body must have identification tags attached to it. If the customer wears dentures, they should be placed in the mouth. The body should be positioned flat, with straight arms and legs.

(59) (C) A surgical mask.This patient must wear a surgical mask while being transported. Gloves or a gown will not stop the spread of droplets. Anyone who enters the room of a TB patient must wear an N95 respirator as part of airborne precautionary measures.

(60) (A) Balance metrics.

Balance metrics are used to analyze how effectively different healthcare system components operate together. Outcome metrics are used to determine how well a patient is doing in terms of hospitalization and the risk of postoperative infections. A structural metric counts how many patients are released within one day. In-process metrics include how long it takes for a doctor to visit a patient and how long it takes a patient to be admitted and released.

(61) (D) Fistula palpation shows a thrill.

To check the fistula's patency, the nurse should auscultate for a bruit or palpate for a thrill. A capillary refill time of fewer than two seconds and the left wrist radial pulse cannot help a nurse determine whether a fistula is open or closed.

(62) (D) All of the above.

Preprinted orders include drug safety recommendations, prescription information, and formatting considerations like type and layout. Additionally, the content of the orders must be well-organized, accurate, and comprehensive.

(63) (D) Protamine sulfate.

Protamine sulfate is a heparin antidote, and it should always be on hand in case of heavy bleeding or hemorrhage. For a potassium deficiency, potassium chloride is given. Thrombolytic treatment's antidote is aminocaproic acid. Warfarin sodium's antidote is vitamin K.

(64) (B) Sulfa allergy, hyperglycemia, and hypokalemia.

Thiazide diuretics like hydrochlorothiazide are sulfa-based drugs, which put patients at risk for an allergic response if they have a sulfa allergy. Hyperuricemia, hyperlipidemia, hypercalcemia, hyperglycemia, and hypokalemia are additional hazards.

(65) (B) Hemoglobin = 8.

Pica often results from iron deficiency anemia, which lowers hemoglobin levels.

(66) (B) Tell the patient those contractions are normal throughout pregnancy.

Braxton-Hicks contractions are painless, irregular, intermittent contractions and occur throughout pregnancy.

(67) (D) Stop feeding.

If there are residual quantities of more than 100 mL, the feeding must be stopped.

(68) (C) Immobilize and elevate the limb.

After surgery, lower extremities or joint autografts are raised and immobilized for three to seven days to reduce swelling and enable the autograft to adhere and connect to the wound bed.

(69) (B) Elevate the affected limb.

To improve blood flow, lower venous pressure, and reduce edema and discomfort, the patient's affected limb should be elevated. It is advised that the patient stay in bed to avoid emboli and the pressure changes that come with movement in the venous system.

(70) (D) Contextual attention.

Contextual attention includes a focus on the interpersonal elements that impacted the event. A key component of self-awareness is reflection on one's temperament, prejudices, and emotions in each distinct nurse-patient encounter.

(71) (B) Battery.

Battery is deliberate contact with another person's body without their permission. Assault occurs when one person threatens another with dangerous or offensive touch. Fraud is purposeful deceit designed to create illegal profits. Defamation is misleading speech that harms someone's reputation, whether in writing or vocally.

(72) (D) All of the above.

Registered nurses may face disciplinary measures from nursing boards if they exhibit unprofessional behavior, jeopardize public health and safety, violate patient privacy, or have inadequate nursing knowledge or judgment. Similarly, nurses who mistreat patients, delegate nursing tasks to unlicensed individuals, falsify records, or neglect nursing duties are all liable for legal action.(73) (C) Plan-do-study-act.

PDSA, Six Sigma, and lean techniques are the most often used quality improvement approaches. The most often utilized strategy is the PDSA.

(74) (A) Glaucoma.

To facilitate intraocular fluid flow, the pupil is constricted as part of the therapy for glaucoma. Atropine is an anticholinergic that increases heart rate and produces mydriasis (dilation of pupils).

(75) (C) History of cardiac disease.

Between 20 and 37 weeks of gestation, preterm labor may occur. Risk factors include age over 40 or younger than 18, anemia that reduces the uterus's oxygen supply, multifetal pregnancies that cause uterine overdistension, drug abuse, and an obstetric medical history.

(76) (B) No injections.

A patient with thrombocytopenia (low platelet count) is at risk for bleeding. Therefore, the patient shouldn't receive injections. The other options have nothing to do with thrombocytopenia.

(77) (D) Meta-analysis.

Systematic reviews or meta-analyses of randomized controlled trials and excellent, single, randomized controlled studies are Level 1 (the highest quality). Cohort studies are considered level 2. Case-control studies are considered level 3. Case studies are considered level 4.

(78) (A) Artificial passive immunity.

When someone is given antibodies produced by another person, this is called artificial passive immunity. Natural passive immunity occurs when newborns receive antibodies from their immune mother through the placenta or colostrum. Artificial active immunity is created when a vaccination or toxin stimulates an immune response. Natural active immunity is when the body produces antibodies in response to a live infection.

(79) (A) Apple juice.

The clear liquid is apple juice. Sherbet and milkshakes are prohibited on a clear liquid diet since they include milk. A clear liquid diet allows gelatin without fruit. Gelatin with fruit is not a transparent substance.

(80) (D) Lower extremity pain, paresthesia, and pulses.

The strain on the popliteal region, where both arteries and veins are near the surface, caused by a prolonged lithotomy position may hinder blood flow to the lower limbs.

(81) (D) All of the above.

The nurse must carefully examine the client at first contact to learn any known sensitivities to latex, radiocontrast used in diagnostic testing, foods, or drugs. Nurses must properly understand the signs and symptoms of an allergic reaction to any medication.

(82) (D) It is an expected, normal finding.

Following a colostomy, a patient will start passing malodorous flatus as peristalsis begins again. This is a predictable occurrence that indicates the resumption of bowel function. Within 72 hours after the operation, the patient should be able to pass stool again.

(83) (D) Diarrhea.

Four to five non-bloody diarrheal stools per day are a feature of Crohn's disease. The diarrhea attacks become more frequent, more intense, and last longer with time.

(84) (B) NG tube irrigation.

The proximal remnant of the stomach is anastomosed to the proximal jejunum during a Bill Roth II surgery. To avoid the retention of gastric secretions, the NG tube must be patent. After gastric surgery, the nurse should never irrigate or move the tube unless the doctor instructs that it be done.

(85) (B) Inform the doctor.

When a patient has a significant amount of drainage (700 mL) with an unusual color (green) in the T-tube (especially after gallbladder removal surgery), it is important for the nurse to inform the doctor. This could be an indication of a complication or an issue that requires medical evaluation and potential intervention. The doctor can then provide guidance on the next steps, whether it involves adjusting the patient's treatment plan, conducting further tests, or taking other medical actions.

(86) (D) Hepatitis A.

Hepatitis virus A–contaminated food or infected food workers may spread the disease through the fecal-oral pathway. The main transmission route for hepatitis B, C, and D is contaminated blood or bodily fluids.

(87) (C) Remove the patient from the room.

The patient should be removed from the room by the nurse, who should also raise the alarm. The nurse should only shut the door when everyone has been taken out of the room.

(88) (B) Confusion, restlessness, and headache.

A patient with respiratory acidosis will have dysrhythmia, an irregular, fast heartbeat, hyperkalemia, cyanosis, diaphoresis, visual abnormalities, confusion, restlessness, and headaches.

(89) (C) Keep the weights off the floor.

Weights must hang freely with knots kept away from the pulleys to produce appropriate traction. It is not advisable to leave weights sitting on a hard surface. The head of the bed should be set low to provide counter traction.

(90) (D) Inform the doctor.

If a nurse observes an edematous (swollen) and red stoma in an infant with a colostomy due to an imperforate anus, the appropriate next step is to inform the doctor. These symptoms could indicate a complication such as an infection or ischemia of the stoma, which requires immediate medical assessment and potential intervention.

(91) (C) On a cushion and elevated.

The patient's arm should be raised on a cushion but not higher than shoulder level to encourage the best drainage from the limb without arm circulation compromise. Because surgery disrupts the lymphatic system, if the arm is flat or dependent, this might worsen the edema.

(92) (C) Decrease the warfarin dose.

Warfarin became more effective because levothyroxine hastens the breakdown of vitamin K–dependent coagulation components. The dose of warfarin should be decreased if thyroid hormone replacement treatment is started.

(93) (B) Confusion.

A histamine 2 receptor antagonist is cimetidine. Confusion is the most prevalent CNS side effect. Headaches, sleepiness, dizziness, and hallucinations are less frequent CNS adverse effects.

(94) (C) Assess the bowel movement's consistency and frequency.

Diarrhea and stomach discomfort are Crohn's disease's main symptoms. An immunomodulator called infliximab lowers the level of inflammation in the colon, which lessens diarrhea.

(95) (B) Food intake relieves the pain.

A mid-epigastric, localized, acute, heavy, or burning pain relieved by food is a sign of a duodenal ulcer. Patients with duodenal ulcers do not lose weight or feel nausea and vomiting. These signs and symptoms are more prevalent in stomach ulcer patients.

(96) (D) Pallor and sweating.

Within half an hour after eating, dumping syndrome begins to show its early symptoms. The need to lie down, palpitations, pallor, sweating, syncope, tachycardia, and vertigo are among the symptoms.

(97) (A) Board-like and rigid abdomen.

A hard and board-like abdomen with acute pain that starts in the mid-epigastric region and extends throughout the abdomen is a sign of a peptic ulcer perforation. As hypovolemic shock may occur, tachycardia can manifest.

(98) (C) Turn the patient every two hours.

To avoid skin deterioration, a patient who uses a cooling blanket should be rotated every two hours.

(99) (B) Incision tension reduction.

When an abdominal surgery patient sits up partially, this eases the stress on the incision. It doesn't stop breathing difficulties. Exercise and elevation of the legs may help avoid venous stasis.

(100) (C) Prothrombin time.

The liver produces a clotting agent known as prothrombin. The physician must determine whether the patient has enough prothrombin levels to avoid bleeding at the biopsy site.

(101) (C) Monitor the patient's swallowing and gag reflexes before he eats.

Myasthenia gravis patients have dysphagia and upper body impairments. Thus, a nurse must assess gag and swallowing reflexes before the patient eats. It is not necessary to promote regular bathing. Myasthenia gravis patients are often active in the morning and progressively deteriorate over the day.

(102) (A) A cane can be used to help the patient balance.

Use of a cane shows the patient has begun to adjust to his difficulties and disabilities.

(103) (B) Move the patient's head to the left side.

To avoid aspiration, the nurse should move the patient's head to the left side. The patient should not be restrained or have anything placed in their mouth by the nurse. It's important to do this and ensure the patient's safety before the doctor is notified.

(104) (B) Request the patient do a shoulder shrug.

The spinal accessory nerve, or cranial nerve XI, is examined when the patient shrugs the shoulders. To test the olfactory nerve, release a clove vial and ask the patient to name the aroma. To test the oculomotor nerve, shine a flashlight in the patient's eyes and watch the pupils. To examine the optic nerve, use the Snellen chart.

(105) (D) Stop smoking.

Smoking addiction is common in people with chronic obstructive pulmonary disease.

(106) (C) Ensure good nutrition and bed rest.

Antibiotics won't be given since the patient has infectious mononucleosis from a virus. Good nutrition and rest should be advised. An individual with chicken pox might benefit from advice about blisters.

(107) (C) Light brown stool.

Supplemental iron results in dark stools.

(108) (D) Multiple previous pregnancies.

Due to venous stasis, pregnancy raises intra-abdominal pressure and the risk of varicose veins. The patient has a sitting profession, but standing for a long time raises the risk of varicose veins. She is not overweight, a risk factor for varicosities. Running boosts venous return.

(109) (D) Neck vein distension.

Venous symptoms of right heart failure include hepatomegaly, pitting edema in the legs, and swollen neck veins. Right heart failure does not often present as constipation, renal failure, or facial edema.

(110) (C) Acute renal failure.

Renal insult is signaled by serum creatinine and BUN increase and urine output decrease. The patient may need hemodialysis, peritoneal dialysis, and medications to increase renal perfusion.

(111) (C) Crackles.

Dyspnea and tachypnea, as well as excessive amounts of frothy, pink-tinged sputum, are symptoms of pulmonary edema. Chest auscultation indicates crackles. Stridor is a crowing noise connected to laryngospasm or upper airway edema.

(112) (A) Metformin.

To ensure safety during cardiac catheterization, it is important to have the patient avoid metformin 48 hours before and after the procedure when the contrast medium is injected. This is because the presence of metformin in the body and any harm caused by the contrast medium could increase the risk of lactic acidosis.

(113) (C) ALT and AST.

Liver function tests encompass ALT (alanine transaminase) and AST (aspartate transaminase), which are important to monitor as INH can lead to liver damage. A complete blood count (CBC) and hematocrit tests may be suggested if the primary toxicities are bleeding or bone marrow suppression. Kidney function indicators, such as serum creatinine and BUN (blood urea nitrogen), are important to detect potential harm from medications like kanamycin or streptomycin.

(114) (A) Use a cotton swab to clean his mouth.

Stomatitis is a common side effect of leukemia treatment. Due to low platelet count, the patient will often bleed, and tooth flossing might exacerbate this. Cotton swabs are a gentle way to clean the patient's mouth. His mouth cannot handle an astringent mouthwash.

(115) (D) High elevation will not affect the patient.

Because of the low oxygen saturation at high elevation, an asthma attack might occur in a sickle cell anemia patient. Aspirin, which may result in acidosis, is not recommended. Juice consumption is advised since it helps prevent dehydration.

(116) (C) It causes a decrease in the blood supply to the legs by vasoconstriction.

This response correctly links the patient's sickness to his behavior. All the other answers are accurate, but they do not apply to patients with peripheral vascular disease.

(117) (D) The nurse should inform the doctor.

A shrimp allergy is a sign of an iodine allergy. The nurse should immediately inform the doctor if an allergic response occurs since the dye used in a cardiac catheterization is iodine.

(118) (B) Inform the doctor.

If there is a pulse deficit, the blood flow is insufficient to start a peripheral pulse. The doctor must be informed right away.

(119) (C) Procedure explanation.

The patient should have the process clearly explained. No preparation is required for this surgery, and the patient does not need to be catheterized or maintained NPO.

(120) (B) Tremors.

Alcohol withdrawal is often accompanied by tremors. Blood loss and shock are consistent with hypotension, lightheadedness, and pallor.

(121) (D) Use a bulb syringe for airway suction.

The most important thing is to maintain a patent airway. The nurse will keep the infant warm and put identification bands on it, but it's important to first open the airway. Legally, the nurse is not allowed to determine the Apgar rating.

(122) (C) Gloves and gown.

When a patient has wound drainage, a colostomy, ileostomy, or diarrhea, a gown and gloves are essential. No matter how much wound drainage is present, a gown and gloves are required. If droplet or airborne precautions are not needed, masks are not required.

(123) (C) Vitamin B12.

The parietal cells cease to function because of chronic gastritis, which causes the stomach lining to deteriorate and atrophy. Vitamin B12 absorption causes pernicious anemia.

(124) (D) Malaise.

Weight loss, clay-colored stools (because conjugated bilirubin cannot exit the liver due to inflammation or blockage of the bile ducts), right upper quadrant pain, nausea, and anorexia are the gastrointestinal symptoms of hepatitis A.

(125) (D) Bowel inflammation suppression.

Prednisone, a steroid, is used to treat intestinal inflammation. To lower the number of gut bacteria, antibiotics are administered. In patients with ulcerative colitis, there is no need to decrease GI tract acidity. Anticholinergics decrease peristalsis.

(126) (B) A patient with acute appendicitis.

It is critical to perform surgery before the appendix bursts. A patient with an inguinal hernia that can't be pushed back into place will require surgery soon, but it's not an immediate necessity. However, if the hernia becomes strangulated, the need for surgery becomes an emergency. A week of moderate vaginal bleeding doesn't necessitate immediate attention. Similarly, cholecystitis doesn't require immediate surgical intervention.

(127) (D) Emphysema.

The diaphragm flattens, and the emphysema patient has hyperinflated alveoli, which cause a barrel chest or an increase in anteroposterior diameter. In addition, the patient has hyperresonant lungs and dyspnea with prolonged expiration.

(128) (B) Paradoxical chest movements.

Multiple rib fractures result in a floating portion of ribs, which causes a flail chest. This segment causes paradoxical chest movement since it is not connected to the remaining bony rib cage. This indicates that when the remainder of the chest expands, the force of inspiration drags the fragmented portion inward.

(129) (B) Patients should only take the medication with water.

This is not true. Patient compliance is difficult due to the taste and palatability of cholestyramine, a bile acid sequestrant used to decrease cholesterol levels. Fruit juices and other flavored goods may improve the medication's flavor. Bile acid sequestrants may cause constipation and a reduction in vitamin absorption.

(130) (D) Blood product expiration date.

To ensure the blood is still fresh, the nurse must note the blood unit's expiration date. It takes time for blood cells to degrade. Thus, safe storage is often only allowed for 35 days.

(131) (A) Decreased blood oozing from gums and puncture sites.

A patient with inadequate platelets may have blood oozing from mucous membranes, wounds, puncture sites, or open bleeding, as platelets are essential for healthy blood coagulation.

(132) (D) If he has a history of transfusions.

To educate patients about transfusion treatment, a nurse should ask about their personal experiences. This can provide the nurse with information about any previous transfusion complications.

(133) (D) Obtain new IV tubing.

The nurse must obtain new IV tubing since the old one has become contaminated and might infect the patient systemically. Because the tubing will be directly connected to a catheter in the patient's vein, it is inadequate or dangerous to wipe it with Betadine or alcohol.

(134) (C) Slow the IV infusion rate.

The patient's symptoms indicate possible circulatory overload. The nurse's initial step must be to slow the infusion. The IV catheter is left in place since it could be required once the issue has been remedied.

(135) (A) Increased urine output, thirst, and weakness.

The high glucose content of parenteral nutrition increases the risk of hyperglycemia. Diuresis, Kussmaul respirations, weakness, disorientation, fatigue, and extreme thirst are all indications of hyperglycemia.

(136) (A) Ensure the infant's eyes are covered.

The infant's eyes should be covered to protect them from harm when the light is on. The infant needs plenty of fluids. There is no need to keep the mother and child apart.

(137) (A) Watermelon.

Furosemide is a potassium-wasting diuretic. Hence, the patient requires potassium. The potassium content in watermelon is quite high. The other answer options don't contain a lot of potassium.

(138) (D) Acute rejection.

Acute rejection often manifests as decreased renal function, graft soreness, hypertension, elevated WBC, malaise, and fever in the first two weeks after transplantation. Chronic rejection progressively develops over a few months to many years.

(139) (C) Elevated serum creatinine level.

A common laboratory test to assess renal function is to measure the creatinine level. When at least 50% of renal function is lost, the amount of creatinine rises. If urinary tract bleeding occurs or the kidney's erythropoietic function is compromised, there may be a reduction in hemoglobin level and RBC count.

(140) (A) Decreased urinary stream force.

An early sign of benign prostatic hyperplasia is a decrease in urinary stream force. The patient may have hematuria, nocturia, urge incontinence, urgency, and frequency. Urine retention and complete obstruction may result if untreated.

(141) (B) Blood pressure.

A frequent adverse reaction to bumetanide usage is hypotension.

(142) (A) Face shield, goggles, gown, and gloves.

Colostomy care may result in bodily fluids that splash. The eyes are shielded with goggles and a face shield. Gloves and gowns are needed for contact precautions. There is no need for shoe guards.

(143) (A) Every 30 minutes.

Every 30 minutes, the nurse should evaluate extremity circulatory and neurovascular status and skin integrity in a restrained patient. To encourage circulation, the safety device should also be removed at least every two hours.

(144) (A) WBC.

Due to antibiotic-resistant infections, individuals with neutropenia may need a transfusion of WBCs. To assess the efficacy of the treatment, the nurse should monitor WBC levels and symptoms of infections.

(145) (A) Circulatory overload.

Circulatory overload is a side effect of IV treatment. Crackles, a wet cough, dyspnea, hypertension, and tachypnea are symptoms. The symptoms of a systemic infection include tachycardia, headache, fever, and chills. Symptoms of an air embolism include DCL, cyanosis, dyspnea, and tachycardia. Hematomas are distinguished by ecchymosis, swelling, and leaks at the IV site.

Test 2: Questions

(1) What should an atrial fibrillation patient be assessed for?

(A) Headache and hypertension.

(B) Dizziness and hypotension.

(C) Vomiting and nausea.

(D) Flat neck veins.

(2) What is the appropriate action for a male patient who presents with dizziness, a blood pressure of 80/62 mm Hg, a heart rate of 49 bpm, and sinus bradycardia?

(A) Transcutaneous pacing.

(B) Monitor continuously.

(C) Administer digoxin.

(D) Defibrillation.

(3) A nurse is positioned behind a five-year-old conscious child who has presented with airway obstruction. She places her arms around the child and under the axilla. Where should she place her hands to deliver rescue thrusts?

(A) On the xiphoid process and umbilicus.

(B) On the chest and lower abdomen.

(C) On the groin and umbilicus.

(D) On the groin and abdomen.

(4) What is an important care step for an internal radiation implant patient?

(A) Give the patient a semiprivate room at the end of the hallway.

(B) Ensure the nurse wears a lead apron.

(C) Do not change any linens until the patient's implant is removed.

(D) Wear gloves when caring for the patient.

(5) A patient who has just undergone surgery has significant blood loss. The nurse recognizes the need to monitor the patient closely for signs of shock. Which symptom would be of most immediate concern?

(A) Blood pressure of 130/85 mm Hg.

(B) Heart rate of 58 bpm.

(C) Urine output decreased to 20 mL/hr.

(D) Patient reports a pain level of three on a scale of 1–10.

(6) What is a risk factor for a sodium level of 129 mEq/L?

(A) Corticosteroids.

(B) Hyperaldosteronism.

(C) Diuretics.

(D) Cushing's syndrome.

(7) What is the role of an advance directive?

(A) To decide who will pay hospital bills.

(B) To avoid family member conflicts during treatment plan decision-making.

(C) To protect the patient's preferences if the patient is terminal and cannot make decisions.

(D) To force the patient to choose how he wants to be treated.

(8) What is not the role of a patient advocate?

(A) Present arguments against medical theories.

(B) Provide quality treatment.

(C) Reconcile patients and medical professionals.

(D) Organize patient appointments.

(9) What is essential during the management of post-trans-sphenoidal hypophysectomy for an acromegaly patient?

(A) The patient should cough.

(B) Put the patient in a Trendelenburg position.

(C) Regularly suction the pharynx and mouth.

(D) Monitor the blood pressure regularly.

(10) What can promote a patient's self-advocacy?

(A) Encourage patients to look for a healthcare provider through reliable sources.

(B) Do not create a medical summary for the patient's condition.

(C) If a patient cannot understand the medical terms, explain them.

(D) The patient has no right to ask questions.

(11) What is the correct management for a patient who takes daily warfarin with an INR of 2.5?

(A) Decrease the dose.

(B) Give the prescribed warfarin dose.

(C) Inform the doctor and stop warfarin.

(D) Increase the dose.

(12) What is the diagnostic test for Kaposi's cutaneous sarcoma in an HIV patient?

(A) Skin with blue-reddish lesions.

(B) A punch biopsy of the lesion.

(C) Lower limb swelling.

(D) Genital area swelling.

(13) What is considered the priority during the care of an HIV patient?

(A) Recognize decreased immune function.

(B) Lifestyle changes.

(C) Emotional support.

(D) Infection protection.

(14) What are appropriate instructions for an osteoporosis patient on an alendronate prescription?

(A) Take the drug with a full glass of water.

(B) Lie down for half an hour after taking the drug.

(C) Take the drug with meals.

(D) Take the drug at bedtime.

(15) What are the contraindications to bethanechol chloride?

(A) GERD.

(B) Neurogenic atony.

(C) Urinary strictures.

(D) Gastric atony.

(16) What statement is not true about care plan decision-making?

(A) If a patient is competent, their choices should be respected.

(B) In a medical emergency, the intervention should be done even if the patient would have rejected it.

(C) The healthcare practitioner must inform the patient about his condition.

(D) In a medical emergency, consent can be presumed unless it is evident that the patient would reject the intervention.

(17) A cardiac and hypertensive patient takes chlorothiazide, digoxin, and atenolol. She presents with digoxin toxicity. What are the clinical signs of digoxin toxicity?

(A) Sleep disorder, dry mouth, and constipation.

(B) Nausea, loss of appetite, and double vision.

(C) Paresthesia, hypotension, and chest pain.

(D) Palpitations, edema, and dyspnea.

(18) In which step during nursing planning does the nurse collect the patient's information about spiritual, sociocultural, emotional, physical, and psychological problems?

(A) Diagnosis.

(B) Implementation.

(C) Planning.

(D) Assessment.

(19) Which cardiac dysrhythmia is characterized by a regular rhythm and heart rate of 150 bpm, wide QRS complexes, and no P waves?

(A) Premature ventricular contraction.

(B) Ventricular tachycardia.

(C) Ventricular fibrillation.

(D) Sinus tachycardia.

(20) Which symptom is associated with deteriorating preeclampsia?

(A) Blurred vision and headache.

(B) Blood pressure reading within range.

(C) Edema.

(D) Increased urine output.

(21) What is an appropriate action for a fetal heart rate of 180 bpm at 37 weeks gestation?

(A) Record that the fetal heart rate is normal.

(B) Record the mother's heart rate.

(C) Record the fetal heart rate.

(D) Inform the doctor.

(22) Which position is appropriate for a thoracentesis patient?

(A) Prone, with the head supported by a pillow and turned to the side.

(B) Sims' position with the head of the bed flat.

(C) Lie on the side that is unaffected.

(D) Lie on the side that is affected.

(23) Why do most cholecystectomy patients usually refuse to see the dressing site?

(A) They do not want to see the blood.

(B) They do not want to see the wound.

(C) They have changes in body image.

(D) They deny the surgery.

(24) What are the benefits of an interprofessional team?

(A) A decrease in safe, quality care.

(B) An increase in adverse outcomes.

(C) A decrease in positive outcomes.

(D) Decreased duplication and fragmentation of care.

(25) What could put a patient on phenytoin at risk?

(A) Alcohol consumption.

(B) Phenytoin serum level of 15 mcg/mL.

(C) Swollen gums.

(D) Pinkish urine.

(26) What indicates a cholinergic crisis in myasthenia gravis patients after administration of edrophonium?

(A) Transient condition worsens.

(B) Strength decreases.

(C) Muscle spasms.

(D) No changes occur.

(27) When managing a conflict, which of these statements is not true?

(A) You should arrange a time and location for a private conversation with the other party.

(B) You should remember that you and your coworker are both in nursing because you want to care for patients.

(C) You should actively listen while the other person is speaking.

(D) You should cross your arms and maintain eye contact to help maintain pleasant body language.

(28) A hemodialysis patient suddenly becomes anxious, pale, tachycardic, and complains of chest pain and dyspnea. What is the correct action if the nurse suspects an air embolism?

(A) Give 700 mL of IV saline.

(B) Check for air in the lines, then continue the dialysis at half the rate.

(C) Monitor vital signs.

(D) Inform the doctor and stop the dialysis.

(29) What are severe and life-threatening complications of propranolol?

(A) Bradycardia.

(B) Hypotension.

(C) Expiratory wheezes.

(D) Insomnia.

(30) What has been proven to have little to no effect on learning results during staff education?

(A) Feedback.

(B) Interaction.

(C) Case-based learning.

(D) Reading or lectures.

(31) What should be checked for if a myocardial infarction patient develops cardiogenic shock?

(A) CVP that falls.

(B) Increased diastolic blood pressure.

(C) Ventricular dysrhythmia.

(D) Bradycardia.

(32) What is true about rifampin's long-term drug administration?

(A) It can be stopped if the symptoms are relieved after three months.

(B) It can cause orange feces, urine, tears, and sweat.

(C) If the patient forgets a dose, a double dose should be taken.

(D) It should not be taken on an empty stomach.

(33) Which statement is true about guaifenesin?

(A) The patient should decrease daily fluid intake.

(B) The drug should be taken with a full glass of water.

(C) The drug should be taken with meals.

(D) If there is a fever, the patient should take another tablet.

(34) Which resource can provide synthesized research?

(A) Printed publications.

(B) Electronic publications.

(C) Organizational intranet.

(D) All of the above.

(35) A nurse notes a high-pressure alarm on the ventilator of an intubated 30-year-old male. Chest auscultation reveals that the upper right lobe of his lung has no air entry. What is the diagnosis?

(A) ARDS.

(B) Endotracheal tube displacement.

(C) Pulmonary embolism.

(D) Right pneumothorax.

(36) A patient has a peptic ulcer caused by a Helicobacter pylori infection. Which statement is true about treatment with amoxicillin, esomeprazole, and clarithromycin?

(A) They decrease stomach acid production and coat the ulcer.

(B) They decrease stomach acid production and kill the bacteria.

(C) They are only taken when there is pain.

(D) They kill the bacteria and heal the ulcer.

(37) What can be treated with omeprazole?

(A) Constipation.

(B) Flatulence.

(C) Heartburn.

(D) Diarrhea.

(38) What could reduce the risk of cardiac dysrhythmias from rapid multiple blood unit transfusions in a shock patient?

(A) Blood-warming device.

(B) Infusion controller.

(C) Cardiac monitor.

(D) Pulse oximetry.

(39) What do the Five Rights of Delegation not include?

(A) Situation.

(B) Person.

(C) Task.

(D) Research.

(40) What action should a patient perform when changing the tubing and bag of parenteral nutrition?

(A) Inhale deeply, hold their breath, and bear down.

(B) Exhale evenly and slowly.

(C) Turn their head to the right.

(D) Breathe normally.

(41) What are good dietary choices for hemodialysis renal failure patients?

(A) Orange juice, strawberries, grits, and cured pork.

(B) Tomato juice, cantaloupe, and bacon.

(C) Orange juice, banana, eggs, and sausage.

(D) Coffee, blueberries, and cream of wheat.

(42) Which statement is true about a diabetic patient with a glycosylated hemoglobin A1c level of 8.7%?

(A) It's important to prevent hyperglycemia.

(B) It's important to prevent hypoglycemia.

(C) It's important to drink plenty of fluids.

(D) It's important to avoid infection.

(43) A patient takes warfarin as a maintenance therapy due to AF. He does a PT test, with a result of 36 seconds. Which next step is appropriate?

(A) Administer the next dose of warfarin.

(B) Increase the next dose of warfarin

(C) Withhold the next dose of warfarin.

(D) Add a dose of heparin sodium.

(44) What can be used to prevent the inappropriate disclosure of a patient's information?

(A) Encryption.

(B) Passwords.

(C) Antivirus software.

(D) All of the above.

(45) Psycho-mental privacy does not require a nurse to:

(A) Provide correct instructions upon discharge.

(B) Respect the patient's values and beliefs.

(C) Speak to the patient respectfully and politely.

(D) Touch the patient's body when unnecessary.

(46) What is a form of follow-up?

(A) Phone calls.

(B) Home visits.

(C) Appointments.

(D) All of the above.

(47) What is the diagnosis for a female four hours post-delivery whose fundus has deviated left, is 3 cm above the umbilicus, and is soft?

(A) Normal involution.

(B) Urinary retention.

(C) Perineal laceration.

(D) Retained fragment of the placenta.

(48) What is an action of phenazopyridine in a cystitis patient?

(A) It protects the kidneys from damage by the infection.

(B) It is an anesthetic and decreases the pain until antibiotic action occurs.

(C) It is an antibiotic and analgesic.

(D) It is an antibiotic.

(49) What refers to the end of care from a healthcare organization?

(A) Transfer.

(B) Discharge.

(C) Follow-up.

(D) Nursing care plan.

(50) A patient with an injury to the spinal cord at the level of C6 complains of hypertension, headache, and blurred vision. What is the appropriate management?

(A) Measure blood pressure.

(B) Give analgesics.

(C) Put the patient in the Trendelenburg position.

(D) Assess the patient for distention of the bladder.

(51) What does the nursing care plan of the radiation site for an external radiation therapy patient include?

(A) The radiation site should not be cleaned.

(B) Pain at the radiation site should be decreased by application of ice.

(C) The patient should be bathed daily.

(D) A loose dressing should be taped to the radiation site.

(52) What does a nursing report include?

(A) Dietary restrictions.

(B) Patient's allergies.

(C) Pain management strategies.

(D) All of the above.

(53) What are some signs of hypovolemic shock?

(A) Decrease in RR.

(B) Decrease in urine output.

(C) Decrease in HR.

(D) Low diastolic and high systolic blood pressure.

(54) What symptom should concern a nurse about a 33-week gestational female?

(A) Foot and ankle edema.

(B) Eye edema.

(C) Weight gain of about four pounds in a month.

(D) Glucose in the urine.

(55) What symptom should concern a nurse about a kidney transplant patient who takes prednisone and cyclosporine?

(A) Mood swings.

(B) Painful throat.

(C) Acne.

(D) Moon face.

(56) Which of these statements is incorrect during HIV patient care?

(A) It's important to wear a mask.

(B) A nurse does not need to wear gloves when rubbing the patient's back.

(C) Nurses can use chlorine bleach to clean up blood spills.

(D) Nurses should wear gloves around fecal incontinence waste products.

(57) What is an individual's sense of value and self-worth by themselves and others?

(A) Self-actualization.

(B) Self-esteem.

(C) Love.

(D) Safety.

(58) What is respect for an individual's right to self-determination?

(A) Nonmaleficence.

(B) Paternalism.

(C) Autonomy.

(D) Justice.

(59) What is a contraindication of cyclobenzaprine hydrochloride administration for a muscle spasm patient?

(A) Diabetes mellitus.

(B) Hypothyroidism.

(C) Emphysema.

(D) Glaucoma.

(60) What is a contraindication for a colchicine prescription?

(A) Diabetes mellitus.

(B) Hypothyroidism.

(C) Renal failure.

(D) Myxedema.

(61) Which nursing intervention is appropriate if a compression bandage comes off on an above-knee amputation that is three days postoperative?

(A) Elevate the limb on a pillow and put on a sterile dry dressing.

(B) Use a compression bandage to rewrap the stump.

(C) Put ice on the stump.

(D) Inform the doctor.

(62) What indicates fat embolus resolution in a patient with multiple fractures?

(A) Arterial oxygen of 82.

(B) Oxygen saturation of 75.

(C) Intact mental state.

(D) Dyspnea.

(63) A closed-arm fracture patient has a cast but complains of severe pain. The nurse gives him an analgesic, applies an ice bag, and elevates the limb, but the patient is still in pain. What is the possible cause?

(A) The fracture is new.

(B) There is tissue perfusion impairment.

(C) The patient is anxious.

(D) The cast is infected.

(64) What is true about Buck's traction for a hip fracture patient?

(A) It helps with fracture immobilization and decreases muscle spasms.

(B) It decreases blood vessel impairment and lengthens the leg.

(C) It helps with fracture site immobilization.

(D) It helps with bone healing.

(65) Which statement is true about phenytoin?

(A) The dose should be administered before drawing a sample for a serum level test.

(B) If side effects occur, the patient should decrease the dose by half.

(C) It is important to brush and floss.

(D) Avoid alcohol.

(66) When a patient cannot sign the consent for surgery due to opioid analgesic sedation, from whom should the consent be obtained?

(A) A family member.

(B) The hospital chaplain.

(C) The surgery should be done without consent.

(D) A court order must be obtained before the surgery.

(67) What is used to analyze how long it takes to admit a patient?

(A) Balance metrics.

(B) Outcome metrics.

(C) In-process metrics.

(D) Structural metrics.

(68) What is not true about preprinted physician orders?

(A) It is a high-cost service.

(B) It provides a straightforward way to change how the healthcare system functions.

(C) It allows flexibility and the capability to swiftly shift and adapt to changes in specific hospital procedures.

(D) It positively affects patient outcomes.

(69) What builds a thorough understanding of nursing tasks and responsibilities and helps to distinguish between ethical and unethical practices?

(A) Conscious attention.

(B) Professional sensibility.

(C) Personal attention.

(D) Contextual attention.

(70) Which test assesses the pain peripheral response in an unconscious patient?

(A) Sternocleidomastoid squeezing.

(B) Orbital rim pressure.

(C) Pressure on the nail bed.

(D) Rub the sternum.

(71) What is the appropriate management step for an abruptio placentae case?

(A) Coagulation studies performed weekly until delivery date.

(B) Bed rest until delivery date.

(C) Output and input monitoring.

(D) Initiate delivery.

(72) What is a risk factor for HIV in pregnant women?

(A) One sexual partner for the past seven years.

(B) History of a sexually transmitted disease.

(C) Heterosexual partner.

(D) History of IV drug use.

(73) What can reduce breast tenderness in pregnant women during the first trimester?

(A) Use lotion to massage the breasts and wash them with soap and water.

(B) Support the breasts with tight dresses and blouses.

(C) Keep the breasts dry and only wash them with warm water.

(D) Do not wear a bra.

(74) What is the correct action to care for a pneumothorax patient who develops bubbling inside the suction control chamber?

(A) Increase the pressure of the suction.

(B) Check for air leaks if the bubbling is intermittent.

(C) Clamp the chest tube and inform the doctor.

(D) This is an expected finding, so you should do nothing.

(75) Which position is used during NG tube insertion?

(A) Head flat and supine.

(B) High Fowler's.

(C) Low Fowler's.

(D) Right side.

(76) What is the nursing care priority for physical abuse victims?

(A) Directly stop the aggressor.

(B) Remove the patient out of the abusive environment.

(C) Check if there is domestic abuse at home.

(D) Report the problem to the appropriate authorities.

(77) Which precaution prevents transmission in a meningitis case?

(A) The staff wears masks whenever the patient leaves the room.

(B) Assign the patient to a private room with negative airflow pressure.

(C) Nurses should wear a personal respiratory protection device.

(D) Assign the patient to a private room or cohort patient.

(78) What is an example of disciplinary actions that could result in the suspension of a nursing license?

(A) Unprofessional behavior.

(B) Behavior that may harm the health and welfare of the public.

(C) Failure to keep proper records for each patient.

(D) All of the above.

(79) What is a cause of hyperkalemia in a patient with a potassium level of 5.8 mEq/L?

(A) A traumatic burn.

(B) Overuse of laxatives.

(C) Cushing's syndrome.

(D) Colitis.

(80) What can be used to graph events to determine their performance over time?

(A) Control chart.

(B) Data collection.

(C) Process mapping.

(D) Data analysis.

(81) What are appropriate dietary instructions for a female with iron deficiency anemia?

(A) Hot chocolate, pickles, and cheese.

(B) Orange juice, tomatoes, spinach, and broccoli.

(C) Milk, carrots, and peanut butter.

(D) Butter, bread, green beans, and applesauce.

(82) Which studies have a Level 2 evidence-based ranking?

(A) Case studies.

(B) Case-control studies.

(C) Cohort studies.

(D) Meta-analysis.

(83) A 64-year-old man fractures his left hip. Which fracture could be present?

(A) Pathological fracture.

(B) Open fracture.

(C) Greenstick fracture.

(D) Comminuted fracture.

(84) Which drugs have a lower occurrence of allergy?

(A) Cephalosporin.

(B) Sulfonamides.

(C) Penicillin.

(D) Aspirin.

(85) During a pan-hysterectomy abdominal surgery, what is removed?

(A) The vagina, ovaries, fallopian tubes, cervix, and the body and fundus of the uterus.

(B) The ovaries, fallopian tubes, cervix, and the body and fundus of the uterus.

(C) The cervix and the body and fundus of the uterus.

(D) The body and fundus of the uterus.

(86) What are some complications of a nephrectomy?

(A) Footdrop.

(B) Atelectasis.

(C) Wound infection.

(D) Thrombophlebitis.

(87) Which patient history could indicate hepatitis A?

(A) History of cholecystectomy.

(B) History of blood transfusion.

(C) History of travel to India.

(D) History of blood donation.

(88) A patient takes cyclophosphamide for multiple sclerosis. She asks the nurse why she is on the same medication her mother took for Hodgkin's disease. Which details should the nurse provide?

(A) The same organism causes Hodgkin's disease and multiple sclerosis.

(B) Multiple sclerosis affects the same neurological system as Hodgkin's disease.

(C) Immunosuppression is a side effect of the cancer medication cyclophosphamide. The immune system attacks the patient's nerves in multiple sclerosis.

(D) Because multiple sclerosis is cancer, the same medications work for both diseases.

(89) What is a cause of histoplasmosis?

(A) Raw milk.

(B) Contaminated water.

(C) Raw shellfish.

(D) Employment as a chicken farmer.

(90) Why is it important to keep oxygen humidified?

(A) Humidification prevents organisms' growth.

(B) It prevents the nasal passages from drying out.

(C) It increases oxygen concentration.

(D) It prevents fires.

(91) What is appropriate management for a patient scheduled for a bronchoscopy?

(A) Stop all medications.

(B) Do a cleansing enema.

(C) Keep the patient in an NPO state.

(D) Give plenty of fluids.

(92) Which finding would indicate the doctor should be informed about a patient with a transurethral prostate resection for benign prostatic hyperplasia?

(A) Pulse of 135 bpm and blood pressure of 90/60 mm Hg.

(B) Fluid intake is less than urinary output.

(C) Bladder spasms.

(D) Red urine.

(93) Bladder trauma pain can be referred to the:

(A) Costovertebral angle.

(B) Umbilicus.

(C) Shoulder.

(D) Hip.

(94) Which dietary product can be offered when a patient is switched from a clear liquid diet to a full liquid diet?

(A) Popsicles.

(B) Custard.

(C) Gelatin.

(D) Tea.

(95) What are dietary sources of iron for iron deficiency anemia cases?

(A) Dark green leafy vegetables and oranges.

(B) Fish and cooked rolled oats.

(C) Tea and coffee.

(D) Milk and nuts.

(96) What is a normal total protein level in a cirrhotic patient on a diet with adequate protein intake?

(A) 9.8 g/dL.

(B) 6.4 g/dL.

(C) 3.7 g/dL.

(D) 0.4 g/dL.

(97) Which BUN levels reflect an adequate volume replacement in a patient with a UTI and dehydration?

(A) 35 mg/dL.

(B) 29 mg/dL.

(C) 15 mg/dL.

(D) 3 mg/dL.

(98) What can occur with an NG tube?

(A) Respiratory alkalosis.

(B) Respiratory acidosis.

(C) Metabolic alkalosis.

(D) Metabolic acidosis.

(99) A nurse discovers his patient's sodium levels are 152 mEq/L. What food items must the patient now avoid?

(A) Processed cereals.

(B) Cauliflower.

(C) Nuts.

(D) Peas.

(100) A five-year-old boy presents with otitis media. The doctor prescribes an antibiotic and a follow-up. What is the reason for the follow-up appointment?

(A) If the infection recurs, the doctor will prescribe another antibiotic.

(B) To make sure the antibiotic cured the infection.

(C) To make sure the patient took the antibiotic.

(D) To test if the child's hearing is affected or not.

(101) Which complication may occur after a hysterectomy?

(A) Aortic aneurysm.

(B) Cerebral embolism.

(C) Varicose veins.

(D) Thrombophlebitis.

(102) What are the possible complications of a radium rod insertion for a cervical cancer patient?

(A) Uterine cramps.

(B) Constipation.

(C) Urinary retention.

(D) Headache.

(103) How can an anorexia nervosa patient manage his anxiety?

(A) He should make decisions and not dwell on them.

(B) He should observe rigid regulations and rules.

(C) He should regularly reinforce his self-approval.

(D) He should engage in immoral acts.

(104) A patient who takes lithium carbonate presents with tremors, tinnitus, blurred vision, diarrhea, abdominal pain, and vomiting. When measured, her lithium carbonate level is 3 mEq/L. What is true about this level?

(A) It's below normal.

(B) It's above normal.

(C) It's normal

(D) It's toxic.

(105) When is an adequate therapeutic level of imipramine reached?

(A) After two months.

(B) After the second week.

(C) After the third week.

(D) After the first week.

(106) Which laboratory test should be monitored for HIV patients with CMV retinitis who take foscarnet?

(A) Lymphocyte count.

(B) Serum creatinine level.

(C) Serum albumin level.

(D) CD4 cell count.

(107) What should be assessed in a patient who takes stavudine for HIV?

(A) GIT function.

(B) Consciousness level.

(C) Appetite.

(D) Gait.

(108) A male patient comes to the ER with a history of a tick bite. He tells the nurse that he has removed the tick. What is the next management step?

(A) The patient should wait six weeks to be tested.

(B) Testing is not essential unless arthralgia occurs.

(C) Lyme disease has no tests.

(D) Do a Lyme disease blood test now.

(109) SLE patients should avoid:

(A) Exercises such as walking when the patient is not exhausted.

(B) Joint stiffness with massage.

(C) Extended periods of rest to save energy.

(D) Hot showers.

(110) What are some instructions for baclofen administration?

(A) If diarrhea occurs, stop the drug.

(B) If fatigue occurs, inform the doctor.

(C) Do not drink alcohol.

(D) Decrease intake of fluids.

(111) What are some instructions a nurse should give patients on allopurinol?

(A) It is normal to have a swollen lip.

(B) An immediate effect will occur.

(C) It should be taken on an empty stomach.

(D) The patient should increase daily water intake to three liters.

(112) What is an adverse effect of intranasal desmopressin?

(A) Flushed skin.

(B) Runny nose.

(C) Vulval pain.

(D) Headache.

(113) What is a contraindication of sildenafil administration in an erectile dysfunction patient?

(A) Multivitamins.

(B) Nitroglycerin.

(C) Insomnia.

(D) Neuralgia.

(114) What is a life-threatening complication of parathyroidectomy?

(A) Incision pain.

(B) Difficulty voiding.

(C) Abdominal cramps.

(D) Laryngeal stridor.

(115) A diabetic 50-year-old female presents with confusion, diaphoresis, and nausea three days postoperatively after an abdominal hysterectomy. She is on regular insulin four times a day. What is the appropriate management step?

(A) Administer 30 g of a carbohydrate snack to the patient.

(B) Administer IV 50% dextrose.

(C) Do a focused assessment of RBS.

(D) Call for help immediately.

(116) What is a symptom of primary hyperparathyroidism?

(A) Weight gain.

(B) Polyphagia.

(C) Polyuria.

(D) Fatigue.

(117) When a nurse inspects a bottle of fat emulsion and discovers clear fat globules at the top of the solution, what should she do?

(A) Pour warm water over the bottle.

(B) Shake the bottle.

(C) Get another bottle of emulsion.

(D) Gently roll the solution bottle.

(118) What is a correct action for a patient on parenteral nutrition with a rate of 100 mL/hr who is being weaned to solid food?

(A) Continue the current parenteral nutrition infusion rate.

(B) Start 0.9% normal saline at 25 mL/hr.

(C) Decrease parenteral nutrition rate to 50 mL/hr.

(D) Discontinue the parenteral nutrition entirely.

(119) A patient has insensible fluid loss of approximately 900 mL daily. Through what route does insensible fluid loss occur?

(A) GIT.

(B) Wound drainage.

(C) Urinary output.

(D) Skin.

(120) What should a nurse ask before antibiotics are administered to a streptococcus-positive patient?

(A) Is the patient allergic to penicillin?

(B) Does the patient drink alcohol?

(C) Does the patient take vitamins?

(D) Does the patient have a history of sulfa drug reactions?

(121) What is a cause of a valve replacement in a mitral stenosis patient?

(A) Rubella.

(B) Rheumatic fever.

(C) Syphilis.

(D) Meningitis.

(122) What is the ideal position for a liver biopsy patient after the procedure?

(A) Semi-recumbent.

(B) Semi-sitting.

(C) On the right side.

(D) On the left side.

(123) What laboratory tests are monitored for long-term diabetes management?

(A) Glycosylated hemoglobin.

(B) Finger-stick glucose test

(C) Glucose tolerance test.

(D) Fasting blood sugar.

(124) What are some signs of Addison's disease?

(A) Ecchymosis.

(B) Hypotension.

(C) Puffy face.

(D) Supraclavicular fat pad.

(125) What is the ideal position for a lumbar laminectomy patient?

(A) Semi-reclining.

(B) Side-lying.

(C) Prone.

(D) Supine.

(126) What is true about Epoetin alfa prescribed to a dialysis patient?

(A) It can improve athletic activity.

(B) The kidneys cannot produce erythropoietin, and the drug replaces it.

(C) The kidneys cannot remove toxins, and the drug replaces this function.

(D) It can help with urine production.

(127) What is the most important test for a UTI patient?

(A) Urine strain for calculi.

(B) Cystoscopy.

(C) CBC.

(D) Urine culture and sensitivity.

(128) What increases the danger for a patient with ulcerative colitis?

(A) Poor health management.

(B) Skin impairment.

(C) Altered body image.

(D) Fluid volume depletion.

(129) What are the manifestations of stage one of Lyme disease?

(A) Neurological disorders.

(B) Inflamed joints.

(C) Flu-like symptoms.

(D) Arthralgias.

(130) What should be assessed in a patient with an implantable cardioverter defibrillator?

(A) The programmed shock numbers, heart rate threshold, and device activation status.

(B) Physical activity that is restricted postoperatively.

(C) Positions that are restricted postoperatively.

(D) Family and patient's level of anxiety.

(131) A male patient has coarse, wavy lines of varying amplitude, no definable QRS complexes, and no P waves. What is the correct interpretation?

(A) Ventricular tachycardia.

(B) Ventricular fibrillation.

(C) Atrial fibrillation.

(D) Asystole.

(132) Which laboratory tests should be done before isoniazid anti-tuberculosis treatment?

(A) Coagulation time.

(B) Serum creatinine level.

(C) Liver enzyme levels.

(D) Electrolyte levels.

(133) What is the appropriate care for a patient in the active labor stage when the monitor strip shows late deceleration of the fetal patterns?

(A) Monitor the fetal patterns.

(B) Increase IV oxytocin rate.

(C) Keep the pregnant female in a supine position.

(D) Use a face mask for oxygen administration.

(134) A 36-year-old pregnant woman is diagnosed with TB after complaints of fatigue, weight loss, and loss of appetite. A sputum culture reveals Mycobacterium tuberculosis. What is an appropriate management step?

(A) Use rifampin and isoniazid for nine months.

(B) Start TB medication after labor.

(C) Advise the patient not to leave home until the completion of the treatment.

(D) It is necessary to do a therapeutic abortion.

(135) Which cardiovascular system changes can occur during pregnancy?

(A) Decreased RBC production.

(B) Frequent bowel elimination.

(C) Hypertension.

(D) Tachycardia.

(136) A nurse educates a patient due for surgery about potential blood loss complications. What is a possible consequence of significant blood loss?

(A) Hypertension.

(B) Bradycardia.

(C) Acute kidney injury.

(D) Hyperthermia.

(137) A patient has experienced significant blood loss after an accident. Her heart rate is 110 bpm, respirations are 24 per minute, and her skin is cool and clammy. What do these findings indicate?

(A) An allergic reaction.

(B) A hyperglycemic episode.

(C) Hypovolemic shock.

(D) A panic attack.

(138) Which body parts, if burned, could create a life-threatening situation?

(A) Perineum.

(B) Feet and hands.

(C) Upper body.

(D) Lower body.

(139) A 55-year-old male presents with a swollen red big toe. What is the appropriate management?

(A) Urinary catheterization.

(B) Use a heat lamp.

(C) Bed rails.

(D) Bed cradle.

(140) What does management of a patient with chronic late-stage renal failure include?

(A) Increase protein intake to promote healing.

(B) Assess the patient for pulmonary edema by lung sounds auscultation.

(C) To increase the venous return, elevate the patient's legs.

(D) Put in a urinary catheter.

(141) What do complications of renal colic include?

(A) Oliguria.

(B) Hypertension.

(C) Polyuria.

(D) Anemia.

(142) A six-year-old boy had recent nocturnal enuresis in the hospital but has voluntary bladder control at home. What is the appropriate management?

(A) Ensure he makes regular trips to the bathroom.

(B) Give him chocolate if he goes to the bathroom.

(C) Do not change the wet linens to discourage him from doing it again.

(D) Make the boy wear diapers.

(143) What is the purpose of voiding encouragement in a postoperative hemorrhoidectomy patient?

(A) The voiding will be difficult if the patient has had multiple pregnancies.

(B) The voiding will be difficult if the patient has had prolonged hemorrhoids.

(C) Urine retention is common after hemorrhoidectomy.

(D) The patient was NPO before and during the operation.

(144) What is the purpose of a semi-sitting position in a patient with a Penrose drain after an appendectomy?

(A) Suture line tension reduction.

(B) Pressure sore prevention.

(C) Abdominal cavity drainage.

(D) Enhance ventilation.

(145) A 45-year-old female patient presents with acute abdominal pain, mainly in the right lower quadrant, nausea, and a low-grade fever. During the physical exam, the nurse notes rebound tenderness in the same area. Which condition should the nurse suspect, and what action should be a priority?

(A) Gastritis; administer antacids.

(B) Pancreatitis; administer pain medication.

(C) Appendicitis; prepare for a possible surgical consultation.

(D) Cholecystitis; apply a warm compress on the abdomen.

Test 2: Answers and Explanations

(1) (B) Dizziness and hypotension.

Loss of atrial kick puts a patient with uncontrolled atrial fibrillation and a ventricular rate of more than 100 bpm at risk for low cardiac output. Evaluate the patient for neck vein distension, shortness of breath, syncope, dizziness, weakness, exhaustion, pulse deficit, hypotension, chest discomfort, and palpitations.

(2) (A) Transcutaneous pacing.

Dizziness and hypotension are symptoms of reduced cardiac output. A temporary solution to raise the heart rate and perfusion is transcutaneous pacing. Use defibrillation to treat ventricular fibrillation and pulseless ventricular tachycardia. The patient's heart rate will fall further after digoxin is administered.

(3) (A) On the xiphoid process and umbilicus.

The nurse should stand behind the patient and put her arms around the victim and under the axilla. She should press the thumb side of one fist into the victim's belly at the midline, above the umbilicus, and below the tip of the xiphoid process. With the other hand, the nurse should grab her fist and apply up to five inward thrusts.

(4) (A) Give the patient a semiprivate room at the end of the hallway.

If a patient has an internal radiation implant, a private room with a private bathroom is necessary to avoid unintentional exposure of more patients to the radiation.

(5) (C) Urine output decreased to 20 mL/hr.

This patient shows signs of hypovolemic shock due to significant blood loss. An important sign of shock is decreased urine output of less than 30 mL/hr. This occurs because the body diverts blood flow from the kidneys and toward vital organs like the heart and brain. The other options (A, B, D) are within normal parameters and do not indicate a problem related to blood loss.

(6) (C) Diuretics.

A serum sodium level of less than 135 mEq/L indicates hyponatremia. A patient who takes diuretics may develop hyponatremia. Corticosteroids, Cushing's syndrome, and hyperaldosteronism put patients at risk for hypernatremia.

(7) (C) Protect the patient's preferences if the patient is terminal and cannot make decisions.

Advanced directives help when patients become critically ill or unable to express their preferences. They should discuss their choices and decide on appropriate medical care.

(8) (D) Organize patient appointments.

Patient advocates uphold a patient's rights, ensure appropriate standards of care, defend human dignity, advance patient equality, and guarantee that patients can make their own health-related decisions. They do not organize patient appointments.

(9) (D) Monitor the blood pressure regularly.

After hypophysectomy, a rapid drop in growth hormone levels occurs. This causes insulin levels to increase, which results in hypoglycemia. Coughing puts more pressure on the surgical site and causes CSF leakage. The Trendelenburg position is inappropriate because the patient's head should be lifted to relieve pressure on the surgical site. The suction can traumatize the mucosa of the mouth and nose.

(10) (A) Encourage patients to look for a healthcare provider through reliable sources.

There are several strategies to encourage patients to advocate for themselves. A patient can request clear communication, decide on a medical team through the assessment of various providers found with reliable sources, ask for a medical summary, and request help to access services both in and outside the hospital. Educate patients and be present for them.

(11) (B) Give the prescribed warfarin dose.

For patients on warfarin, the ideal INR is between 2–3. The nurse should administer the medication as directed since a level of 2.5 is within the recommended range. If the INR is more than three, the nurse should stop the medication and contact the doctor.

(12) (B) A punch biopsy of the lesion.

Kaposi's sarcoma lesions appear on the lower legs as purple or dark blue macules that develop into plaques. They eventually ulcerate or break open and discharge. The lesions may metastasize to the GIT, lungs, lymphatic system, oral mucosa, face, and upper body. A punch biopsy is used to diagnose cutaneous lesions, whereas a biopsy is used to diagnose pulmonary and gastrointestinal abnormalities.

(13) (D) Infection protection.

A patient with immunodeficiency has insufficient or no immune system. Thus, the primary concern is to protect the patient from infection. Although the other choices may be components of care, they are not the immediate concern.

(14) (A) Take the drug with a full glass of water.

It is necessary to take alendronate with a full glass of water. After the drug is administered, the patient should not lie down or eat anything for 30 minutes to increase absorption.

(15) (C) Urinary strictures.

Patients with weak bladder walls or a urinary tract blockage may be at risk if they take bethanechol chloride. The drug may cause bladder contractions, which will raise the pressure within the urinary system.

(16) (B) In a medical emergency, the intervention should be done even if the patient would have rejected it.

This statement is not true regarding care plan decision-making. In a medical emergency, if it is known that a patient would reject a particular intervention (for instance, due to previously expressed wishes, an advance directive, or a do-not-resuscitate order), those wishes should be respected.

(17) (B) Nausea, loss of appetite, and double vision.

Early symptoms of digoxin poisoning include nausea, lack of appetite, and double vision. Impotence, lowered libido, vomiting, diarrhea, disorientation, halos or spots, yellow and green eyesight, difficulties reading, and bradycardia are further symptoms of digoxin toxicity.

(18) (D) Assessment.

The nurse should identify the patient's information and needs and prioritize them with their permission. To establish the correct objectives, needs should be categorized as high, intermediate, or low.

(19) (B) Ventricular tachycardia.

Ventricular tachycardia is characterized by a regular rhythm and a heart rate between 140 and 180 bpm, wide QRS complexes (more than 0.11 seconds), and absent P waves.

(20) (A) Blurred vision and headache.

The doctor should be informed if the patient complains of headaches and impaired vision since these are symptoms of deteriorating preeclampsia.

(21) (D) Inform the doctor.

The heart rate of a developing fetus varies with gestational age. It ranges from 160-170 bpm in the first trimester before it slows to 120–160 bpm close to or at term. The fetus may be in distress if the HR is lower than 120 bpm at or near term or more than 160 bpm with the uterus at rest. The nurse should inform the doctor if the FHR exceeds the reference range.

(22) (C) Lie on the side that is unaffected.

The patient should be positioned on the unaffected side with the head of the bed raised to 45 degrees or sit at the edge of the bed leaned over the bedside table with their feet propped up on a stool.

(23) (C) They have changes in body image.

A surgical incision alters the appearance of the body. Some patients find it difficult to adjust to the look of their altered body. (24) (D) Decreased duplication and fragmentation of care.

Interprofessional teams have many benefits. These include decreased errors, fragmentation, duplication of care, and risk of adverse outcomes. Additionally, HCP retention and job satisfaction increase, as well as promotion of quality care and positive patient outcomes.

(25) (A) Alcohol consumption.

Phenytoin's efficacy is decreased by alcohol. 10–20 mcg/mL level of phenytoin is considered normal. The most frequent non-life-threatening adverse effects of phenytoin are pink urine and swollen gums.

(26) (A) Transient condition worsens.

A decrease in weakness is a sign of a myasthenia crisis. An edrophonium injection momentarily worsens the patient's cholinergic crisis.

(27) (D) You should cross your arms and maintain eye contact to help maintain pleasant body language.

Pleasant body language, like relaxed arms (not crossed) and steady eye contact, shows respect for the other person. Remember that the ultimate goal is to care for patients. Go into the talk with this in mind.

(28) (D) Inform the doctor and stop the dialysis.

When a patient has an air embolus while receiving hemodialysis, the nurse should give them oxygen, inform the doctor, and stop the procedure immediately.

(29) (C) Expiratory wheezes.

Particularly in individuals with asthma or COPD, audible expiratory wheezes may indicate a dangerous adverse response called bronchospasm. Although not life-threatening, bradycardia, hypotension, or sleeplessness are to be anticipated.

(30) (D) Reading or lectures.

Passive teaching methods like reading or lectures deliver information, and the facilitator decides on the topic, organization, and speed. This has been proven to have little to no effect on learning results.

(31) (C) Ventricular dysrhythmias.

Classic symptoms of cardiogenic shock include tachycardia, low blood pressure, and a rise in CVP. Common causes of dysrhythmias include reduced oxygenation and severe injury to more than 40% of the myocardium.

(32) (B) It can cause orange feces, urine, tears, and sweat.

The patient should not stop rifampin unless ordered by the doctor. Doses should not be skipped or missed. The drug rifampin turns bodily secretions an orange color. It should be given on an empty stomach unless it causes stomach upset.

(33) (B) The drug should be taken with a full glass of water.

Guaifenesin is an expectorant. It should be taken with a full glass of water to reduce the viscosity of the secretions. It is not necessary to take the drug with food. If the cough persists for over a week or is accompanied by a persistent headache, sore throat, rash, or fever, the patient should inform the doctor, and no more doses should be administered.

(34) (D) All of the above.

Synthesized research is available through organizational intranets, electronic publications, and printed publications to provide the workforce with high-quality research-based knowledge.

(35) (D) Right pneumothorax.

Pneumothorax is characterized by absent or decreased air entry, asymmetrical chest expansion on the afflicted side, discomfort with breathing, dyspnea, and tachycardia. It may raise airway pressure due to resistance when the lung inflates. Due to the curvature between the right and left main stem bronchi, a dislodged endotracheal tube will likely be on the left side.

(36) (B) They decrease stomach acid production and kill the bacteria.

Amoxicillin and clarithromycin are antibiotics, and esomeprazole is a proton pump inhibitor. Together, they make up a triple treatment for Helicobacter pylori infection. These drugs kill the bacteria and lessen the formation of acid.

(37) (C) Heartburn.

A proton pump inhibitor, omeprazole is categorized as an antiulcer drug. The medicine is used to relieve heartburn discomfort as it reduces stomach inflammation.

(38) (A) Blood-warming device.

Blood warmers should be used when many units of blood are administered. The patient is at risk for cardiac dysrhythmia after a quick transfusion of cold blood. Electronic infusion systems, which regulate flow rate, are ineffective since the infusion must be fast. Cardiac monitoring devices do not lower the incidence of cardiac dysrhythmia.

(39) (D) Research.

The Five Rights of Delegation should be followed when tasks are assigned. They include the proper person, situation, task, monitoring and assessment, and communication.

(40) (A) Inhale deeply, hold their breath, and bear down.

When tubing is changed, the patient should be encouraged to execute the Valsalva maneuver. This helps prevent air embolism. The nurse should instruct the patient to inhale deeply, hold their breath, and bear down. The patient should turn their head to the left if the intravenous line is on the right.

(41) (D) Coffee, blueberries, and cream of wheat.

Patients with renal failure who are on hemodialysis should eat a diet low in fluids, potassium, calcium, phosphorus, and sodium. Potassium, phosphorus, and salt content are high in options A, B, and C.

(42) (A) It's important to prevent hyperglycemia.

A glycosylated hemoglobin A1c test determines how much glucose from circulating glucose has permanently attached to red blood cells. A value of 7% or less suggests excellent control, 7%–8% shows acceptable control, and 8% or more indicates poor control.

(43) (C) Withhold the next dose of warfarin.

The therapeutic PT level is 1.5–2 times higher than the normal level. The normal PT ranges from 9.6 to 11.8 seconds. Because 36 seconds is an extended period, the nurse should plan for the patient to stop receiving dosages at this point.

(44) (D) All of the above.

Medical information should be disposed of, transmitted, and stored with strict precautions to protect confidentiality. Use antivirus software, firewalls, passwords, and encryption to prevent unauthorized access, alteration, or destruction of the data.

(45) (D) Touch the patient's body when unnecessary.

Psycho-mental privacy needs include respect for a patient and their privacy. Speak respectfully and politely. Use the person's first and last name when addressing them. Do not make fun of their appearance, pain, or fear. Respect their values and beliefs. Be available when they are discharged and provide proper instructions. Do *not* touch a patient when unnecessary and/or without permission.

(46) (D) All of the above.

A follow-up requires a medical professional to call a patient at a predetermined date to check on their progress. A follow-up can take many forms, such as phone calls, home visits, and hospital appointments.

(47) (B) Urinary retention.

Urinary retention most often occurs when the fundus is left deviated, elevated above the umbilicus, and soft. If the patient cannot empty their bladder, the nurse should schedule a catheterization and encourage the patient to void.

(48) (B) It is an anesthetic and decreases the pain until antibiotic action occurs.

A urinary tract anesthetic called phenazopyridine will relieve discomfort until the antibiotics have had the chance to take effect. It does not stop renal damage, nor is it an antibiotic or an analgesic.

(49) (B) Discharge.

The end of care from a healthcare organization is called discharge. A transfer involves the direct release of a patient from one unit to another.

(50) (D) Assess the patient for distention of the bladder.

The patient should be placed in the semi-Fowler's position rather than the Trendelenburg position since the symptoms point to autonomic hyperreflexia, often brought on by bladder distention. The doctor must be informed, and the patient must undergo catheterization.

(51) (A) The radiation site should not be cleaned.

The patient should not wash the skin around the radiation site in an attempt to remove the purple stains. There will be no need for a dressing since the skin will be dry. The skin near the site will be delicate, and an ice bag might cause harm.

(52) (D) All of the above.

Nursing reports include recent changes in symptoms or conditions, pain management strategies, level of consciousness, allergies, dietary restrictions, medication information such as the time of last dose and dosage amount, the reason for hospital admission, and medical history.

(53) (B) Decrease in urine output.

The urine output, systolic and diastolic blood pressure, pulse width, and pulse pressure are all decreased. A person who is in shock and has a reduced blood volume has a rise in respiratory and heart rates.

(54) (B) Eye edema.

Edema around the eyes in a pregnant woman can be a sign of concern, especially if it occurs suddenly or is severe. It could indicate a more serious condition, such as preeclampsia, which is a complication characterized by high blood pressure and often involves swelling in various parts of the body.

(55) (B) Painful throat.

Due to immunosuppressants, a painful throat is often a sign of immunosuppression. Prednisone therapy's anticipated adverse effects include mood swings, acne, and moon face.

(56) (A) It's important to wear a mask.

There is no need to wear a mask when you enter an HIV patient room or to wear gloves when you give a back rub on unbroken skin. When any bodily fluids are involved, gloves should be used. Blood spills should be cleaned up with the use of a 1:10 dilution of chlorine bleach.

(57) (B) Self-esteem.

Self-esteem is the need to be appreciated and acknowledged as a valuable individual by oneself and others. Self-actualization aims to inspire people to realize their fullest potential. Love is the individual's intrinsic need for affection, a sense of community, and acceptance from others.

(58) (C) Autonomy.

Autonomy is the respect for an individual's right to self-determination.

(59) (D) Glaucoma.

Cyclobenzaprine should be used with care in patients with a history of elevated intraocular pressure, glaucoma, or urine retention due to its anticholinergic properties. Additionally, it should only be taken for two to three weeks.

(60) (C) Renal failure.

Patients who have GIT, renal, or cardiac conditions, or who are elderly or debilitated should take colchicine with caution. Administration of this drug is not an issue with myxedema, hypothyroidism, or diabetes mellitus patients.

(61) (B) Use a compression bandage to rewrap the stump.

The nurse must quickly wrap the stump with another compression bandage if the patient's bandage comes off after an amputation. Otherwise, excessive edema could quickly build, which might significantly slow the recovery process.

(62) (C) Intact mental state.

Intact mentation is a favorable sign of fat embolus resolution since an altered mental state is an early sign of a fat embolus. Oxygen saturation should be greater than 95%. Arterial oxygen levels should be between 80–100 mm Hg, and dyspnea is not a normal finding.

(63) (B) There is tissue perfusion impairment.

Most fracture-related pain can be reduced with analgesics, cold therapy, elevation, and rest. Pain that does not go away after these remedies are implemented should be discussed with a doctor since it can be a sign of neurovascular impairment.

(64) (A) It helps with fracture immobilization and decreases muscle spasms.

Buck's skin traction is often used after hip fractures before they are surgically reduced. It lessens muscle spasms and prevents the start of bone repair. Traction does not make the leg longer.

(65) (C) It is important to brush and floss.

When they take phenytoin, patients should use good oral hygiene and maintain regular dental care. They should avoid activities that call for alertness and coordination and must consult the doctor before they take over-the-counter medications. It is important to avoid alcohol and continue prescribed medications while phenytoin is taken. Blood samples must be drawn to check the serum drug level before the morning dose is taken. Patients should take the recommended daily dosage to maintain blood levels.

(66) (A) A family member.

When consent is signed by a patient on sedatives, mentally unable, unconscious, or disoriented, it is not informed consent. If the patient cannot sign the consent form, every attempt should be made to acquire consent from a responsible family member.

(67) (C) In-process metrics.

In-process metrics such as how long it takes for a doctor to visit a patient, a patient to be admitted, and a patient to be released are used to track patients.

(68) (A) It is a high-cost service.

Preprinted physician orders have the flexibility and capability to shift and adapt to changes in specific hospital procedures swiftly. They provide a low-cost and straightforward way to change how the healthcare system functions and the standard of treatment, which results in improved patient care.

(69) (A) Conscious attention.

Conscious attention is the knowledge of ethical and unethical nursing practices and how they relate to nursing tasks and responsibilities.

(70) (C) Pressure on the nail bed.

When you examine an unconscious patient's reaction to painful stimuli, this allows for motor testing. A basic peripheral response is tested with pressure on the nail bed. The other choices test the cerebral reaction to pain.

(71) (D) Initiate delivery.

The early detachment of the placenta from the uterine wall is known as abruptio placentae. Fetal delivery and hemorrhage control are the two main objectives of care in abruptio placentae. Delivery is recommended if the fetus is at term or if the bleeding is moderate to severe.

(72) (D) History of IV drug use.

HIV may transfer from an infected mother to her unborn child and is spread via exposure to contaminated blood, the exchange of bodily fluids, and intimate sexual contact. Patients who have several sexual partners, recurrent and chronic STDs, or use IV drugs are at a higher risk of HIV contraction.

(73) (C) Keep the breasts dry and only wash them with warm water.

Pregnant women should avoid the use of soap and only wash their breasts with warm water to prevent dryness. A supportive bra helps lessen breast soreness, and tight-fitting tops can be uncomfortable.

(74) (D) This is an expected finding, so you should do nothing.

The suction control chamber should have persistent, mild bubbling. Only the rate of water evaporation in the drainage system is accelerated by the increase of suction pressure. Continuous rather than sporadic bubbling is desired in the suction control chamber. Chest tubes should only be clamped to replace drainage devices or check for air leaks.

(75) (B) High Fowler's.

The patient is put in a seated or high Fowler's position to lessen the possibility of pulmonary aspiration if the patient vomits.

(76) (B) Remove the patient from the abusive environment.

The priority must be to determine if the victim is at imminent risk in the abusive setting. If so, immediate steps must be taken to remove the patient to a safe location. Other options are important, but they are not the priority.

(77) (D) Assign the patient to a private room or cohort patient.

Meningitis is spread via infected droplets. The standard precaution mask and a private room or cohort patient are precautions for this illness. Airborne diseases require separate rooms with negative airflow pressure. When the patient exits the room, he must wear the mask, not the healthcare provider.

(78) (D) All of the above.

A state board of nursing can refuse, revoke, or suspend any license for many reasons. Unprofessional behavior, harm to the public's health and welfare, and disregard for patient confidentiality are cause for action. Additionally, inadequate knowledge, skills, preparation, or nursing judgment, abuse of a patient either physically or verbally, knowledge that unlicensed workers were assigned nursing care tasks, failure to keep proper records, the creation of false records, or the abandonment of a nursing duty can result in disciplinary measures.

(79) (A) A traumatic burn.

Hyperkalemia is indicated by serum potassium levels of more than 5.1 mEq/L. Patients who encounter potassium cellular shifting during the first phases of extensive cell death, such as respiratory or metabolic acidosis, sepsis, burns, or trauma, are at risk for hyperkalemia. Other options are at risk of hypokalemia.

(80) (A) Control chart.

Changes to healthcare processes and policies are often included in quality improvement programs, as is the use of quality improvement tools and methodologies such as data collecting and analysis, process mapping, and root cause analysis. A control chart may be used to graph events to determine performance over time.

(81) (B) Orange juice, tomatoes, spinach, and broccoli.

Iron is present in both spinach and broccoli. Vitamin C is found in foods like orange juice and tomatoes. A person should consume foods that contain Vitamin C to improve absorption when iron-rich foods are consumed.

(82) (C) Cohort studies.

Cohort studies are considered Level 2 evidence-based ranking.

(83) (A) Pathological fracture.

In this case, an underlying disease, not trauma, caused the pathological fracture. An open fracture has soft tissue that connects the fracture. One side of the bone fractures in a green-stick fracture, while the other splinters like a stick of green wood.

(84) (D) Aspirin.

Compared to the other options, aspirin generally has a lower occurrence of true allergic reactions. Penicillin, sulfonamides, and cephalosporin allergies are common allergies. They may be very harmful or even fatal. The sensitizing dose, or initial contact with penicillin, sensitizes the body for reaction to subsequent exposure or dosage.

(85) (B) The ovaries, fallopian tubes, cervix, and the body and fundus of the uterus.

An abdominal pan-hysterectomy involves the removal of the ovaries, fallopian tubes, cervix, and the body and fundus of the uterus, while the vagina is unaffected.

(86) (B) Atelectasis.Nephrectomy procedures include a high abdominal incision in the back, which raises the risk of respiratory problems such as atelectasis in those who do not willingly take deep breaths.

(87) (C) History of travel to India.

Sewage-contaminated water spreads hepatitis A. The hepatitis A virus is often present in the water of less developed nations. The patient is not at risk for hepatitis A after a cholecystectomy, blood transfusion, or blood donation.

(88) (C) Immunosuppression is a side effect of the cancer medication cyclophosphamide. The immune system attacks the patient's nerves in multiple sclerosis.

Due to the autoimmune nature of multiple sclerosis, the patient's immune system attacks the nervous system. Immunosuppression is an adverse effect of cancer chemotherapy medicines like cyclophosphamide. The medication does not treat multiple sclerosis but does decrease the disease's progression.

(89) (D) Employment as a chicken farmer.

A fungus in bat and bird stool causes histoplasmosis and damages the lungs. The consumption of raw milk can cause Brucellosis. Consumption of tainted water or raw shellfish can cause hepatitis A.

(90) (B) It prevents the nasal passages from drying out.

Oxygen should be humidified to avoid drying out the nasal passages. It does not lessen the possibility of organism development in the tubing, make oxygen more concentrated, or prevent fires.

(91) (C) Keep the patient in an NPO state.

After midnight, the patient should be NPO. A local anesthetic will be administered to the patient to stop the gag reflex. No enema is required. It is unnecessary to stop the medication the day before the surgery.

(92) (A) Pulse of 135 bpm and blood pressure of 90/60 mm Hg.

A doctor should be informed if the patient has hypotension and rapid pulse since this might indicate excessive blood loss. After surgery, hematuria and bladder spasms are common side effects.

(93) (C) Shoulder.

Lower abdominal discomfort may radiate to one of the shoulders because of phrenic nerve stimulation. It is a sign of bladder damage or injury. The discomfort from a bladder injury does not affect the hip, costovertebral angle, or umbilicus.

(94) (B) Custard.

Strained vegetable juices, refined cooked cereals, strained soups, custard, pudding, milk, breakfast drinks, sherbet, and plain ice cream are all fully liquid foods. Answers A, C, and D are for a clear liquid diet.

(95) (A) Dark green leafy vegetables and oranges.

Oranges are a rich source of vitamin C, which helps the body absorb iron, and dark green leafy vegetables are an excellent source of iron.

(96) (B) 6.4 g/dL.

Total serum protein levels should be between 6 and 8 g/dL. Due to poor diet, patients with cirrhosis often have low total protein levels. However, cirrhosis can make this process inefficient since the liver metabolizes protein.

(97) (C) 15 mg/dL.

A BUN level of 15 mg/dL is within the normal range (usually around 7-20 mg/dL) and would reflect adequate volume replacement in a patient that suffers from dehydration due to a urinary tract infection (UTI). Elevated BUN levels can indicate dehydration among other conditions, so a value within the normal range suggests effective rehydration. In contrast, values such as 35 mg/dL (A) and 29 mg/dL (B) are elevated and might indicate ongoing dehydration or other renal issues. A BUN level as low as 3 mg/dL (D) is unusually low and generally not associated with dehydration.

(98) (C) Metabolic alkalosis.

Hyperaldosteronism, whole blood transfusions, excessive bicarbonate intake, gastric fluid loss, or hypovolemia cause metabolic alkalosis, characterized by a loss of hydrogen ions or excess bicarbonate.

(99) (A) Processed cereals.

A serum sodium level of 152 mEq/L indicates hypernatremia. The normal serum sodium level is 135–145 mEq/L. The sodium amount in processed foods is high, whereas the phosphorus content of peas, cauliflower, and almonds is high.

(100) (B) To make sure the antibiotic cured the infection.

Following the course of antibiotics, the patient should be evaluated to see whether the infection has subsided. If there is recurrent otitis media, hearing tests should be performed.

(101) (D) Thrombophlebitis.

Patients who have pelvic surgery are susceptible to thrombophlebitis. Pregnancy-related complications include varicose veins. The removal of the uterus is not linked to a cerebral or aortic aneurysm.

(102) (A) Uterine cramps.

Constant uterine cramping is common. A catheter will be installed to prevent urine retention. A clear liquid or low-residue diet can reduce the likelihood of constipation. A bowel preparation should be administered before surgery.

(103) (B) He should observe rigid regulations and rules.

Anorexics' obsession with being flawless impairs their ability to make sensible decisions. They can regulate their anxiety through rules and routines.

(104) (D) It's toxic.

Maintenance levels are 0.6–1.2 mEq/L of lithium in the blood. Toxicity signs start at concentrations of 1.5–2 mEq/L. Lithium poisoning requires prompt medical intervention, like peritoneal dialysis, hemodialysis, or lavage.

(105) (C) After the third week.

After the commencement of antidepressant medication, the maximal therapeutic benefits of imipramine may not begin to show for two to three weeks.

(106) (B) Serum creatinine level.

Foscarnet is toxic to kidneys. Additionally, foscarnet may lower potassium, phosphorus, magnesium, and calcium levels. The blood creatinine level is checked before the start of treatment and weekly maintenance therapy.

(107) (D) Gait.

Antiretroviral stavudine treats HIV infection in resistant patients or those unable to take standard medication. The patient's gait and paresthesia should be monitored since the medicine can induce peripheral neuropathy.

(108) (A) The patient should wait six weeks to be tested.

A blood test is available to diagnose Lyme disease. It is unreliable until six weeks after the tick bite since IgM antibodies develop within four weeks, and IgG antibodies develop three months after infection and may stay high for years.

(109) (D) Hot showers.

Patients with systemic lupus erythematosus should follow a balanced diet, engage in low-impact exercise when not exhausted, avoid hot showers, and limit their extended rest periods since this may exacerbate joint stiffness.

(110) (C) Do not drink alcohol.

Baclofen is a skeletal muscle relaxant. Because it amplifies the depressive effects of alcohol and other CNS depressants, the patient should be advised against using these substances. Fatigue occurs in the early stages of treatment and lessens with continuing pharmaceutical usage. Fluid restriction is not required. Rather than diarrhea, a side effect is constipation.

(111) (D) The patient should increase daily water intake to three liters.

Allopurinol users are advised to consume three liters of liquids each day. It may take up to a week for the full therapeutic impact to manifest. Allopurinol should be administered with or just after milk or meals. The patient should see a doctor if they experience a swollen mouth or lips, eye discomfort, or a rash, which may be signs of hypersensitivity.

(112) (B) Runny nose.

A runny or stuffy nose may result from the intranasal use of desmopressin. The adverse effects mentioned in other options can occur if the medicine is given intravenously.

(113) (B) Nitroglycerin.

Sildenafil strengthens nitric oxide's ability to dilate blood vessels in the corpus cavernosum of the penis to maintain an erection. It is not advised to take the drug at the same time as organic nitroglycerin or nitrates because of how it affects the body. The drug has the adverse effects of insomnia and neuralgia.

(114) (D) Laryngeal stridor.

When the trachea is compressed, it causes respiratory distress and a high-pitched, harsh sound called laryngeal stridor. It is audible during inspiration and expiration. The airway may become obstructed entirely if not treated.

(115) (C) Do a focused assessment of RBS.

Diaphoresis and disorientation are symptoms of hypoglycemia. In this situation, it was caused by giving the patient insulin before food consumption. However, the capillary blood glucose level is required to determine if hypoglycemia is present.

(116) (C) Polyuria.

Polyuria, or excessive urination, is a common symptom of primary hyperparathyroidism. Hyperparathyroidism is characterized by hypercalcemia. Osmotic diuresis and polyuria are produced when serum calcium levels are elevated. This can cause dehydration, which can lead to weight loss. Constipation, anorexia, and vomiting are GIT signs of hyperparathyroidism.

(117) (C) Get another bottle of emulsion.

The fat emulsion, a white, opaque fluid, is infused intravenously during parenteral nutrition treatment to avoid fatty acid insufficiency. The nurse should inspect the fat emulsion bottle for the formation of froth or separation into layers of fat globules. If any of these occur, the nurse should return the solution to the pharmacist and not use it.

(118) (C) Decrease parenteral nutrition rate to 50 mL/hr.

The rate should be progressively reduced when a patient switches to a regular diet after a time of receiving parenteral nutrition. When the infusion rate is gradually reduced, the patient can maintain an acceptable level of nutrition as they transition to a regular diet. This avoids hypoglycemia, which can result when parenteral nutrition is suddenly stopped. The glucose required for the transition is not present in a saline solution.

(119) (D) Skin.

Insensible losses occur daily through the lungs and skin without a person's knowledge. Sensible losses are those via urine, gastrointestinal tract losses, and wound drainage.

(120) (A) Is the patient allergic to penicillin?

The most common treatment for streptococcal infection is penicillin. Given the prevalence of penicillin allergies, the nurse should inquire. When used with metronidazole rather than penicillin, alcohol will have an effect like that of Antabuse. Vitamins do not contraindicate penicillin. Sulfa medications are not recommended for streptococcal infections.

(121) (B) Rheumatic fever.

Rheumatic fever is the cause of mitral valve stenosis. The outcome of meningitis or rubella is not mitral stenosis. Cardiovascular issues like aortic aneurysms may be brought on by tertiary syphilis.

(122) (C) On the right side.

The liver is located on the right side. A patient who had a liver biopsy should be positioned so that pressure is applied to the liver to prevent possible hemorrhage.

(123) (A) Glycosylated hemoglobin.

Blood sugar is measured by glycosylated hemoglobin. It examines baseline blood and urine glucose levels and how they change to a given quantity of glucose. The glucose tolerance test is the gold standard to diagnose diabetes mellitus.

(124) (B) Hypotension.

Hypotension, or low blood pressure, is one of the signs of Addison's disease. This condition results from the insufficient production of cortisol and aldosterone by the adrenal glands. These hormones help regulate blood pressure, and their deficiency can cause hypotension. Other signs not listed in the options but commonly associated with Addison's disease include fatigue, weight loss, hyperpigmentation of the skin, and a craving of salt.

(125) (D) Supine.

The patient should lie on their back during the first 24 hours after a lumbar laminectomy. As a result, the spine remains straight. The patient may be shifted from side to side after eight hours.

(126) (B) The kidneys cannot produce erythropoietin, and the drug replaces it.

Healthy kidneys produce erythropoietin and promote the growth of red blood cells. Epogen is recombinant human erythropoietin.

(127) (D) Urine culture and sensitivity.

The patient must have a fresh sample for urine sensitivity and culture. The other tests are unsuitable for first testing in a patient with symptoms of a urinary tract infection.

(128) (D) Fluid volume depletion.

Inadequate fluid volume requires prompt, continuous management. Psychological nursing diagnoses such as reduced skin integrity, poor health management, and altered body image are significant but not concerning.

(129) (C) Flu-like symptoms.

A rash that appears between 2–30 days after infection is a sign of Lyme disease stage one. The rash takes on a bull's-eye look as it grows into a concentric ring. Most infected people get flu-like symptoms in stage one, which lasts 7–10 days. Stage two is characterized by neurological impairments. Stage three is characterized by arthralgias and joint enlargement.

(130) (A) The programmed shock numbers, heart rate threshold, and device activation status.

Device settings must be evaluated while a patient is assessed after the implantable cardioverter defibrillator has been installed. The nurse specifically needs to know whether the device is on, the heart rate threshold at which it will fire, and how many shocks it is set to administer.

(131) (B) Ventricular fibrillation.

Ventricular fibrillation is distinguished by chaotic, irregular undulations of variable amplitudes, QRS complexes, no discernible P waves, no measurable rate, and results from electrical chaos in the ventricles.

(132) (C) Liver enzyme levels.

Hepatic enzyme levels may rise due to hepatitis because of isoniazid (INH) medication. Liver enzyme levels are checked before medication is started and throughout the first three months. If the patient is above 50 or consumes alcohol, they could be watched for a more extended period.

(133) (D) Use a face mask for oxygen administration.

Late decelerations caused by uteroplacental insufficiency happen because the fetus receives less oxygen and blood as uterine contractions occur. A face mask and 8–10 L/min of oxygen are required. Intravenous oxytocin infusion should stop due to the increase of uteroplacental insufficiency brought on by the medication's stimulation of contractions. Avoid the supine position as it reduces uterine blood supply to the fetus.

The patient should be rolled onto her side to relieve pressure on the IVC caused by the gravid uterus.

(134) (A) Use rifampin and isoniazid for nine months.

Rifampin and isoniazid are recommended as the primary therapy for pregnant women for nine months. To avoid fetal neurotoxicity, pyridoxine (vitamin B6) is often given together with isoniazid. The patient is not obliged to stay at home, nor is a therapeutic abortion necessary.

(135) (D) Tachycardia.

The pulse rate rises by 10–15 bpm between 14 and 20 weeks of pregnancy and stays elevated until delivery. Constipation caused by reduced gastrointestinal motility and increased RBC production are common during pregnancy. Until 20 weeks, blood pressure remains at pre-pregnancy levels, then systolic and diastolic pressures drop by 5–10 mm Hg.

(136) (C) Acute kidney injury.

Acute kidney injury can result from significant blood loss. Reduced blood flow to the kidneys can lead to kidney damage. Hypertension and hyperthermia are not normally associated with blood loss. Bradycardia would be unexpected. Instead, tachycardia would be common due to compensatory mechanisms trying to maintain cardiac output.

(137) (C) Hypovolemic shock.

These are classic signs of hypovolemic shock. This occurs when the body loses about one-fifth or more of the normal amount of blood or fluid. This severe fluid loss doesn't allow the heart to pump sufficient blood to the body, which leads to organ failure.

(138) (C) Upper body.

People with burns to the upper body commonly have respiratory disorders, and the death rate is higher due to airway issues. The alternative possibilities do not include danger to one's life.

(139) (D) Bed cradle.

Gout pain is very painful. A bed cradle will prevent the bedclothes from touching his toe. Gout treatment does not include the use of a heat lamp or a urinary catheter. Bed rails are advised for back issues.

(140) (B) Assess the patient for pulmonary edema by lung sound auscultation.
To detect pulmonary edema, a side effect of chronic renal failure, lung sounds should be evaluated. In chronic renal failure, protein consumption is reduced. When you elevate the feet, it causes the heart to work harder because the blood supply to the organ is increased. Catheter insertion does not improve kidney function.
(141) (A) Oliguria.
When a stone irritates the ureter, it may cause ureteral spasms and intense pain, known as renal colic. A stone may obstruct the ureter, prevent urine excretion, and cause hydronephrosis. This problem may result in renal necrosis.
(142) (A) Ensure he makes regular trips to the bathroom.
In hospitalized children, regression is common. It will be easier for the boy to recover control if the nurse regularly takes him to the bathroom. Giving him chocolate as a reward is not constructive. It is not helpful to put him in diapers and leave him in his wet bed. These actions are punitive.
(143) (C) Urine retention is common after a hemorrhoidectomy.
Urinary retention is a prevalent side effect after a hemorrhoidectomy due to the closeness of the bladder and the anus. A patient's past pregnancies or an extensive history of hemorrhoids are not primary causes of bladder retention. Despite her NPO status before and throughout surgery, the patient received IV fluids.
(144) (C) Abdominal cavity drainage.
The semi-seated position is usually used to encourage abdominal cavity drainage. Additionally, this position could ease suture line strain and improve ventilation. Turning will help to avoid pressure sores.
(145) (C) Appendicitis; prepare for a possible surgical consultation.
The symptoms described are indicative of appendicitis. Appendicitis is a medical emergency that often requires surgical intervention to remove the inflamed appendix.

Test 3: Questions

(1) After spinal cord trauma, the patient complains of hypertension, headache, and blurred vision. What should you do?

(A) Put the patient on the left side.

(B) Give the patient analgesics.

(C) Put the patient in the Trendelenburg position.

(D) Monitor the patient for bladder distention.

(2) What is true about a living will?

(A) It states the patient's preferred medical procedures.

(B) It states the patient's preferred burial attire.

(C) It states the patient's preferred funeral song.

(D) It states the patient's preference for an open-casket funeral.

(3) What is not the role of the patient advocate?

(A) Engage the legal system on the patient's behalf.

(B) Provide clarification or object to advice or a therapy.

(C) Implement a nutritional plan for the patient.

(D) Communicate with the patient's relatives.

(4) What is an indication of an effective nitroglycerin treatment in an angina patient?

(A) Increase in physical activity.

(B) Pain is relieved.

(C) Increased heart rate.

(D) Under-the-tongue tingling.

(5) Before the patient makes a decision, what should a healthcare provider inform them about?

(A) Intervention risks.

(B) Intervention goals.

(C) The safe choices.

(D) All of the above.

(6) What is not true during the oral nursing care of an unconscious patient?

(A) The patient should be kept in a lateral position.

(B) Place a towel under the patient's chin.

(C) The patient should be kept in an upright position.

(D) Place the patient with a turned head in the lateral position.

(7) Which nursing care steps involve a review of an intended intervention to determine if it was successful or not?

(A) Intervention planning.

(B) Evaluation.

(C) Goal setting.

(D) Assessment.

(8) Which statement does not describe an interprofessional team?

(A) A good grasp of others' roles and responsibilities.

(B) Clear communication.

(C) Provision of patient care.

(D) Mutual respect.

(9) What is a symptom of concern in a barbiturate withdrawal patient?

(A) Seizures.

(B) Hallucinations.

(C) Anxiety.

(D) Vomiting and nausea.

(10) What is the action mechanism of alteplase, which is prescribed for a myocardial infarction case?

(A) It repairs the heart muscle.

(B) It prevents clot formation.

(C) It dissolves the coronary artery clot.

(D) It decreases pain.

(11) Which of these steps is essential to prepare a patient for cardiac catheterization?

(A) Decrease high-fat food.

(B) Inquire about a shellfish allergy.

(C) Decrease caffeine intake.

(D) Do an enema before the surgery.

(12) A patient presents with tingling in the toes, fingers, and around the mouth. His RR is 41, pulse is 117, and blood pressure is 138/79. What should you do?

(A) Tell the patient to start deep breathing exercises.

(B) Inform the doctor.

(C) Tell the patient to use a paper bag.

(D) Give the patient oxygen.

(13) An adult presents with severe diarrhea, vomiting, and nausea. The patient reports consumption of 1,000 mL of IV fluid and 100 mL of ice in the previous eight hours. The patient had four diarrheal stools, 350 mL of urine, and 600 mL of vomit in the last eight hours. What is the patient at risk for?

(A) Fluid overload.

(B) Dehydration.

(C) Normal urine output.

(D) Normal fluid intake and output.

(14) What is one of the instructions for a leg plaster cast?

(A) Use a padded hanger end for scratching inside the cast.

(B) Lift the legs with your fingertips.

(C) Use warm blankets to cover the cast.

(D) Do not wet the cast.

(15) What is a sign of infection in a casted extremity?

(A) Extremity pallor and coolness.

(B) Cast hot spot.

(C) Distal pulses affected.

(D) Dependent edema.

(16) During conflict management, a nurse should:

(A) Maintain pleasant body language.

(B) Be aggressive.

(C) Use "you" messages.

(D) Start emotion-based discussions.

(17) Which postpartum patient is at the greatest risk of hemorrhage?

(A) A multiparous patient who had an oxytocin induction and delivered a large fetus.

(B) A primiparous patient who used epidural anesthesia.

(C) A multiparous patient delivered in the past five hours.

(D) A primiparous patient delivered in the last five hours.

(18) What indicates jacket safety device restraints were applied unsafely?

(A) Two fingers can slide easily between the patient's skin and the safety device.

(B) The safety device straps do not tighten when force is applied against them.

(C) The safety device straps are secured to the side rails.

(D) There is a knot in the safety device straps.

(19) What is the appropriate action after it is determined that the patient has had a transfusion reaction?

(A) Do a culture of the catheter tip.

(B) Run normal saline.

(C) Run a 5% dextrose solution.

(D) Remove the IV line.

(20) Which IV solution is prescribed to increase blood pressure, replace immediate blood loss volume, and increase intravascular volume in an unresponsive and hypotensive patient after a motor vehicle accident?

(A) 1/2 normal saline.

(B) 1/4 normal saline.

(C) 1/3 normal saline.

(D) 5% dextrose in lactated Ringer's.

(21) Which IV line complication is suspected when infusion ceases and there is swelling, pallor, and coolness at the infusion site?

(A) Thrombosis.

(B) Infiltration.

(C) Phlebitis.

(D) Infection.

(22) Which vitamin is essential in a vegan diet?

(A) Vitamin E.

(B) Vitamin C.

(C) Vitamin B_{12}.

(D) Vitamin A.

(23) Which WBC count requires the implementation of neutropenic precautions in an immunosuppressed cancer patient?

(A) 12,500 cells/mm^3.

(B) 9,400 cells/mm^3.

(C) 6,700 cells/mm^3.

(D) 2,530 cells/mm^3.

(24) Which serum potassium levels should be considered in a cardiac patient who takes Lasix (furosemide)?

(A) 4.7 mEq/L.

(B) 4.5 mEq/L.

(C) 3.9 mEq/L.

(D) 3.1 mEq/L.

(25) What is true about Kussmaul respirations in diabetic ketoacidosis patients?

(A) Patients have abnormal regular and deep respiration.

(B) Patients have increased respiration in terms of rate and depth.

(C) Patients have abnormally slow and regular respirations.

(D) Patients have repeated cessation of respiration.

(26) What statement is true about an ABG that shows HCO_3 = 21, PCO_2 = 29, and pH = 7.47?

(A) It reflects uncompensated respiratory acidosis.

(B) It reflects uncompensated metabolic alkalosis.

(C) It reflects compensated respiratory alkalosis.

(D) It reflects compensated metabolic acidosis.

(27) What is true about the role of cimetidine in the treatment of an acute lymphocytic leukemia patient?

(A) It decreases prednisone's negative effects.

(B) It promotes peristalsis.

(C) It increases methotrexate's effect.

(D) It decreases pancreatic enzyme secretions.

(28) Which medication should be administered to a patient with herpes zoster?

(A) Benadryl.

(B) Tetracycline.

(C) Acyclovir.

(D) Penicillin.

(29) What is the long-term purpose of case management for a woman who has been beaten by her husband?

(A) To place the blame on the abuser.

(B) To talk to her about her behavior.

(C) So the woman can feel like a survivor.

(D) To provide a long-term support team.

(30) What is the aim of continuous bladder irrigation in a postoperative transurethral prostatectomy?

(A) Prevent a urethral stricture.

(B) Prevent a bladder clot.

(C) Maintain bladder tone.

(D) Prevent a UTI.

(31) In which position should the urinary bag be placed after an indwelling catheter insertion?

(A) At the patient's bedside.

(B) At the head of the bed.

(C) Below the bladder.

(D) In line with the taut drainage tubing.

(32) What is a contraindication for laxative use in appendicitis patients who complain of constipation?

(A) It can cause appendix rupture.

(B) It can cause high blood pressure.

(C) It is contraindicated before the surgery.

(D) It decreases the infection spread.

(33) Misleading speech that harms someone's reputation, whether in writing or orally, is known as:

(A) Assault.

(B) Battery.

(C) Defamation.

(D) Fraud.

(34) What should be prescribed for a congestive heart failure patient who takes furosemide and digoxin?

(A) Coumadin.

(B) Aspirin.

(C) Calcium.

(D) Potassium.

(35) What is a reason for the use of parenteral heparin?

(A) It causes therapeutic levels to be reached more rapidly.

(B) It causes gastric upset.

(C) It causes respiratory distress.

(D) It is broken down by gastric acids.

(36) What example below does not demonstrate an invasion of privacy?

(A) Patient information that is disclosed to unauthorized individuals.

(B) An intrusion on private patient or family affairs.

(C) A patient who is informed of the truth about his condition.

(D) A breach of confidentiality.

(37) What is ranked as a Level 3?

(A) Case studies.

(B) Case-control studies.

(C) Cohort studies.

(D) Meta-analysis.

(38) What is not a risk factor for contrast media anaphylaxis?

(A) AIDS.

(B) Old age.

(C) Beta-blocker use.

(D) Heart failure.

(39) What is not important to be assessed for in a patient with lost short-term memory?

(A) English language comprehension.

(B) Person, place, and time orientation.

(C) Ambulatory difficulty.

(D) Visual state.

(40) Which behavior is of concern when a patient's coping strategies and emotional state are assessed?

(A) Self-mutilation.

(B) Social isolation.

(C) Family dysfunction.

(D) Anxiety.

(41) The main goal of standard precautions is to:

(A) Prevent the spread of disease.

(B) Prevent nosocomial infections.

(C) Prevent the spread of AIDS.

(D) Help protect patients with weak immune systems.

(42) For a patient with a portable drainage wound system, what is the best action during ambulation?

(A) Stop the system before ambulation.

(B) Empty the collection device before ambulation.

(C) Fasten the collection device to the wounds beneath.

(D) Remove the apparatus during ambulation.

(43) What is the most important assessment in a blood transfusion patient?

(A) Pulse.

(B) Respiration.

(C) Blood pressure.

(D) Temperature.

(44) A UTI patient complains of dysuria, urgency, and frequency. What is the appropriate next step?

(A) Give the patient phenazopyridine.

(B) Give the patient sulfisoxazole.

(C) Check if the patient has a sulfa drug allergy.

(D) Ensure the patient gives a clean urine sample.

(45) Which immunization should be given to a 75-year-old female who has received previous pneumonia immunizations?

(A) Haemophilus influenzae type B.

(B) Pneumovax.

(C) MMR.

(D) DPT.

(46) What could increase the danger for a patient who takes warfarin for DVT?

(A) A history of taking thyroid drugs.

(B) A history of cholecystectomy.

(C) Daily walks.

(D) Osteoarthritis.

(47) Which of these nursing assessments should be done on a patient prescribed atropine sulfate and diphenoxylate hydrochloride?

(A) Neurological examination.

(B) Urine output.

(C) Respiratory rate.

(D) Blood pressure.

(48) What is included in the instructions for the administration of sulfisoxazole to a UTI patient?

(A) Do a daily urinalysis and culture.

(B) Decrease daily fluid intake.

(C) Avoid sun exposure.

(D) Stop the drug if the symptoms improve.

(49) A 14-month-old baby presents with puffy, warm, and red spots at the area of the skin where the MMR vaccine was injected. What should you do to manage the situation?

(A) No management is needed.

(B) Give the baby aspirin.

(C) Use a warm compress at the injection site.

(D) Inform the doctor.

(50) When he assesses an alcohol detoxification patient, the nurse notices the patient's gait is unsteady. He bumps into doorframes and has slurred speech. What should the nurse do?

(A) Use diazepam.

(B) Do a CNS consultation.

(C) Do a blood alcohol level test.

(D) Check for Wernicke-Korsakoff syndrome.

(51) Which of these steps should be taken when a dressing is removed?

(A) Put the dressing on the patient's bed.

(B) Put the dressing on the chair near the patient's bed.

(C) Open the initial flap of the dressing towards the nurse.

(D) Open the initial flap of the dressing away from the nurse.

(52) Which laboratory test result will be found in an acute appendicitis patient?

(A) A shift to the left in leukopenia.

(B) A shift to the left together with leukocytosis.

(C) A rightward shift in leukocytosis.

(D) Leukopenia with a rightward shift.

(53) When can a tuberculosis patient return to work?

(A) If the Mantoux test and sputum culture are negative.

(B) If the chest X-ray and sputum culture are negative.

(C) If four sputum cultures are negative.

(D) If three sputum cultures are negative.

(54) What should be done for a retinal detachment patient who had scleral buckling surgery?

(A) Have the patient wear dark glasses if he reads or watches TV.

(B) Put a patch on the damaged eye.

(C) Elevate the head of the bed.

(D) Give the patient bathroom privileges.

(55) What should be done before a cuffed tracheostomy tube is plugged?

(A) Make sure that the patient can speak.

(B) Make sure that the patient can swallow.

(C) Deflate the tube cuff.

(D) Put the inner cannula into the tube.

(56) What should be done after half of an enema solution is administered to a patient who complains of cramping and pain?

(A) Inform the doctor and remove the enema.

(B) Continue the enema flow.

(C) Decrease the flow rate and clamp the tube.

(D) Elevate the bag of the enema.

(57) A doctor must be informed when the NG tube drainage is:

(A) Green-tinged.

(B) Dark brown.

(C) Dark red.

(D) Yellowish-brown.

(58) Which foods should a woman breastfeeding a lactose-intolerant child avoid?

(A) Egg yolk.

(B) Beans.

(C) Leafy green vegetables.

(D) Cheese.

(59) Which of these positions could increase dyspnea in emphysema patients?

(A) Leaned against the table and seated.

(B) Low Fowler's position on the back.

(C) Leaned on the wall and upright.

(D) Elbows on knees while seated.

(60) What is the purpose of glucagon treatment for a diabetes mellitus patient?

(A) Lipo-hypertrophy due to inadequate absorption of insulin.

(B) Lipoatrophy due to injections.

(C) Hyperglycemia.

(D) Hypoglycemia.

(61) What is a clomipramine noncompliance sign?

(A) Use of hot, soapy water to wash the hands frequently.

(B) Heart rate below 60.

(C) Fatigue and hunger.

(D) Insomnia.

(62) What best describes the treatment regimen for a tricyclic antidepressant–using patient?

(A) The patient sleeps five hours during the day and 13 hours at night.

(B) The patient has an inability to do any activities.

(C) The patient has an appropriate appearance.

(D) The patient doesn't work for a week.

(63) Which foods should be avoided when taking cyclosporine drugs?

(A) Leafy green vegetables.

(B) Grapefruit juice.

(C) Orange juice.

(D) Red meat.

(64) Which of these statements is true about the administration of phenazopyridine hydrochloride for a UTI?

(A) Orange-red urine may occur.

(B) If a headache occurs, the patient should stop the drug.

(C) The drug should be taken before a meal.

(D) The drug should be taken at bedtime.

(65) A male patient presents with a UTI and a history of taking warfarin sodium daily. The doctor prescribes nalidixic acid. What should be done next?

(A) The nalidixic acid dose should be decreased.

(B) The warfarin sodium dose should be increased.

(C) The warfarin sodium dose should be decreased.

(D) The warfarin sodium should be stopped.

(66) What is a sign of male urethritis?

(A) Penile discharge and dysuria.

(B) Urgency and hematuria.

(C) Proteinuria and dysuria.

(D) Pyuria and hematuria.

(67) A patient with cardiac dysrhythmia received IV procainamide and developed dizziness. What is the correct action?

(A) Measure the blood pressure and apical pulse.

(B) Do an ECG immediately.

(C) Measure the heart rate.

(D) Give nitroglycerin tablets.

(68) What is an indication that a pericardiocentesis done to treat cardiac tamponade was unsuccessful?

(A) There is a CVP increase.

(B) The patient feels relief from symptoms.

(C) There are audible heart sounds.

(D) The patient's blood pressure increases.

(69) A male 47-year-old presents with chest pain. On examination, blood pressure is 85/62, respiratory rate is 34 breaths/min, and pulse is 119 beats/min. Myocardial infarction is excluded. What is the most likely diagnosis?

(A) Dissecting thoracic aortic aneurysm.

(B) Pulmonary embolism.

(C) Cardiac tamponade.

(D) Cardiogenic shock.

(70) Before the prescription of zafirlukast, which of these laboratory tests should be done?

(A) CBC.

(B) Liver function tests.

(C) Neutrophil count.

(D) Platelet count.

(71) What are some ways emphysema patients can improve breathing effectiveness during dyspneic periods?

(A) Lean on the nightstand.

(B) Sit in a recliner.

(C) Lie on the side of the bed.

(D) Sit up in bed.

(72) What is a sign of pulmonary embolism?

(A) Deep breaths that cause dyspnea.

(B) Sudden chest pain.

(C) Fever and chills.

(D) Flushing and hot feeling.

(73) When a low-pressure alarm goes off on a ventilator and the nurse cannot determine the cause, what is the correct action?

(A) Start CPR.

(B) Start manual ventilation for the patient.

(C) Monitor the patient's vital signs.

(D) Give the patient oxygen.

(74) What statement is correct about the necessary measures to protect the fetus of a patient with genital herpes?

(A) During labor, if vaginal lesions are present, a Cesarean section is required.

(B) During pregnancy, acyclovir must be administered.

(C) Sitz baths should be done every three hours.

(D) During pregnancy, sexual intercourse must be stopped.

(75) What is the best position for a patient who underwent a total hip replacement?

(A) External rotation of the limb while the patient lies on his side.

(B) Internal rotation of the limb while the patient lies on his side.

(C) Abduction of the limb while the patient lies on his nonoperative side.

(D) On his back.

(76) A nurse reviews the lab results of a patient who is suspected of having diabetes. Which laboratory finding is most consistent with a diagnosis of diabetes mellitus?

(A) Fasting blood glucose level of 90 mg/dL.

(B) Oral glucose tolerance test result of 130 mg/dL at 2 hours.

(C) Hemoglobin A1c level of 7.5%.

(D) Random blood glucose level of 140 mg/dL.

(77) What is the right action for a patient with a serum digoxin level of 2.6 ng/mL?

(A) Administer the next dose.

(B) Record the normal value on the patient's sheet.

(C) Check the patient's last pulse rate.

(D) Notify the physician.

(78) What is a sign of bethanechol chloride toxicity?

(A) Dehydration.

(B) Bradycardia.

(C) Dry mouth.

(D) Dry skin.

(79) What should be done for a patient who is prescribed sulfisoxazole?

(A) When symptoms improve, the dose should be decreased to prevent allergy.

(B) The doctor should be informed if dark urine occurs.

(C) The patient should drink a lot of fluids.

(D) The patient should decrease fluid intake.

(80) What is a sign of arterial steal syndrome in a new hemodialysis patient with a fistula in the left arm?

(A) Left arm edema, pallor, and angina pain.

(B) Left arm red discoloration and edema.

(C) Left arm pain, decreased pulse, and pallor.

(D) Left arm pain, redness, and warmth.

(81) What is the first management step for a patient with a serum potassium level of 7.2 mEq/L?

(A) Give the patient 1,000 mL IV fluids.

(B) Have the patient eat vegetables.

(C) Monitor the patient's heart rate.

(D) Monitor the patient's serum sodium level.

(82) To follow heparin's therapeutic effect, what should be monitored?

(A) PTT.

(B) PT.

(C) Hemoglobin.

(D) Hematocrit.

(83) What is the first thing that should be monitored in case of premature ventricular contractions?

(A) Oxygen saturation and blood pressure.

(B) Infection.

(C) Caffeine.

(D) Palpitations.

(84) A patient who has taken isoniazid for two months complains of tingling, paresthesia, and numbness in the extremities. What is the cause?

(A) Impaired peripheral circulation.

(B) Small blood vessel spasm.

(C) Peripheral neuritis.

(D) Hypercalcemia.

(85) For a COPD patient, which oxygen delivery system should be used?

(A) Tracheostomy collar.

(B) Aerosol mask.

(C) Venturi mask.

(D) Face tent.

(86) An HIV-positive male presents with an 8-mm induration area after the Mantoux skin test. What is the result of the test?

(A) Repeat testing.

(B) Inconclusive.

(C) Negative.

(D) Positive.

(87) A postpartum patient presents with increased respiratory rate, tachycardia, dyspnea, and sharp and sudden chest pain. She is suspected of having a pulmonary embolism. What is the appropriate step to take?

(A) Give the patient a face mask and oxygen.

(B) Give the patient morphine sulfate.

(C) Monitor the patient's blood pressure.

(D) Insert an IV line.

(88) What is the first step when a nurse finds an umbilical cord that protrudes during the vaginal assessment of a pregnant patient?

(A) Inform the delivery room to initiate the delivery.

(B) Inform the doctor immediately.

(C) Put the patient in the Trendelenburg position.

(D) Reintroduce the cord into the vagina.

(89) What is not a management step for a placenta previa case patient who presents with vaginal bleeding?

(A) Monitor the fetal HR with external electronic equipment.

(B) Do hematocrit and hemoglobin tests.

(C) Perform a digital examination.

(D) Perform an ultrasound.

(90) Which finding is associated with the second stage of labor?

(A) Clear vaginal fluid.

(B) Complete dilation of the cervix.

(C) Ruptured membranes.

(D) Regular contractions.

(91) What should be assessed to determine preeclampsia complications in a severe case during the last trimester?

(A) Purpura, petechiae, and bleeding gums.

(B) Quiet fetal movements.

(C) The patient feels hot when the room is cool.

(D) The patient's breasts are enlarged.

(92) What is true about a negative contraction stress test?

(A) A cesarean section is needed.

(B) There is a high risk of fetal demise.

(C) The test result is abnormal.

(D) The test result is normal.

(93) A patient with a three-day history of nausea and vomiting had an RR of 12 bpm, HR of 130, and a fever of 37.5°C. What is true about his ABG?

(A) Increased HCO_3 and increased pH.

(B) Decreased HCO_3 and decreased pH.

(C) Decreased CO_2 and increased pH.

(D) Increased CO_2 and decreased pH.

(94) What is the appropriate assistive device for an osteoarthritis patient who has a broken left arm?

(A) Tripod cane.

(B) Walker.

(C) Crutches.

(D) Quad cane.

(95) How can you decrease the chances of seizures in a meningitis patient?

(A) The patient's room should be darkened.

(B) A blade tongue blade should be available.

(C) The patient must be stimulated every three hours.

(D) The patient's favorite music must be played.

(96) Which value is suggestive of shock?

(A) Pulse = 70.

(B) Blood pressure = 126/82.

(C) Pulse = 120.

(D) Blood pressure = 118/64.

(97) What is the adequate procedure to obtain a patient's pedal pulses?

(A) Press the top of the foot with the fingers.

(B) Press the side of the neck with the fingers.

(C) Position the stethoscope above the heart's apex.

(D) Press the wrist bone with the fingers.

(98) How can you transfer a hemiplegia patient to a wheelchair from the bed?

(A) Use a trapeze bar.

(B) Place the wheelchair near the bed on the unaffected side of the patient at a 45-degree angle.

(C) Place the patient's arm around a family member's neck.

(D) Place the wheelchair on the patient's affected side in a parallel position.

(99) What is the cause of high-grade fever in a postoperative patient after five hours?

(A) Bladder infection.

(B) Wound infection.

(C) Atelectasis.

(D) Dehydration.

(100) What is a contraindication for oral contraceptives?

(A) Cystitis.

(B) History of diabetes.

(C) Thrombophlebitis.

(D) Gonorrhea infection.

(101) What should be done during the Schilling test?

(A) An enema.

(B) An X-ray.

(C) A 24-hour urine sample collection.

(D) A blood sample collection.

(102) A five-month-old baby presents with a generalized bumpy rash. What is the management step?

(A) Elimination diet.

(B) CBC.

(C) Stool analysis.

(D) Cutaneous biopsy.

(103) What is the action mechanism of propranolol?

(A) A heart rate that slows.

(B) Metabolism control.

(C) Replacement of the deficient hormone.

(D) Thyroid function regulation.

(104) For a patient who must have an IV pyelogram, gallbladder X-ray, cardiac catheterization, and thyroid scan, which should be done first?

(A) IV pyelogram.

(B) Gallbladder X-ray.

(C) Cardiac catheterization.

(D) Thyroid scan.

(105) What conflict occurs when two persons have very different personalities or communication styles?

(A) Task-based conflict.

(B) Value-based conflict.

(C) Interpersonal conflict.

(D) None of the above.

(106) What should be assessed in a cervical laminectomy patient?

(A) Urine output.

(B) Radial pulse.

(C) Hand grip.

(D) Pedal pulses.

(107) What dietary instructions should cholecystitis patients follow?

(A) Avoid fatty foods.

(B) Avoid caffeine.

(C) Avoid carbonated beverages.

(D) Sit up after eating.

(108) Which ostomy will have the most formed stools?

(A) Descending colon.

(B) Transverse colon.

(C) Ascending colon.

(D) Ileum.

(109) What is the best way to manage a patient who presents with chronic constipation?

(A) Restrict fluid intake.

(B) Use atropine sulfate and diphenoxylate hydrochloride.

(C) Eat vegetables and fruits.

(D) Eat rice.

(110) What is not true about efficient staff learning?

(A) Repeated lessons provide better learning results.

(B) Single lessons provide better learning results.

(C) Passive teaching methods have been proven to have little to no effect on learning results.

(D) If efficient methods are applied, computer-based learning may be just as successful as live instruction.

(111) What is not true about the activities of assistive nursing staff?

(A) All care given by assistive nursing staff should be assigned to and overseen by an RN.

(B) All care given by assistive nursing staff should be assigned by the level of competence.

(C) All care given by assistive nursing staff should be assigned to and overseen by the physician.

(D) All care given by assistive nursing staff should be according to the patient's documented plan of care.

(112) To prevent the disclosure of a patient's information during an interaction with other professionals, what can be avoided?

(A) Individualized apps.

(B) Individualized platforms.

(C) Public laptops and phones.

(D) Antivirus software.

(113) A blood transfusion patient complains of shivers and feels cold 10 minutes after the transfusion. What should be done?

(A) Stop the transfusion.

(B) Elevate the patient's feet.

(C) Measure the patient's vital signs.

(D) Use a warm blanket.

(114) A patient presents to the ER with severe chest pain that rates 10 out of a 10-point scale. What should the patient do first?

(A) Rest in bed.

(B) Take deep breaths.

(C) Lie flat.

(D) Take aspirin.

(115) What is the appropriate action to take for a female scheduled to have external radiation therapy but who is annoyed by the purple marks and wants to remove them?

(A) Inform the doctor before she tries to remove the marks.

(B) Ask her why she is annoyed by the marks.

(C) Use alcohol to help her remove the marks.

(D) Tell her it is important to keep those marks to inform the doctor about the radiation site.

(116) What could cause problems for a patient who takes lithium carbonate?

(A) Increased water intake.

(B) Weight gain.

(C) Low-sodium diet.

(D) A 0.7 mEq/L serum lithium level.

(117) While assessing a post-enucleation patient, the nurse finds bright red drainage. What should he do next?

(A) Observe if the bleeding increases.

(B) Monitor for any increase in drainage.

(C) Locate the patient's medical records.

(D) Inform the doctor.

(118) Which laboratory test results indicate a side effect from the use of tacrolimus?

(A) WBC count = 8,000 cells/mm^3.

(B) Platelet count = 410,000 cells/mm^3.

(C) Serum potassium level = 4.1 mEq/L.

(D) Random blood sugar = 250 mg/dL.

(119) When in the emergency department, what could cause a violation of a patient's privacy?

(A) Limited bed space.

(B) The beds are crammed together with just a few curtains separating them.

(C) Information overheard by patients nearby.

(D) Very large patient rooms.

(120) If a follow-up appointment will be difficult or sensitive, who should do it?

(A) The nurse.

(B) The pharmacist.

(C) The primary care doctor.

(D) Office personnel.

(121) Which finding in postpartum patients would require immediate intervention?

(A) Foul odor and red lochia.

(B) Colostrum discharge from both breasts.

(C) HR = 70 bpm.

(D) Mild afterpain.

(122) What should be done when a postpartum female presents with a fever of 37.8°C five hours after delivery?

(A) Increase oral fluid intake.

(B) Measure her temperature after 30 minutes.

(C) Document the findings.

(D) Inform the doctor.

(123) What is the labor dystocia type when the pregnant patient complains of weak, irregular, and short contractions at 39 weeks gestation?

(A) Preterm.

(B) Hypertonic.

(C) Precipitous.

(D) Hypotonic.

(124) What is true about feeding options for the infant of an HIV patient?

(A) Switch to bottle-feeding after 10 months of breastfeeding.

(B) Switch to bottle-feeding after seven months of breastfeeding.

(C) Use NG tube feeding.

(D) Use bottle-feeding from day one.

(125) Which of the findings does not indicate a surgical incision site infection?

(A) Warm, tender skin.

(B) Purulent drainage

(C) Serous drainage.

(D) Hard, red skin.

(126) What is the first step in cases of numerous casualties due to a tornado that hit a local residential area, so multiple victims will be coming to the ER at once?

(A) Request additional nursing staff.

(B) Request additional supplies.

(C) Activate the emergency response plan.

(D) Prepare the triage rooms.

(127) What is essential after the insertion of a central venous catheter and before the flow rate of the IV solution is started?

(A) Measure urine output.

(B) Do a portable chest X-ray.

(C) Measure serum electrolyte levels.

(D) Measure serum osmolality.

(128) What does not indicate the need for a patient transfer?

(A) A more specialized treatment is provided in a life-threatening emergency.

(B) Healthcare expenses will be reduced.

(C) Less intense nursing care is required.

(D) The end of healthcare occurs.

(129) What is involved in a nursing report?

(A) The patient's wounds or pressure injuries and the care required.

(B) The specific medical tests that must be performed during the next nursing shift.

(C) The type and rate of IV fluids.

(D) All of the above.

(130) Which blood type can be administered to a patient with an unknown blood type?

(A) AB-negative.

(B) AB-positive.

(C) O-negative.

(D) O-positive.

(131) A patient presents with coal-tar-covered psoriasis lesions. What should be done?

(A) If the skin is dark during the treatment, inform the doctor.

(B) Wash the solution within eight hours.

(C) Protect the area from sunlight.

(D) If nausea or vomiting occurs, inform the doctor.

(132) What is not a physical and biological demand?

(A) Urination.

(B) Personal care.

(C) Nourishment.

(D) Emotional support.

(133) Which of these drugs will be prescribed initially for a patient with alcohol withdrawal?

(A) Dilantin.

(B) Ascorbic acid.

(C) Antabuse.

(D) Thiamine.

(134) A nurse calls for help after she finds a patient with no pulse and who is not breathing. What is the initial action she should take?

(A) Perform defibrillation.

(B) Call the ER team.

(C) Start chest compression.

(D) Start giving breaths.

(135) Which term refers to the fair distribution of benefits among potential patients?

(A) Nonmaleficence.

(B) Paternalism.

(C) Autonomy.

(D) Justice.

(136) What is the consent that is acquired at the time of admission and outlines the healthcare agency's obligations to the patient?

(A) Research consent.

(B) Admission consent.

(C) Special consent.

(D) Surgical consent.

(137) What is used to analyze the risk of postoperative infection?

(A) Balance metrics.

(B) Outcome metrics.

(C) In-process metrics.

(D) Structural metrics.

(138) What could be the cause of fatigue in a chemotherapy patient?

(A) RBC count decrease.

(B) Depression.

(C) Stress.

(D) WBC count decrease.

(139) A patient presents with a swollen ankle that causes severe pain when it is moved. What is the first management step?

(A) Have the patient try to move the ankle.

(B) Have the patient do ROM ankle exercises.

(C) Have the patient elevate the ankle.

(D) Have the patient use a warm compress on the ankle.

(140) Which information cannot be present in the preprinted physician orders?

(A) Evidence-based algorithms to assist treatment and decision-making.

(B) Reportable core measurements for a specific condition.

(C) List of eligible formulary drugs.

(D) Patient's history and examination.

(141) A 38-week pregnant patient arrives at the ER in the early stages of labor. She tells the nurse she needs to go to the toilet, and she leans forward as if to push out a stool. What should the nurse do?

(A) Inquire about recent defecation.

(B) Call the charge nurse.

(C) Get the patient to pant.

(D) Get the patient to push.

(142) What are personal behaviors, thoughts, and actions directed toward patients, their families, and other healthcare professionals?

(A) Conscious attention.

(B) Professional sensibility.

(C) Personal attention.

(D) Contextual attention.

(143) What is an indication of magnesium sulfate toxicity in a preeclampsia patient?

(A) Serum level of magnesium of 5.

(B) Deep tendon reflexes.

(C) Respiratory rate of 12 bpm.

(D) Proteinuria.

(144) When will normal bowel elimination resume after delivery?

(A) Within three weeks of postpartum.

(B) On the first day of delivery.

(C) A week after delivery.

(D) Within three days of delivery.

(145) What is a red flag finding of dysfunctional maternal or fetal labor?

(A) Persistently abnormal fetal HR.

(B) Progressive cervical changes.

(C) Coordinated contractions of the uterus.

(D) Maternal fatigue.

Test 3: Answers and Explanations

(1) (D) Monitor the patient for bladder distention.

The symptoms of hypertension, headache, and blurred vision after a spinal cord injury may indicate autonomic dysreflexia, which is a condition that can occur in individuals with spinal cord injuries above T6. Autonomic dysreflexia is usually triggered by a noxious stimulus below the level of injury, where bladder distention is a common cause. The nurse should monitor for bladder distention and address any urinary retention to alleviate the triggering stimulus.

(2) (A) It states the patient's preferred medical procedures.

A living will is a legal document that specifies how a patient wishes to be treated if unable to make choices for themselves on emergency care.

(3) (C) Implement a nutritional plan for the patient.

Patient advocacy is a component of healthcare that upholds a patient's rights to appropriate standards of care, human dignity, patient equality, and guarantees that patients have the freedom to make their own healthcare-related decisions. The creation of a nutritional plan is not a patient advocate's role.

(4) (B) Pain is relieved.

When nitroglycerin is administered, pain alleviation is anticipated because the dilation of coronary veins will enhance the blood flow to the heart muscle and lessen discomfort brought on by ischemia. When the discomfort is alleviated, the patient's heart rate should drop.

(5) (D) All of the above.

The healthcare practitioner must inform the patient about the nature of the patient's medical condition and the goals, choices, potential results, and risks associated with suggested therapy.

(6) (C) The patient should be kept in an upright position.

This is not true. An unconscious patient should be positioned in a lateral position with the head tilted to the side. After oral care, the patient should remain in a lateral position for 30 minutes to avoid fluid aspiration and secretion pooling.

(7) (B) Evaluation.

In evaluation, the intended intervention is reviewed to determine whether it was successful. This may be a continuous process, and the intervention should define the frequency and length of the assessment.

(8) (C) Provision of patient care.

Interprofessional teams involve the ability to change viewpoints when given new information, have an openness to learn and understand others' roles and responsibilities, share decision-making and goals, focus on the client, have clear communication, and demonstrate mutual respect.

(9) (A) Seizures.

The most hazardous sign of barbiturate withdrawal is a seizure, which may be fatal. Anxiety, hallucinations, nausea, and vomiting may be terrifying but are not life-threatening.

(10) (C) It dissolves the coronary artery clot.

A thrombolytic medication called alteplase dissolves the clot that obstructs a coronary artery. It doesn't aid in the recovery of the heart muscle, stop the development of new clots, or reduce pain.

(11) (B) Inquire about a shellfish allergy.

A nurse should ask about an iodine allergy because cardiac catheterization uses an iodine dye.

(12) (C) Tell the patient to use a paper bag.

The patient is in respiratory alkalosis and is hyperventilating. It is fine to have the patient breathe into a paper bag as a solution. The patient will get worse with oxygen. Exercises that require the patient to breathe deeply probably won't be as beneficial as paper bag breathing.

(13) (B) Dehydration.

The output is four large diarrheal stools and 950 mL fluids, whereas the input is 1,100 mL. So, the risk of dehydration is increased.

(14) (D) Do not wet the cast.

To maintain the cast strength, it must stay dry. The palms of the hands, not the fingers, should be used to handle the cast. The patient may use a hair dryer on the cold setting to soothe an itch, but the patient should never scratch beneath the cast.

(15) (B) Cast hot spot.

Hot spots, or parts of the cast that are warmer than others, and purulent leakage are indicators of infection under a cast. Edema, decreased arterial pulse, skin pallor, and coldness are indications of poor circulation in the distal limb.

(16) (A) Maintain pleasant body language.

Uncross your arms and maintain eye contact to help you maintain pleasant body language and show respect to the other person.

(17) (A) A multiparous patient who had an oxytocin induction and delivered a large fetus.

The causes of postpartum hemorrhage are intrauterine manipulation, cesarean or forceps delivery, dystocia, multiparity, infection, large fetus, polyhydramnios, uterine overdistension, abruptio placentae, placenta previa, history of postpartum-hemorrhage-retained placental fragments, perineum or cervical hematoma, and uterine atony.

(18) (C) Safety device straps are secured to the side rails.

To prevent harm because the side rail is loosened, the safety device straps are always fastened to the bedframe. One or two fingers should be able to move freely between the safety device and the patient's jacket and skin. Because it does not tighten when pressure is applied to it, and it is possible to remove the safety device quickly in an emergency, a knot should be used when attaching a safety device.

(19) (B) Run normal saline.

If a nurse fears a transfusion response, she should pause the transfusion and keep the vein open with an infusion of normal saline. This helps preserve the patient's intravascular volume and a patent IV access line.

(20) (D) 5% dextrose in lactated Ringer's.

The patient's blood pressure will rise because of the hypertonic solution of 5% dextrose in lactated Ringer's, which also increases the intravascular volume and replaces lost fluid volume until a transfusion can be given. Other options are hypotonic solutions, which move into the cells via osmosis rather than increasing intravascular space.

(21) (B) Infiltration.

A dislodged IV that rests in the subcutaneous tissue and exhibits swelling, coldness, and pallor has infiltrated. Warmth, not coolness, is more likely to accompany infection, phlebitis, and thrombosis at the IV site.(22) (C) Vitamin B_{12}.

Because vitamin B_{12} is a component of animal products, a vegan is most likely deficient in this vitamin. Fresh fruits and vegetables, which are part of a vegan diet, provide vitamins A, C, and E.

(23) (D) 2,530 cells/mm^3.

The normal WBC count ranges from 4,500 to 11,000/mm^3. The patient with a decreased WBC count is immunosuppressed. The nurse must implement neutropenic precautions when the patient's values fall below normal.

(24) (D) 3.1 mEq/L.

A blood potassium level of 3.5 to 5.1 mEq/L is considered normal. Only Option D is below the therapeutic range. Ventricular dysrhythmias may develop if furosemide is given to a cardiac patient with a low potassium level.

(25) (A) Patients have abnormal regular and deep respiration.

Kussmaul respirations are abnormally increased in rate for both regular and deep respiration.

(26) (C) It reflects compensated respiratory alkalosis.

Normal pH ranges from 7.35 to 7.45. The pH is above the normal range in this instance, which means it is alkalosis. The PCO_2 is low due to respiratory causes. Compensation occurs when the pH levels off and returns to normal.

(27) (A) It decreases prednisone's negative effects.

Cimetidine, methotrexate, and prednisone are the drugs recommended for acute lymphocytic leukemia. Gastric ulcers are a prednisone adverse effect. Cimetidine use aids in the prevention of ulcer growth.

(28) (C) Acyclovir.

Acyclovir is the most common antiviral medication prescribed for herpes zoster, which is a chicken pox virus infection that damages the nerves. Benadryl may assist with itching. For bacterial infections, tetracycline or penicillin are prescribed.(29) (C) So the woman can feel like a survivor.

The victim's primary long-term objective is to feel that she has endured the suffering and can restore her self-esteem. Although a long-term support group is beneficial, it is not this patient's priority.

(30) (B) Prevent a bladder clot.

The development of bladder clots may be avoided through regular bladder irrigation. Continuous bladder irrigation does not help maintain bladder tone, stop the development of urethral strictures, or protect against UTIs.

(31) (C) Below the bladder.

Urine continuously drains into the bag, which is positioned underneath the bladder. The tubing is slanted to facilitate this. Ascending infection is less likely to occur in this position.

(32) (A) It can cause appendix rupture.

Laxatives enhance peristalsis, which increases the risk of appendix rupture. Although this is not the main reason why laxatives are not administered to someone who has appendicitis, the patient has pressure rather than constipation. Before colon, rectal, or gynecological surgery, laxatives may be administered.

(33) (C) Defamation.

Defamation is misleading speech that harms someone's reputation, whether in writing or orally. Assault refers to a threat of dangerous or offensive physical contact. Battery refers to deliberate contact with another person's body without their permission. Fraud is purposeful deceit with the intent of creating illegal profits.

(34) (D) Potassium.

Digoxin poisoning occurs more rapidly because Lasix is a diuretic that depletes potassium. When a patient is on a potassium-depleting diuretic, supplements are often prescribed.

(35) (D) It is broken down by gastric acids.

Heparin is broken down by stomach secretions. That is why it is administered subcutaneously or intravenously so that it doesn't disturb the stomach or intestines.
(36) (C) A patient who is informed of the truth about his condition.
Invasion of privacy involves a breach of confidentiality, an intrusion on the patient or family's private affairs, and disclosure of patient information to unauthorized individuals.
(37) (B) Case-control studies.
Case-control studies reviewed systematically are considered Level 3.
(38) (A) AIDS.The risk factors for radiocontrast media allergies include cardiac or kidney illness, female gender, older age, and use of beta-blockers. Patients with asthma and eczema or immunosuppressive disorders such as AIDS are at the most risk for latex allergies.
(39) (C) Ambulatory difficulty.
Ambulatory issues are unimportant in this case. To identify the patient's capacity for learning, the nurse should evaluate orientation status. The directions must be clear enough for the patient to comprehend.
(40) (A) Self-mutilation.
Self-mutilation is a more significant concern than social isolation, a dysfunctional household, or anxiety. It is a cry for help that demands quick attention because it reveals inadequate mechanisms of coping.
(41) (A) Prevent the spread of disease.
The main goal of standard precautions is to stop the spread of illness. To safeguard patients with a weakened immune system, protective or reverse measures are used. A nosocomial infection may be avoided through the use of the usual precautions.
(42) (C) Fasten the collection device to the wounds beneath.
Always keep portable suction below the wound level. It won't drain otherwise. The system won't be drained if the collecting chambers are full. It will only be replaced. You shouldn't remove the drainage catheter until the doctor orders it.
(43) (D) Temperature.

The first indication of a transfusion response is an increase in temperature. The temperature must be checked every 15 minutes and then every hour throughout the remainder of the transfusion.

(44) (D) Ensure the patient gives a clean urine sample.

To confirm the diagnosis and enable the identification of the causative organism, the nurse should first collect clean-catch urine for culture. Sulfisoxazole is a sulfa medication, whereas phenazopyridine is an anesthetic for the urinary system.

(45) (B) Pneumovax.

Because pneumonia is dangerous for the elderly, Pneumovax is advised. Infants are administered Haemophilus influenzae type B to avoid meningitis. MMR is less significant than Pneumovax. Patients over 65 are not eligible for the pertussis vaccination. The patient could get a booster injection if it has been more than 10 years since her previous tetanus vaccine.

(46) (D) Osteoarthritis.

Aspirin and NSAIDs are often used to treat osteoarthritis. However, warfarin is contraindicated with any of these medications. The patient's arthritis management should be discussed with the nurse.

(47) (C) Respiratory rate.

As a class-V opioid, atropine sulfate has the potential to lower respiration. Before administration, the nurse must check the patient's respiration. No blood pressure, urine output, or neurological tests are required.

(48) (C) Avoid sun exposure.

Prolonged sun exposure results in skin problems for patients prescribed sulfisoxazole. To avoid the formation of kidney stones, the patient should consume lots of water. A urine sample is required both before and after the course of treatment, not on a daily basis. Antimicrobials need to be taken as directed.

(49) (A) No management is needed.

Most immunizations may result in a minor skin response, and this is anticipated. The mother can use a cold compress, but it is not required. Children should not be given aspirin. A warm compress would not be recommended.

(50) (C) Do a blood alcohol level test.

The nurse should inquire about the patient's blood alcohol level and search the room for alcohol if this behavior points to drunkenness. For withdrawal symptoms such as increased blood pressure and heart rate, anxiety, or tremors, diazepam is prescribed. If all potential reasons are ruled out, a CNS consultation or Wernicke-Korsakoff syndrome can be explored.

(51) (D) Open the initial flap of the dressing away from the nurse.

If the final flap is opened away from the nurse and the first flap is opened toward the nurse, the nurse will have to reach across the field. This will contaminate the wound.

(52) (B) A shift to the left, together with leukocytosis.

The presence of leukocytosis (elevation of WBC count) and a shift to the left (increase in immature WBC) in the laboratory may indicate the presence of acute appendicitis. However, it is not always present.

(53) (D) If three sputum cultures are negative.

After starting antituberculosis medication treatment, the TB patient must have sputum cultures done every four weeks. When three sputum cultures provide negative findings, the patient is noninfectious and may resume work.

(54) (B) Put a patch on the damaged eye.

To minimize eye movement, the nurse should cover the patient's damaged eye with a patch. Activity limits can be required right away based on where and how big the retinal tear is. These limitations are required to facilitate drainage of any subretinal fluid and to stop additional tears or separation.

(55) (C) Deflate the tube cuff.

Tracheostomy plugs are inserted into the outer cannula aperture to block tracheostomy tubes so breathing and airflow proceed normally through the mouth and the nose. A cuffed tracheostomy tube must first be deflated before being plugged. There is no connection between weaning and plugging the tube and the capacity to talk or swallow.

(56) (C) Decrease the flow rate and clamp the tube.

The risk of intestinal spasms and premature ejection of the solution is reduced when the enema is administered slowly. If required, the flow is paused for 30 seconds and then reintroduced slowly if the patient complains of fullness or discomfort.

(57) (C) Dark red.

The discharge from the NG tube may be dark brown to dark red during the first 12 hours after gastric surgery. A green tint might be caused by bile. The drainage should eventually become a pale yellowish-brown color. If dark red discharge is seen 24 hours after surgery, let the doctor know.

(58) (D) Cheese.

It's important to urge lactose-intolerant newborn moms to consume less dairy. Molasses, cauliflower, beans, green leafy vegetables, and egg yolk are some substitute calcium-rich foods that the mother may eat.

(59) (B) Low Fowler's position on the back.

Choices A, C, and D should be used to achieve maximum expansion of the chest. Because it restricts the mobility of a significant portion of the chest wall, the patient shouldn't lie on their back. A seated position is better than standing.

(60) (D) Hypoglycemia.

Insulin overdose–related hypoglycemia is treated with glucagon. Arousal normally occurs within 20 minutes after glucagon administration in an unconscious patient. It is best to provide oral carbs after the patient regains consciousness.

(61) (A) Use of hot, soapy water to wash hands frequently.

A tricyclic antidepressant called clomipramine is used to treat obsessive-compulsive disorder. This medicine has the adverse effects of tachycardia and weight gain. Sleeplessness and sedation are rare occurrences.

(62) (C) The patient has an appropriate appearance.

People who are depressed feel like they are unable to do anything except lie in bed all day. When these patients get some therapeutic benefit, they report that many of their concerns have been resolved and that their look has improved.

(63) (B) Grapefruit juice.

A substance in grapefruit juice prevents the metabolization of cyclosporin. The consumption of grapefruit juice may therefore increase the amount of cyclosporine, which raises the risk of toxicity.

(64) (A) Orange-red urine may occur.

The patient should be warned that urine may become orange-red in color, and it can stain clothing. To lessen the chance of stomach distress, the drug should be taken after meals. Headaches are infrequent side effects and require the prescription to be stopped.

(65) (C) The warfarin sodium dose should be decreased.

Because it displaces oral anticoagulants from their binding sites on plasma protein, nalidixic acid may increase the effects of oral anticoagulants. This is why the anticoagulant dose will need to be reduced.

(66) (A) Penile discharge and dysuria.

Male urethritis is characterized by clear mucopurulent penile discharge and dysuria, which results from chlamydial infection. Because this condition often coexists with gonorrhea, fast assays and cultures are used as diagnostic tools for both.

(67) (A) Measure the blood pressure and apical pulse.

Tachydysrhythmia, vomiting, nausea, reduced urination, drowsiness, dizziness, and disorientation are symptoms of procainamide toxicity. When a patient complains of dizziness, the nurse should immediately check vital signs before any other alternatives are considered.

(68) (A) There is a CVP increase.

Following successful pericardiocentesis, the patient should feel instant relief. CVP drops, blood pressure rises, and the heartbeat is neither muffled nor distant and becomes audible. If the surgery fails, the CVP will increase.

(69) (D) Cardiogenic shock.

When the left ventricle is severely damaged (greater than 45%), cardiogenic shock develops. Signs include hypotension, tachypnea, a rapid, weak pulse, cool, clammy skin, reduced urine output, and metabolic acidosis.

(70) (B) Liver function test.

A leukotriene receptor antagonist called zafirlukast is used to prevent and treat bronchial asthma attacks. In patients with compromised hepatic function, zafirlukast should be administered with caution. To establish a baseline, the liver function test should be done, and the values should be checked during the treatment course.

(71) (A) Lean on the nightstand.

When a patient with emphysema leans against a wall when upright, rests the elbows on the knees while seated, and leans on a nightstand while sitting up, these positions will facilitate respiration.

(72) (B) Sudden chest pain.

Symptoms of pulmonary embolism include sudden chest pain, tachypnea, dyspnea, cyanosis, cough, and tachycardia.

(73) (B) Start manual ventilation for the patient.

The patient is withdrawn from the ventilator, and manual resuscitation is employed to sustain respiration until the issue can be resolved.

(74) (A) During labor, if vaginal lesions are present, a Cesarean section is required.

To avoid infection of the fetus with genital herpes, deliveries should be performed by Cesarean section on patients who have active lesions at the time of labor, whether recurring or primary. Keep the genital region dry and clean to facilitate healing. Acyclovir's safety during pregnancy has not been determined.

(75) (C) Abduction of the limb while the patient lies on his nonoperative side.

When the patient is positioned on the nonoperative side or in a supine position, abduction is maintained. Adduction, external or internal rotation, and lying on the surgical side should be avoided.

(76) (C) Hemoglobin A1c level of 7.5%.

A hemoglobin A1c level of 6.5% or higher indicates diabetes. The test provides an average of blood sugar levels over the past two to three months. A fasting blood glucose level should be 126 mg/dL or higher to diagnose diabetes. An oral glucose tolerance test result would need to be 200 mg/dL or higher at 2 hours to be indicative of diabetes. A random blood glucose level of 200 mg/dL or higher suggests diabetes.

(77) (D) Notify the physician.

Digoxin's therapeutic range is between 0.5 and 2 ng/mL. A 2.6 ng/mL level is toxic. The nurse should inform the doctor.

(78) (B) Bradycardia.

Indicators of excessive muscarinic stimulation brought on by bethanechol chloride toxicity include hypotension, bradycardia, involuntary urine and feces, sweating, and salivation. Atropine sulfate is given intravenously or subcutaneously as part of the treatment.

(79) (C) The patient should drink a lot of fluids.

Sulfisoxazole should be taken with a full glass of water, and the patient should continue to drink plenty of fluids. Some sulfisoxazole formulations produce dark brown urine, but this is normal and does not require the doctor to be informed. The patient shouldn't be given instructions to taper or stop the medication.

(80) (C) Left arm pain, decreased pulse, and pallor.

After a fistula, steal syndrome is brought on by vascular insufficiency. The patient displays pallor, a decreased pulse, and discomfort distal to the fistula brought on by tissue ischemia. An infection would be characterized by warmth and redness.

(81) (C) Monitor the patient's heart rate.

The hyperkalemia patient has a danger of cardiac arrest or dysrhythmias. Therefore, the patient should be cardiac monitored. The nurse should check the patient's sodium level because this is often checked together with potassium levels, but it is not a priority. The consumption of vegetables, which are natural sources of potassium in the diet, does not need to be increased. Fluid intake should not be increased.

(82) (A) PTT.

Warfarin sodium's therapeutic effect will be evaluated by the PT, whereas heparin's therapeutic effect will be evaluated by the PTT. Red blood cell concentrations are evaluated by hematocrit and hemoglobin levels.

(83) (A) Oxygen saturation and blood pressure.

Hemodynamic compromise may be brought on by premature ventricular contractions. When an ectopic beat occurs, the ventricular filling time is reduced, which results in smaller stroke volume and cardiac output. Premature ventricular contractions may be brought on by alcohol, nicotine, coffee, hypoxemia, and cardiac disorders.

(84) (C) Peripheral neuritis.

Peripheral neuritis, which causes paresthesia, tingling, and numbness in the extremities, is a frequent adverse effect of isoniazid, which is a drug used to treat tuberculosis. Pyridoxine (vitamin B_6) can prevent this.

(85) (C) Venturi mask.

The Venturi mask provides the most precise concentration of oxygen for a patient with chronic airflow restriction.

(86) (D) Positive.

A patient without HIV has an induration that is more than 10 mm in size. An HIV patient who is immunosuppressed is positive on Mantoux skin testing if the region of induration is bigger than 5 mm. Due to the immunosuppressive component, it is conceivable for an HIV patient to have a false-negative result.

(87) (A) Give the patient a face mask and oxygen.

Pulmonary embolism is a potentially life-threatening condition, so the immediate priority is to ensure adequate oxygenation. Administer oxygen via a face mask to help alleviate hypoxemia and reduce the strain on the heart and lungs.

(88) (C) Put the patient in the Trendelenburg position.

Immediately after a cord prolapse, reduce cord compression and improve fetal oxygenation. To move the fetus toward the diaphragm, the patient should be positioned with the hips higher than the head.

(89) (C) Perform a digital examination.

A poorly placed placenta in the lower uterine segment near or over the internal cervical OS is called a placenta previa. Ultrasound is used to diagnose it, and cervical digital examination is contraindicated because it may result in bleeding. The electronic fetal HR is essential to determine the fetus's condition. Hematocrit and hemoglobin levels may be checked.

(90) (B) Complete dilation of the cervix.

When the cervix has fully dilated, the second stage of labor starts, and it finishes with the delivery of the newborn.

(91) (A) Purpura, petechiae, and bleeding gums.

Because of the extensive vascular integrity damage caused by severe preeclampsia, DIC may develop. Bleeding is a precursor of DIC.

(92) (D) The test result is normal.

Results from contraction stress tests may be equivocal, positive (abnormal), or negative (normal). Despite the fetus being strained by three contractions that last at least 40 seconds over 10 minutes, a negative test result means no late decelerations in the fetal heart rate.

(93) (A) Increased HCO_3 and increased pH.

Most patients who experience nausea and vomiting have metabolic alkalosis caused by the loss of stomach acid, which raises pH and HCO_3, as seen in the ABG.

(94) (B) Walker.

A walker is the best option for a patient who has arthritis, a fractured arm, or underwent foot surgery.

(95) (A) The patient's room should be darkened.

Triggers that cause seizures are less likely to occur in a dark room. The patient's room should also have as little audio and visual stimulation as possible.

(96) (C) Pulse = 120.

The pulse pressure falls, the blood pressure falls, and the pulse rate accelerates in a patient in shock.

(97) (A) Press the top of the foot with the fingers.

When you press the top of the foot with the fingers and gently push the artery against the bone, you can feel the pedal pulse. Press the side of the neck to test the carotid pulse. To take the apical pulse, position the stethoscope above the heart's apex.

(98) (B) Place the wheelchair near the bed on the unaffected side of the patient at a 45-degree angle.

Hemiplegic patients will find it difficult to wrap their arms around another person's neck or use a trapeze. The wheelchair should be positioned at a 45-degree angle on the patient's unaffected side. The patient may stand on the unaffected leg in this position before settling into the wheelchair.

(99) (C) Atelectasis.

Atelectasis appears 24–48 hours after surgery. Wound infection takes at least 72 hours to result in a fever. The 48–72-hour time period after surgery is the most probable for a bladder infection–related fever to develop. In the first 24 hours after surgery, a low-grade temperature with dehydration is common.

(100) (C) Thrombophlebitis.

Oral contraceptives are contraindicated because they may induce clotting issues, such as thrombophlebitis. Oral contraceptives should not be used if the patient smokes or has migraines. The use of oral contraceptives is not contraindicated in cases of diabetes, gonorrhea, or bladder infections.

(101) (C) A 24-hour urine sample collection.

To determine if vitamin B_{12} is absorbed from the GIT into the bloodstream and is eliminated in the urine, the patient is administered radioactive vitamin B_{12} orally, and a 24-hour urine sample is taken.

(102) (A) Elimination diet.

An elimination diet can be an appropriate management step, especially if there is a suspicion that the rash might be related to an allergic reaction or food intolerance. At this age, the introduction of new foods can sometimes trigger allergic reactions, which can manifest as skin rashes. An elimination diet removes potential allergens and then gradually reintroduces them to identify the culprit.

(103) (A) A heart rate that slows.

The heart rate of a Graves's disease patient is high. Propranolol is a beta-blocker and will lower the heart rate. It does not control metabolism, it is not a hormone, and it does not affect thyroid function.

(104) (D) Thyroid scan.

The way the thyroid gland absorbs iodine affects the thyroid scan. The findings won't be correct if the patient had a different test that used an iodine dye.

(105) (C) Interpersonal conflict.

There are multiple causes for conflicts, such as conflict based on interpersonal relationships, conflict that arises when nurses have different personal values, and task-based conflict that arises when two medical experts disagree on a method.

(106) (C) Hand grip.

An upper extremity neurological examination should be performed on cervical laminectomy patients. To gauge the patient's grip strength, the nurse should ask them to grab her hand. Urinary output, pedal, and radial pulses are unrelated.

(107) (A) Avoid fatty foods.

The gallbladder is inflamed in cholecystitis. The gallbladder's purpose is to hold bile and then release it to aid in the digestion of fat. The patient should stay away from fatty meals.

(108) (A) Descending colon.

The reabsorption of liquids is the colon's function. The more water is absorbed and the more solid the stool, the longer fecal material remains in the colon. Semi-solid to solid drainage occurs from a descending colon ostomy. Transverse colon discharge is mushy. Liquid occurs from the ascending colon and ileum ostomies.

(109) (C) Eat vegetables and fruits.

Vegetables and fruits include fiber, which gives the stool more weight. Fiber also softens and facilitates defecation. Constipation is often caused by the consumption of a lot of rice. Lomotil, which is used to treat diarrhea, would make the patient's constipation worse.

(110) (B) Single lessons provide better learning results.

This is false. It has been shown that repeated lessons provide better learning results than single ones. (111) (C) All care given by assistive nursing staff should be assigned to and overseen by the physician.

This is false. All care given by assistive nursing staff should be assigned to and overseen by an RN per the patient's documented plan of care and the staff member's level of competence.

(112) (C) Public laptops and phones.

To interact with other professionals, you should use secure apps, platforms, and networks. Avoid unprotected or public devices, such as unsecured phones or laptops.

(113) (A) Stop the transfusion.

Fever is a symptom of a transfusion response, whereas chills indicate a sudden rise in body temperature. After the transfusion is stopped, the nurse should take the patient's vital signs and alert the charge nurse.

(114) (D) Take aspirin.

Due to its anticoagulant properties, aspirin may help prevent clot growth. A seated position will make the patient more comfortable. (115) (D) Tell her that it is important to keep those marks to inform the doctor about the radiation site.

The purple marks show the nuclear doctor where to direct the radiation and highlight the tumor. Throughout the course of the radiation treatment, these marks should remain. If the patient erases the marks, it will impair the delivery of treatment and she may also damage her skin.

(116) (C) Low-sodium diet.

A low-sodium diet may cause the levels of lithium to increase, which may lead to lithium poisoning because lithium is eliminated from the body as a salt. Lithium levels in serum should range from 0.5 to 1.4 mEq/L. Although it is not hazardous, weight gain is an adverse effect of lithium. To reduce GI adverse effects, take the drug after meals and with lots of fluids.

(117) (D) Inform the doctor.

If the nurse observes bright red drainage on the dressing, she must inform the doctor because this is an indication of a hemorrhage.

(118) (D) Random blood sugar = 250 mg/dL.

A blood sugar level of 250 mg/dL indicates a side effect. Other side effects include hyperkalemia, hypertension, vomiting, nausea, diarrhea, insomnia, tremor, and headache.

(119) (C) Information overheard by patients nearby.The hospital's emergency department is a busy area. The beds are crammed together, with a few curtains separating them. Particularly

when staff members disclose patient personal information and the information is overheard by patients nearby, a lack of physical distance is a significant issue.

(120) (C) The primary care doctor.

The primary care doctor may be required to make the call if the follow-up is difficult or sensitive. Nurses and medical assistants examine blood pressure and blood glucose levels, discuss, promote healthy habits, and assess medication adherence. Pharmacists follow up with patients on their medications.

(121) (A) Foul odor and red lochia.

For the first one to three days after delivery, the discharge known as lochia is red and progressively lessens in volume. Typical lochia smells like menstrual discharge. It is abnormal to encounter foul or purulent lochia. This indicates infection.

(122) (A) Increase oral fluid intake.

Every four hours, the patient's temperature should be taken. The dehydration effects of labor are often to blame for temperatures as high as 38°C in the first 24 hours after delivery. Encourage oral fluid intake, which should return the temperature to normal.

(123) (D) Hypotonic.

Hypotonic labor contractions are often weak, irregular, and short. They take place during the active stage of labor. Preterm labor begins between 20 and 37 weeks of gestation. Precipitous labor lasts no more than three hours. Uncoordinated, frequent, and painful contractions are symptoms of hypertonic dystocia.

(124) (D) Use bottle-feeding from day one.

HIV may be transmitted during the postpartum period, labor, and the postpartum period if the mother is breastfeeding, so bottle feeding should be used from day one. There is no physiological justification for using an NG tube to feed the infant.

(125) (C) Serous drainage.

An expected finding at a surgical site is serous drainage. Sensitive, red, and warm skin around the incision or purulent material from drains or the borders of divided wounds may indicate an infection.

(126) (C) Activate the emergency response plan.

Victims of an external disaster may be sent to the ER for treatment. Even if steps A, B, and D may be taken to prepare for the casualties, the emergency response plan must be activated as the first action.

(127) (B) Do a portable chest X-ray.

The chest X-ray indicates whether the central catheter is in the appropriate location before the IV solution is started. This is required to prevent the penetration of IV fluid into the pulmonary or subcutaneous regions.

(128) (D) The end of healthcare occurs.

Transfers are used when less intense nursing care is required, to save healthcare expenses, or to provide more specialized treatment in a life-threatening emergency.

(129) (D) All of the above.

Nursing reports include the patient's wounds or pressure injuries, the specific medical tests that must be performed during the next nursing shift, discharge instructions, whether the patient needs help to get up or use the restroom, the type and rate of the IV fluids received, the catheter used, whether isolation is necessary to stop the spread of illness or diseases, and oxygenation needs if any.

(130) (C) O-negative.

O-negative is the most widely available blood type and may be donated to anybody. The receiver is always AB-positive. There are no other alternatives available.

(131) (C) Protect the area from sunlight.

Coal tar preparations require the patient to keep the affected regions out of direct sunlight for at least 24 hours after application. Vomiting and nausea are uncommon adverse effects of coal tar preparations.

(132) (D) Emotional support.Physical and biological demands include urination, personal care, water, sleep, and nourishment.

(133) (D) Thiamine.

In alcoholism, thiamine deficiency is common, so it will be prescribed upon admission. Alcohol abusers are not prescribed Dilantin (anti-seizure) or ascorbic acid. Antabuse is prescribed upon discharge and helps the patient to abstain from drinking.

(134) (D) Start giving breaths.

At the start, the nurse should give the patient two breaths.

(135) (D) Justice.

Justice is the equal division of prospective advantages.

(136) (B) Admission consent.

Admission consent is acquired at the time of admission. It outlines the healthcare agency's obligations to the patient. Special consent is required for the use of shackles, photographs of the patient, disposal of body parts after surgery, donation of organs after death, or an autopsy. Surgical consent is acquired for any surgical or invasive operations or invasive diagnostic testing. Research consent is necessary to participate in a research project.

(137) (B) Outcome metrics.

Outcome metrics are used to determine how well a patient is doing in terms of hospitalization and the risk of postoperative infection.

(138) (A) RBC count decrease.

Chemotherapy results in a drop in RBC count and bone marrow activity, both of which contribute to fatigue. Cancer treatment reduces WBC counts, but instead of making the patient tired, it increases the risk of infection.

(139) (C) Have the patient elevate the ankle.

According to the examination, the patient may have a fracture or sprain. The nurse should elevate the ankle and use a cold compress to reduce the edema and bleeding. Weight-bearing and exercise are not advised.

(140) (D) Patient's history and examination.

Indicators of appropriate antibiotic use, a list of eligible formulary drugs and doses, reportable core measurements for a specific condition, and evidence-based algorithms to assist treatment and decision-making are examples of the information that may be included.

(141) (B) Call the charge nurse.

The lady is in transition to the second stage of labor if she feels the need to go to the toilet or push. She should be asked to pant by the nurse, who should then call the RN to do a sterile vaginal exam. She shouldn't push if she isn't completely dilated yet.

(142) (B) Professional sensibility.

Professional sensibility involves the identification of personal behaviors, thoughts, and actions directed toward patients, their families, and other healthcare professionals.

(143) (C) Respiratory rate of 12 bpm.

Reduced maternal and fetal blood pressure, respiratory depression, and loss of deep tendon reflexes are symptoms of magnesium sulfate poisoning. A value of 4–7.5 mEq/L is considered therapeutic. Preeclampsia is accompanied by proteinuria.

(144) (D) Within three days of delivery.

To check if bowel sounds have returned after delivery, the nurse should auscultate the patient's abdomen in all four quadrants. Normal bowel movements normally resume two to three days after delivery.

(145) (A) Persistently abnormal fetal HR.

Meconium passing, fetal acidosis, and irregular, abnormal, persistent fetal HR are all indicators of maternal or fetal compromise. Normal labor signs include synchronized uterine contractions and cervical changes.

Test 4: Questions

(1) What is a benefit of shaving before an operation?

(A) Decreased postoperative itching.

(B) Decreased postoperative skin irritation caused by adhesive tape.

(C) Decreased infection risk.

(D) Increased surgical field vision.

(2) What should be administered to a female with burn injuries who was vaccinated against tetanus two years ago?

(A) Dose of DPT vaccine.

(B) Dose of human hyperimmune tetanus globulin.

(C) Dose of tetanus antitoxin.

(D) Booster dose of tetanus toxoid.

(3) What is a hip fracture risk factor?

(A) Osteoporosis.

(B) Increased absorption of calcium.

(C) Immobility due to arthritis.

(D) Decreased secretion of progesterone.

(4) What is true related to the circulatory system in a patient with a cast?

(A) Skin irritation may occur.

(B) Cast integrity should be maintained.

(C) There will be no impairment of circulation.

(D) A cast is not associated with pain in the extremities.

(5) What is the appropriate management when a patient passes a small stone after difficulty urinating?

(A) Administer analgesics.

(B) Perform a glucose test on the stone.

(C) Perform a guaiac test on the stone.

(D) Request an immediate laboratory analysis of the stone.

(6) What is the purpose of warm oatmeal baths for patients with pancreatic cancer?

(A) Decrease fever.

(B) Decrease fullness and bloating after meals.

(C) Decrease pruritus secondary to jaundice.

(D) Improve the paralytic ileus.

(7) What justifies an order of neomycin for a patient with a scheduled colostomy and abdominoperineal resection surgery?

(A) It prevents postoperative pneumonia.

(B) It prevents bowel inflammation.

(C) It decreases colon bacterial content.

(D) It decreases intestinal peristalsis.

(8) What should be avoided by a patient with Parkinson's disease?

(A) The development of hand-motor coordination skills.

(B) Daily care.

(C) ROM exercises.

(D) Decreased daily fluid intake.

(9) What is true about coronary artery disease risk in a patient with low LDL and high HDL?

(A) The risk increases with age.

(B) The risk increases with exercise.

(C) There is no correlation.

(D) The risk is low.

(10) Why should an extra-wide blood pressure cuff be used on an obese patient?

(A) The pulse will increase with the use of a narrow cuff.

(B) The patient will experience discomfort with the use of a narrow cuff.

(C) Blood pressure will increase with the use of a narrow cuff.

(D) A narrow cuff will not wrap around the patient's entire arm.

(11) What is the intent of Kegel exercises?

(A) Preparation for delivery.

(B) Preparation for breastfeeding.

(C) Strengthen the pelvic floor muscles.

(D) Improve the uterus circulation.

(12) What is an objective sign of bulimia?

(A) Feeling of social inadequacy.

(B) Feeling out of control.

(C) Loss of tooth enamel.

(D) Low self-esteem.

(13) What is a common patient response when advised that the cause of their liver cirrhosis is excessive alcohol consumption?

(A) They will admit that they should stop drinking alcohol excessively.

(B) They will ask about how to stop drinking.

(C) They will insist that they are a good person and this should not happen to them.

(D) They will deny excessive alcohol intake.

(14) What is the appropriate management of a postoperative transsphenoidal hypophysectomy patient who complains of mouth drainage?

(A) Start an antiemetic.

(B) Rinse the patient's mouth with water.

(C) Test drainage for glucose.

(D) Have the patient blow his nose.

(15) What should be prepared for a total thyroidectomy operation?

(A) A ventilator.

(B) A sterile dressing set.

(C) A catheterization tray.

(D) A tracheostomy set.

(16) What is a physiological change during pregnancy?

(A) Decreased metabolic rate.

(B) Increased blood volume.

(C) Increased GIT peristalsis rate.

(D) Decreased oxygen consumption.

(17) What is a symptom of placenta previa?

(A) Rigid and tender abdomen with no vaginal bleeding.

(B) Painless, bright red vaginal bleeding.

(C) Painless, dark red vaginal bleeding.

(D) Severe lower abdominal pain.

(18) What is an indication of anorexia nervosa in a 15-year-old female patient?

(A) Acne.

(B) Wheezes.

(C) Amenorrhea.

(D) Tachycardia.

(19) Which of these orders is not reflected on an advance directive?

(A) Do not resuscitate.

(B) Do not intubate.

(C) Do not hospitalize.

(D) Funeral preferences.

(20) Which orders does a nursing plan for a myasthenia gravis patient include?

(A) Detect neuropathy signs.

(B) Encourage the patient to void daily.

(C) Monitor the patient's swallowing reflex before he eats.

(D) Bathe the patient every night.

(21) What is an indication of isoniazid toxicity?

(A) Difficulty differentiating between traffic light colors.

(B) Orange-colored urine.

(C) Sharp pain in the leg(s).

(D) Ringing in the ear(s).

(22) What is the most life-threatening type of jaundice?

(A) All types of jaundice are life-threatening.

(B) Jaundice that appears within 6 to 10 days after birth.

(C) Jaundice that appears more than 48 hours after birth.

(D) Jaundice that appears within 24 hours after birth.

(23) A patient advocate's role is not to:

(A) Maintain moral principles and ethics.

(B) Describe medical terminology or techniques.

(C) Engage the legal system on the patient's behalf.

(D) Create a nursing care plan for the patient.

(24) A six-year-old was treated for flu and fever with chewable acetaminophen and aspirin for five days. What could be the cause of a new generalized, itchy rash?

(A) Flu.

(B) Aspirin.

(C) Acetaminophen.

(D) Diphenhydramine.

(25) What indicates the development of eclampsia in a preeclampsia patient?

(A) No audible heart sounds.

(B) Edema of the face and hands.

(C) Seizure.

(D) Albuminuria.

(26) Which laboratory test should be done before the administration of fludrocortisone acetate?

(A) CBC.

(B) Serum electrolytes.

(C) Renal function tests.

(D) Liver function tests.

(27) What is true about the umbilical cord of a 10-day-old?

(A) It should fall off immediately.

(B) The doctor should be informed if the cord hasn't fallen off.

(C) It will fall off about three weeks after birth.

(D) It will not fall off if the stump was not wiped with alcohol.

(28) What will reduce pain associated with ankle sprains?

(A) Apply steroid ointment.

(B) Avoid elevating.

(C) Apply ice.

(D) Exercise the ankle.

(29) What is a cause for concern in a postoperative cystoscopy patient?

(A) Pink-tinged urine.

(B) Leg cramps.

(C) Tea-colored urine.

(D) Back pain.

(30) What is not a potential complication for bedridden patients?

(A) Thrombophlebitis.

(B) Varicose veins.

(C) Hypostatic pneumonia.

(D) Muscle atrophy.

(31) What could concern a nurse about a pregnant female patient at 33 weeks gestation?

(A) Tender breasts.

(B) Swollen feet.

(C) Feeling hot.

(D) Swollen fingers.

(32) Which assessment is essential during TPN administration?

(A) Daily weight measurement.

(B) Bowel sounds auscultation.

(C) Note if the stomach contains the NG tube.

(D) Bowel movement count.

(33) What should be monitored before digoxin administration?

(A) Apical pulse.

(B) Respirations.

(C) Blood pressure.

(D) Temperature.

(34) Which immunizations will be given to a one-year-old baby girl?

(A) Meningococcal and pneumococcal.

(B) Varicella and HiB.

(C) Polio and Hepatitis B.

(D) Rotavirus and MMR.

(35) When informing a patient about the appropriate intervention for his condition, a nurse should:

(A) Not tell the patient about the intervention risks to prevent loss of hope.

(B) Not tell the patient about the intervention goals so as not to increase his expectations.

(C) Inform the patient about all his treatment options so he can choose between them freely.

(D) Not inform the patient about all his options if the doctor prefers a specific option.

(36) A young type 1 diabetes patient inquires how his situation varies from his grandma's, who was diagnosed with type 2 diabetes. What is the correct answer?

(A) An excessive intake of fats causes type 2 DM, while an excessive intake of sugar causes type 1 DM.

(B) The patient will only have type 1 DM as a child.

(C) Insulin is never used to treat type 2 DM and is always administered to treat type 1 DM.

(D) The cells cannot reuptake insulin in type 2 DM, while the pancreas produces insufficient insulin in type 1 DM.

(37) What does the assessment and monitoring of a sciatica (low back pain) patient include?

(A) Heat application.

(B) Ibuprofen administration.

(C) If the patient can lift or bend.

(D) Bed rest.

(38) What do early signs of compartment syndrome in a patient with an arm cast include?

(A) Tingling and numbness in fingers.

(B) Dependent arm pain.

(C) Severe pain that is disproportionate to the injury.

(D) Bluish discoloration and coldness in fingers.

(39) What could prevent a patient's use of crutches?

(A) ROM impairment.

(B) Axilla breakdown of the skin.

(C) Brachial plexus nerve injury.

(D) Fall and injury.

(40) Which sign is of least concern about a skeletal traction pin site?

(A) Purulent drainage.

(B) Pain.

(C) Serous drainage.

(D) Inflammation.

(41) What are some signs of a phenytoin level of 38 mcg/mL?

(A) This is a normal level, and there are no symptoms.

(B) Slurred speech.

(C) Tachycardia.

(D) Hypotension.

(42) What are the side effects of carbidopa-levodopa?

(A) Voluntary movement impairment.

(B) Hypertension.

(C) Tachycardia.

(D) Pruritus.

(43) Which step in the nursing care plan uses clinical judgment and knowledge to design procedures or treatments to satisfy the requirements of patients?

(A) Intervention planning.

(B) Evaluation.

(C) Goal setting.

(D) Assessment stage.

(44) Nurses on interprofessional teams should not:

(A) Report their observations on patients' health to colleagues.

(B) Direct care to assigned patients throughout the day.

(C) Learn about the patients' living environment.

(D) Play a role in emergency rooms.

(45) What is a sign of persistent spinal shock after spinal cord injury?

(A) Flaccid paralysis.

(B) Bladder-emptying reflex.

(C) Positive reflexes.

(D) Hyperreflexia.

(46) What conflict occurs when two medical experts disagree on a particular method?

(A) Task-based conflict.

(B) Value-based conflict.

(C) Interpersonal-based conflict.

(D) None of the above.

(47) What is true about case-based learning?

(A) It gives the student information about performance.

(B) It is characterized by the interaction between the provider and the learner.

(C) It uses fictitious or real-life clinical scenarios.

(D) It is a passive teaching method.

(48) Basic nursing skills do not include:

(A) Cleanliness.

(B) Feeding.

(C) Daily living.

(D) Endotracheal suction.

(49) Which communication method is appropriate when you talk with a patient who is hard of hearing?

(A) You should talk into the impaired ear.

(B) You should talk at a normal volume.

(C) You should talk frequently.

(D) You should talk loudly.

(50) A patient presents with an eyeball contusion after blunt object trauma. What is the first management step?

(A) Send him to the emergency room.

(B) Clean the eye with water.

(C) Put ice on the eye.

(D) Inform the doctor.

(51) What is not true about patient confidentiality?

(A) Patient information should be disposed of via the deletion of electronic records or the destruction of hard-copy documents.

(B) You should not share patient information with unauthorized individuals.

(C) It is permissible to share patient information with any family member.

(D) You should utilize secure apps and platforms to interact with other professionals.

(52) What could be done to improve patient privacy in an emergency department?

(A) Use private rooms.

(B) Use curtains to separate beds.

(C) Increase the physical distance between rooms.

(D) Make the emergency room less busy.

(53) Which foods should be limited with theophylline administration?

(A) Dairy creamers, cream cheese, and cottage cheese.

(B) Pineapple, oranges, and melon.

(C) Shrimp, lobster, and oysters.

(D) Chocolate, soda, and coffee.

(54) Who should perform the follow-up with patients about their medications?

(A) Nurses.

(B) Pharmacists.

(C) Primary care doctors.

(D) Office personnel.

(55) What PPE should be worn to treat tuberculosis patients?

(A) Eyewear, gown, and surgical mask.

(B) Eyewear and particulate respirator.

(C) Gloves, gown, and particulate respirator.

(D) Gloves and surgical mask.

(56) Which finding in a patient after a biopsy and bronchoscopy would indicate the nurse should inform the doctor?

(A) Blood-streaked sputum.

(B) Bronchospasm.

(C) Hematuria.

(D) Dry cough.

(57) A 35-year-old male patient presents after a blunt chest wall injury. What is a sign of pneumothorax?

(A) A sucking sound at the injury site.

(B) Barrel chest.

(C) Diminished air entry and breath sounds.

(D) Low respiratory rate.

(58) A female patient took NSAIDs for three months and now takes misoprostol. What will be noted after she takes misoprostol?

(A) Decreased WBC count.

(B) Decreased platelet count.

(C) Relieved epigastric pain.

(D) Relieved diarrhea.

(59) What does loperamide hydrochloride treat?

(A) Hematest-positive NG tube drainage.

(B) Diarrhea.

(C) Abdominal pain.

(D) Constipation.

(60) What do the diet instructions for a cirrhotic patient with elevated ammonia level include?

(A) High carbohydrates.

(B) Moderate fat.

(C) High protein.

(D) Low protein.

(61) To prevent dumping syndrome in a postoperative Billroth II procedure patient, a nurse should:

(A) Put the patient in a high Fowler's position when sitting.

(B) Decrease the patient's fluid intake with meals.

(C) Offer high-carbohydrate foods.

(D) Ambulate the patient after meals.

(62) A nurse assesses a patient with severe blood loss. The patient's blood pressure has dropped, and she shows signs of confusion. What is the likely cause for this change in mental status?

(A) An increase in oxygen supply to the brain.

(B) An increase in carbon dioxide levels in the brain.

(C) A decrease in glucose supply to the brain.

(D) A decrease in oxygen supply to the brain.

(63) What is essential to measure before a blood transfusion?

(A) Latest hematocrit level.

(B) Urine output.

(C) Skin color.

(D) Vital signs.

(64) For the care of a patient with liver cirrhosis, which dietary product is rich in thiamine?

(A) Broccoli.

(B) Chicken.

(C) Milk.

(D) Pork.

(65) What is true for a patient with a platelet count of 326,000 cells/mm^3 and who presents with gastrointestinal bleeding?

(A) It is a normal value.

(B) You should start bleeding precautions.

(C) It is an abnormally high value.

(D) It is an abnormally low value.

(66) What is the management for cramps that occur during colostomy irrigation?

(A) Remove the tube.

(B) Pinch the tube to interrupt the flow.

(C) Roll the patient to the other side.

(D) The solution flow should be increased.

(67) What is true after an iliac crest bone marrow biopsy?

(A) You should put the patient in a recumbent position.

(B) The biopsy site should be covered with a bandage.

(C) You should give the patient analgesics.

(D) The biopsy site should be compressed for an hour.

(68) Which PPE should be worn to treat a patient with a major abscess of a mosquito bite?

(A) Gown only.

(B) Gown and gloves.

(C) Face mask and eye protector.

(D) Gloves and N95 respirator.

(69) What is the best management for a patient with short-term memory impairment?

(A) Write down the instructions.

(B) Advise the patient of care details.

(C) Give directions as simply as possible.

(D) Give complex instructions.

(70) When does planning for discharge occur?

(A) Upon admission.

(B) Three days after admission.

(C) Five hours after admission to allow you to assess the patient's condition.

(D) Upon discharge.

(71) What should be assessed in an infant after delivery of a diabetic mother?

(A) Hypoglycemia.

(B) Acidosis.

(C) Hyperglycemia.

(D) Infection.

(72) What does the nursing report involve?

(A) Discharge instructions.

(B) Catheter instructions.

(C) Oxygenation needs.

(D) All of the above.

(73) Which positions are comfortable for a low-back pain patient?

(A) Extension of the legs in a semi-seated position.

(B) Flexion of the knees while the patient lies on his side.

(C) Supine position.

(D) Prone position.

(74) Side effects of IV gentamicin include:

(A) Hypertension.

(B) Orange sputum.

(C) Blurred vision.

(D) Decreased urine output.

(75) A patient's psychological needs do not include:

(A) Comfort.

(B) Emotional support.

(C) Low-level stress and anxiety.

(D) Nourishment.

(76) What is the first action for a postoperative patient who has a chronic cough and eviscerated abdominal wound?

(A) Monitor his vital signs.

(B) Irrigate the wound with sterile water.

(C) Return the intestines to the abdomen.

(D) Use dressings or sterile towels to cover the intestines.

(77) What is the first management step for a cerebrovascular accident patient?

(A) ROM exercises.

(B) Ambulation assessment.

(C) Hygienic care.

(D) Lung auscultation.

(78) What does the obligation to fulfill one's promises fall under?

(A) Nonmaleficence.

(B) Paternalism.

(C) Autonomy.

(D) Fidelity.

(79) What are important instructions for a patient with peritoneal ambulatory continuous dialysis?

(A) Eat a high-potassium and high-sodium diet.

(B) Stop any medications with dialysis.

(C) Train for aseptic technique.

(D) Provide information about the technique, diffusion, and osmosis.

(80) A patient's instructions after a gastrectomy procedure include:

(A) Sit up after meals.

(B) Drink plenty of fluids.

(C) Decrease carbohydrate and sodium consumption.

(D) Eat high-carbohydrate and low-protein foods.

(81) Which condition requires cleansing and oil retention enemas?

(A) Fecal impaction.

(B) Ulcerative colitis.

(C) Melena.

(D) Difficult defecation.

(82) Which consent is required before an autopsy is performed?

(A) Research consent.

(B) Admission consent.

(C) Special consent.

(D) Surgical consent.

(83) What should be done before a tracheostomy tube is suctioned?

(A) Give the patient a pencil and paper to communicate with during the procedure.

(B) Get signed consent before the procedure.

(C) Give oxygen at a high level.

(D) Have the patient drink water to liquefy secretions.

(84) What is an examination of one's ideas, feelings, strengths, weaknesses, and emotions?

(A) Conscious attention.

(B) Professional sensibility.

(C) Personal attention.

(D) Contextual attention.

(85) Elder abuse can occur in:

(A) A patient's home.

(B) Residential care facilities.

(C) Nursing homes.

(D) All of the above.

(86) A nurse reviews the lab results of a patient who has experienced significant blood loss. Which finding would be of most concern?

(A) Elevated hemoglobin level.

(B) Decreased platelet count.

(C) Decreased WBC.

(D) Elevated potassium level.

(87) What purposeful deceit is designed to create illegal profits?

(A) Assault.

(B) Battery.

(C) Defamation.

(D) Fraud.

(88) What is an indication to prescribe atropine sulfate and diphenoxylate hydrochloride?

(A) Tachycardia.

(B) Depression.

(C) Hypertension.

(D) Diarrhea.

(89) What could describe quality improvement initiatives?

(A) Outcomes that are monitored.

(B) Quality improvement activities that are implemented.

(C) Quality concerns that are identified.

(D) All of the above.

(90) What is a normal aging sign not indicative of a disease?

(A) Frequent loose stools.

(B) A preference for warmth.

(C) A preference for dark rooms to sleep in.

(D) Knee and foot pain.

(91) What can describe a normal bowel sound?

(A) Low-pitched sounds audible in one or two quadrants.

(B) Audible gurgles or high-pitched clicks in all four quadrants.

(C) Loud, high-pitched rushes audible in one or two quadrants.

(D) Loud, gurgling waves audible in four quadrants.

(92) A suicidal patient is being cared for by a nurse. What should the nurse do?

(A) Use power, act, and participate.

(B) Display an attitude of detachment, confrontation, and efficiency.

(C) Provide hope and reassurance that the problems will resolve themselves.

(D) Demonstrate confidence in the patient's ability to deal with stressors.

(93) What has a Level 4 evidence-based ranking?

(A) Case studies.

(B) Case-control studies.

(C) Cohort studies.

(D) Meta-analysis.

(94) A patient with an intestinal obstruction was admitted with an NG tube insertion. Before NG tube removal, a nurse should assess:

(A) That gastric aspirates have a normal PH.

(B) That intestinal sounds are audible.

(C) That serum electrolytes are normal.

(D) That the NG tube is in place.

(95) The nursing care plan for a skin traction patient does not include assessment for:

(A) Urinary incontinence.

(B) Skin breakdown.

(C) Infections.

(D) Bowel sounds.

(96) What are the signs of allergy?

(A) Fever.

(B) Hypertension.

(C) Slow pulse.

(D) Respiratory distress.

(97) What is true for iron supplements in a malnourished pregnant female?

(A) She doesn't need them.

(B) They may cause diarrhea.

(C) Meat should be avoided.

(D) They should be taken on an empty stomach.

(98) Which tests indicate that continuous infusion of heparin is at the therapeutic level for a patient with atrial fibrillation?

(A) PTT of more than 120 seconds.

(B) PTT of 30 seconds.

(C) PTT of 61 seconds.

(D) PTT of 13 seconds.

(99) What is a diagnostic test for TB?

(A) Tuberculin skin test.

(B) Sputum culture.

(C) Bronchoscopy.

(D) Chest x-ray.

(100) What is the initial management step of a DCL patient diagnosed with hyperglycemic hyperosmolar nonketotic syndrome?

(A) Sodium bicarbonate administration.

(B) Normal saline administration.

(C) NPH insulin administration.

(D) ET intubation.

(101) What is the nursing diagnosis for a postpartum patient with several hemorrhoids and a midline episiotomy?

(A) Fluid volume could be imbalanced.

(B) Elimination of urine could be impaired.

(C) Body image could be disturbed.

(D) Acute pain.

(102) Which serum amylase level is not consistent with chronic pancreatitis?

(A) 600 units/L.

(B) 300 units/L.

(C) 120 units/L.

(D) 74 units/L.

(103) What should be available close to a patient with bleeding esophageal varices and an NG triple-lumen tube?

(A) Clamp.

(B) Scissors.

(C) Water in a syringe.

(D) Adhesive tape.

(104) What is true about administration orders for a patient who takes Maalox, cimetidine, and omeprazole?

(A) All medications must be given before meals.

(B) Maalox should be taken with meals, cimetidine before meals, and omeprazole after meals.

(C) Maalox should be taken before meals, cimetidine after meals, and omeprazole with meals.

(D) Maalox should be taken after meals, cimetidine with meals, and omeprazole before meals.

(105) What is present in a pyelonephritis patient's history?

(A) High uric acid diet.

(B) Urolithiasis.

(C) Cystitis.

(D) Pharyngitis.

(106) Contraindications of laxative administration include:

(A) Abdominal pain in the lower right quadrant.

(B) Vomiting and nausea.

(C) Fever.

(D) No bowel movement for the past five days.

(107) The nursing care plan for bacterial meningitis patients with opisthotonos posturing includes:

(A) ROM exercises.

(B) Legs and arms restrained.

(C) Lie on the side.

(D) Lie in the supine position.

(108) Which cranial nerve is evaluated when a patient is asked to follow a finger that moves?

(A) CN VI

(B) CN IV.

(C) CN III.

(D) CN II.

(109) An Rh-negative pregnant female in her first pregnancy communicates worry about her baby as her husband is Rh-positive. Which of these statements is true?

(A) If the child is found to be affected, an intrauterine transfusion can be performed.

(B) Erythroblastosis fetalis will occur.

(C) Treatment will be started after the delivery of the second baby.

(D) The first baby will not be affected.

(110) Which ABG results are diagnostic of diabetic ketoacidosis?

(A) HCO3 = 32, pCO2 = 47, and pH = 7.49.

(B) HCO3 = 21, pCO2 = 46, and pH = 7.47.

(C) HCO3 = 10, pCO2 = 31, and pH = 7.31.

(D) HCO3 = 19, pCO2= 41, and pH = 7.33.

(111) A male patient presents with a horizontal pustular rash that extends from the front midline to the spine, back pain, and headache. Which medications should be prescribed?

(A) Benadryl.

(B) Topical hydrocortisone.

(C) Antibiotics.

(D) Antiviral.

(112) A patient complains of black stools and tongue. What could be the cause?

(A) Consumption of red meat.

(B) Iron tablets.

(C) Consumption of broccoli and beets.

(D) Bismuth subsalicylate.

(113) What is not true when a patient takes diphenhydramine?

(A) Avoid activities that need mental alertness.

(B) Use oral rinses, candy, or sugarless gums to avoid dry mouth.

(C) Avoid alcohol.

(D) Take on an empty stomach.

(114) Indications of metoclopramide drug use include:

(A) Chemotherapy-associated vomiting.

(B) Perforated diverticulitis.

(C) Melena in cases of peptic ulcer.

(D) Intestinal obstruction.

(115) What do ileostomy postoperative complications include?

(A) Electrolyte and fluid imbalance.

(B) Intestinal obstruction.

(C) Fat malabsorption.

(D) Folate deficiency.

(116) What is the appropriate management step for an esophagogastroduodenoscopy postoperative patient?

(A) Check the gag reflex.

(B) Relieve the sore throat with warm gargles.

(C) Perform a heartburn assessment.

(D) Do a temperature assessment.

(117) Which actions should be taken when a female diabetic patient who uses NPH insulin daily starts to use prednisone?

(A) Add daily oral hypoglycemic drugs.

(B) Increase the NPH insulin dose.

(C) Decrease the NPH insulin dose.

(D) Add another dose of prednisone.

(118) What should be monitored with desmopressin acetate administration?

(A) Decreased blood glucose.

(B) Decreased peripheral edema.

(C) Decreased blood pressure.

(D) Decreased urinary output.

(119) How should an open insulin vial be stored?

(A) At room temperature.

(B) In a dry and dark place.

(C) In the refrigerator.

(D) In the freezer.

(120) What is a dietary instruction for a Cushing's syndrome patient?

(A) There is no specific diet to follow.

(B) Salty food is not restricted.

(C) Protein should be limited.

(D) Potassium is not restricted.

(121) What is the priority to monitor during preoperative care of adrenalectomy-scheduled pheochromocytoma patients?

(A) Urine ketone and glucose.

(B) BUN level.

(C) Output and input.

(D) Vital signs.

(122) What is the initial management step of a myxedema coma patient?

(A) IV fluid administration.

(B) Thyroid hormone administration.

(C) Maintain a patent airway.

(D) Maintain the patient's temperature by warming him.

(123) Which of these indicators are associated with DKA?

(A) Low plasma bicarbonate and high glucose level.

(B) pH and respiratory rate increase.

(C) Urine output decreases.

(D) DCL.

(124) Which action is appropriate in the management of a postpartum female with dizziness and faintness seven hours after delivery?

(A) Do not bring in the newborn until the mother improves.

(B) Help the patient get out of bed.

(C) Do a hematocrit and hemoglobin test.

(D) Elevate the patient's legs.

(125) What should be the first thing assessed after amniotomy?

(A) Fetal HR.

(B) Maternal BP.

(C) Distention of the bladder.

(D) Dilation of the cervix.

(126) What indicates a pregnant female is at a high risk of developing DIC?

(A) A gravida 4 who lost 300 mL of blood when she delivered in the last seven hours.

(B) A gravida 2 who has dead fetus syndrome.

(C) A primigravida who delivered four hours ago.

(D) A primigravida with mild preeclampsia.

(127) A patient on parenteral nutrition presents with crackles bilaterally, jugular vein distention, bounding pulse, increased blood pressure, and headache. What is the cause?

(A) Hyperglycemia.

(B) Hypervolemia.

(C) Air embolism.

(D) Sepsis.

(128) What is the first action when an unresponsive patient is found with no pulse and not breathing?

(A) Use a mouth-to-mask device.

(B) Perform chest compressions.

(C) Deliver oxygen.

(D) Open the airway.

(129) Which following laboratory studies could postpone surgery?

(A) Serum creatinine is 0.6.

(B) Platelets count is 2500,000.

(C) Hemoglobin is 7.5.

(D) Sodium is 138.

(130) Which of these symptoms occurs in a presbycusis patient?

(A) Sensorineural hearing loss.

(B) Conductive hearing loss.

(C) Nystagmus.

(D) Tinnitus.

(131) Which action is appropriate if an insecticide is sprayed accidentally into a patient's eye?

(A) Use diluted hydrogen peroxide to clean the eye.

(B) Refer to the emergency room.

(C) Clean the eye with water.

(D) Inform the doctor.

(132) What should be assessed in a Cushing's syndrome patient?

(A) Postural hypotension risk.

(B) Polyuria that leads to sodium and water loss.

(C) Cold intolerance.

(D) Osteoporosis.

(133) What could be prevented by the placement of a below-knee amputation patient in a prone position?

(A) Wound infection.

(B) Contracture of the hip flexor.

(C) Thrombophlebitis.

(D) Atelectasis.

(134) What is true of a cardiac murmur in a Down syndrome baby admitted to the hospital due to pneumonia?

(A) Down syndrome children have heart disorders associated with murmurs.

(B) The ductus arteriosus starts to function due to pneumonia.

(C) The murmur has on-and-off characteristics.

(D) Cardiac contractility increases with pneumonia.

(135) Which medications should be available when magnesium sulfate is administered to a patient with proteinuria, edema, and hypertension?

(A) Glucose.

(B) Phenytoin.

(C) Naloxone.

(D) Calcium gluconate.

(136) A patient who takes cyclosporine for post-renal transplantation complains of a headache. Which vital signs may occur?

(A) Pulse oximetry increase.

(B) Hypertension.

(C) Tachypnea.

(D) Tachycardia.

(137) Which laboratory tests should be done on an HIV patient who takes zidovudine?

(A) BUN level.

(B) CBC.

(C) Random blood glucose.

(D) Blood culture.

(138) What is not a risk factor for Kaposi's sarcoma?

(A) Asbestos exposure.

(B) Antineoplastic drugs.

(C) Family history.

(D) Kidney transplantation.

(139) What are the side effects of IV methocarbamol?

(A) Hypertension.

(B) Bradycardia.

(C) Rapid pulse.

(D) Tachycardia.

(140) What are the manifestations of cataracts in the early stages?

(A) Blurred vision.

(B) Floating spots.

(C) Eye pain.

(D) Diplopia.

(141) Which laboratory test results are a side effect of cyclosporine for a post-kidney transplantation patient?

(A) Decreased WBC count.

(B) Increased BUN level.

(C) Decreased hemoglobin level.

(D) Decreased serum creatinine level.

(142) What should be considered for a patient who receives tPA (tissue plasminogen activator) to treat acute myocardial infarction?

(A) Availability of heparin.

(B) Monitor for bleeding signs.

(C) Monitor psychosocial status.

(D) Monitor for renal failure.

(143) Signs of COPD acute exacerbation include:

(A) Chest X-ray shows a diaphragm widening.

(B) Oxygen saturation increases with exercise.

(C) Chest X-ray shows a hyperinflated chest.

(D) Hypocapnia.

(144) Which action can determine ballottement presence?

(A) Cervical upward tap.

(B) Check fetal movement by abdominal palpation.

(C) Check the compressibility of the cervix.

(D) Fetal heart sounds assessment.

(145) What is the appropriate action to administer medication in a suction-connected NG tube?

(A) After administration of the medication, lower the suction settings for half an hour.

(B) After administration of the medication, clamp the NG tube for half an hour.

(C) After administration of the medication, aspirate the NG tube.

(D) To help medication absorption, put the patient in a supine position.

Test 4: Answers and Explanations

(1) (C) Decreased infection risk.

There is some debate about the benefits of shaving before surgery, but the main objective is to lower the risk of infection. Shaving does not decrease postoperative itching or adhesive tape irritation and does not increase surgical field vision.

(2) (D) Booster dose of tetanus toxoid.

In this situation, a booster dose of tetanus toxoid is appropriate. The Centers for Disease Control and Prevention recommend a booster dose of tetanus toxoid in the event of a wound or burn if it has been more than five years since the last dose for dirty wounds or more than ten years for clean wounds. However, since burns can increase the risk of tetanus, it is a good idea to administer a booster dose even if the last vaccination was within five years is a prudent measure.

(3) (A) Osteoporosis.

Osteoporosis, a risk factor for a hip fracture, is brought on by various factors, such as a drop in estrogen after menopause. Progesterone drops are not factors. A decrease (not an increase) in calcium absorption is also a factor.

(4) (B) Cast integrity should be maintained.

If a patient has a cast, it is critical to maintain the integrity of the cast to ensure it effectively immobilizes the affected area and promotes healing.

(5) (D) Request immediate laboratory analysis of the stone.

The stone should be immediately submitted to the laboratory for identification. This will aid in diet plan determination. Although passing the stone might be unpleasant, the patient's discomfort normally subsides afterward. Blood or glucose are not found in stones.

(6) (C) Decrease pruritus secondary to jaundice.

Warm oatmeal baths are used to lessen the intense pruritus (itching) brought on by jaundice from pancreatic cancer. These baths are not recommended to treat paralytic ileus, fever, bloating, or feeling full.

(7) (C) It decreases colon bacterial content.

Neomycin is an antibiotic that kills gut bacteria even if it is poorly absorbed from the GIT. It should be administered before surgery to avoid peritonitis. It does not prevent pneumonia because it is not absorbed from the intestine and does not destroy germs outside of the GIT.

(8) (D) Decreased daily fluid intake.

Because Parkinson's patients tend to drool and lose liquids, fluid intake should be increased.

(9) (D) The risk is low.

Elevated HDL and decreased LDL reduce the chance of developing CAD. Elevated LDL and decreased HDL are positively connected with CAD. Exercise may raise HDL, which reduces a patient's chance of developing CAD.

(10) (C) Blood pressure will increase with the use of a narrow cuff.

An unnaturally high reading is produced by a cuff that is too narrow. An unnaturally low reading is produced by a cuff that is too wide. A cuff's width is of concern, not its length. The heartbeat is not impacted by the cuff.

(11) (C) Strengthen the pelvic floor muscles.

The pubococcygeus muscle is relaxed and tightened during Kegel exercises, which strengthens the pelvic floor. This could help prevent rectocele and cystocele. Kegel exercises have nothing to do with the breasts or the uterus.

(12) (C) Loss of tooth enamel.

Enamel erosion is an objective indication of bulimia. Subjective bulimia symptoms include feeling inadequate in social situations, feeling out of control, and low self-esteem.

(13) (D) They will deny excessive alcohol intake.

Denial is the most common response of alcohol or drug abusers who receive a poor diagnosis. When told they are alcoholics, most people do not immediately inquire about how to receive assistance. Most people do not immediately react in anger when a major disease is diagnosed.

(14) (C) Test drainage for glucose.

In transsphenoidal hypophysectomy, the pituitary gland is removed. The incision is in the mouth's upper gumline, which travels into the sphenoid sinuses. Cerebrospinal fluid that tests positive for glucose might be the cause of the mouth drainage.

(15) (D) A tracheostomy set.

The patient is in danger of airway blockage, so a tracheostomy, suction, and oxygen setup are required. A thyroidectomy patient does not require a bedside ventilator, sterile dressing set, or catheterization tray.

(16) (B) Increased blood volume.

By the conclusion of the second trimester, the pregnant woman's blood volume rises. Pregnancy causes an increase in metabolic rate. Peristalsis happens less often, and there is an increase in oxygen intake.

(17) (B) Painless, bright red vaginal bleeding.

When placenta previa occurs, the patient will experience painless bright red vaginal bleeding. Placental abruptions are characterized by a painful abdomen and uterus without vaginal bleeding or severe lower abdominal discomfort and heavy vaginal bleeding. At this stage of pregnancy, dark vaginal discharge is common.

(18) (C) Amenorrhea.

A person with anorexia nervosa usually exhibits bradycardia, minimal or no menstruation (amenorrhea), and a sluggish metabolic rate.

(19) (D) Funeral preferences.

Advance directives include decisions about the patient's medical care if they become critically sick or unable to express their preferences. They include do not resuscitate, out-of-hospital DNR, do not hospitalize, and do not intubate orders. They do not include funeral preferences.

(20) (C) Monitor the patient's swallowing reflex before he eats.

Myasthenia gravis patients are characterized by weakness in the upper body parts. Eyelid ptosis, double vision, and trouble swallowing are the main symptoms. Before the patient eats, the nurse should ensure that they can swallow and have a gag reflex.

(21) (C) Sharp pain in leg(s).

Isoniazid peripheral neuropathy, characterized by acute leg aches, is one of the drug's most common adverse effects. Ethambutol has the adverse effect of color blindness. Rimactane's side effect is orange-colored urine. Streptomycin's side effect is ototoxicity.

(22) (D) Jaundice that appears within 24 hours after birth.

Pathological jaundice occurs during the first day after birth and is the most hazardous because it results from significant liver abnormalities or blood incompatibility. Physiological jaundice develops after two days and is linked to an immature liver. Breast milk jaundice often appears 6–10 days after delivery.

(23) (D) Create a nursing care plan for the patient.

Patient advocacy is a component of healthcare that encompasses a patient's right to select the appropriate standard of care, uphold human dignity, advance patient equality, and guarantee that patients have the freedom to make their own health-related decisions. Patient advocates do not create nursing care plans.

(24) (B) Aspirin.

The new generalized and itchy rash in a six-year-old who was treated with acetaminophen and aspirin could be due to the aspirin. Aspirin is associated with Reye's syndrome in children who have recently had a viral illness like the flu. One of the symptoms of Reye's syndrome is a rash. Also, aspirin and other salicylates are known to sometimes cause hypersensitivity reactions such as rashes.

(25) (C) Seizure.

Eclampsia denotes seizure activity. The absence of fetal heart sounds is symptomatic of fetal mortality and may be linked to severe eclampsia, although it does not guarantee that eclampsia has occurred. The hallmark signs of preeclampsia include edema of the face and hands and albuminuria.

(26) (B) Serum electrolytes.

Patients with an underactive adrenal cortex or those who have undergone adrenalectomy are administered fludrocortisone acetate. Like aldosterone, it causes potassium excretion and salt and water retention. It is important to monitor serum electrolytes for sodium and potassium levels.

(27) (C) It will fall off about three weeks after birth.

Umbilical cords generally dry out and fall off one to three weeks after birth. Caretakers are advised to maintain a clean, dry cord. The use of alcohol to clean the cord is no longer advised.

(28) (C) Apply ice.

Ice helps to relieve pain in two ways: it has a numbing effect, and it helps prevent internal bleeding and edema. Topical steroids help reduce inflammation and irritation, not pain. It is important to elevate the leg and ankle. It is not advisable to exercise with a sprained ankle.

(29) (D) Back pain.

Back discomfort after a cystoscopy may be a sign of kidney damage. Leg cramps often occur due to the lithotomy position. Urine that is tea-colored or has a pink tint is common after a cystoscopy.

(30) (B) Varicose veins.

Venous stasis results from extended standing and is associated with varicose veins. Varicose veins do not occur due to extended bed rest. Complications of extended bed rest include thrombophlebitis, hypostatic pneumonia, and muscle atrophy.

(31) (D) Swollen fingers.

Edema in the face and hands is indicative of pregnancy-induced hypertension. Pregnant women often experience foot swelling because the growing fetus limits venous return in the latter stages of pregnancy, which leads to swelling of the feet and ankles.

(32) (A) Daily weight measurement.

A patient on TPN requires daily weight assessments from the nurse. A central venous line provides TPN nutrition directly into the right atrium, not the GIT, so bowel sounds, bowel movements, and NG tubes are not essential.

(33) (A) Apical pulse.

The nurse should check the patient's apical pulse before giving digoxin. The nurse should stop the medicine and call the doctor if the patient's pulse is less than 60 bpm.

(34) (B) Varicella and HiB.

The last HiB vaccination is administered between 12–15 months of age. The varicella vaccination is advised around age 12 months. MMR is administered between 12–15 months of age. The pneumonia vaccination is administered at two, four, six months, and 12–15 months.

(35) (C) Inform the patient about all his treatment options so he can choose between them freely.

The healthcare practitioner should tell the patient about the nature of his medical condition and the goals, choices, potential results, and risks associated with the suggested therapy.

(36) (D) The cells cannot reuptake insulin in type 2 DM, while the pancreas produces insufficient insulin in type 1 DM.

In type 2 DM, the cells cannot absorb insulin. In type 1 DM, the pancreas does not release enough insulin. Oral hypoglycemics are used to treat type 2 DM, and insulin is used to treat type 1 DM. However, insulin may sometimes be utilized to treat type 2 DM.

(37) (C) If the patient can lift or bend.

A herniated lumbar disc often causes sciatica, a low back pain that travels down one leg. The nurse must evaluate the patient to determine if activities that raise intraspinal pressure worsen the patient's pain.

(38) (A) Tingling and numbness in the fingers.

Finger numbness and tingling are the first signs of compartment syndrome. Other symptoms include pallor and coldness in the distal limb, pain that worsens with elevation of the limb, and pain that is unresponsive to painkillers. A late indicator is cyanosis.

(39) (C) Brachial plexus nerve injury.

The crutch tops are measured to be three finger widths apart from the axillae. This prevents the patient's axillae from resting on the crutch or carrying its weight, which might cause damage to the brachial plexus nerves.

(40) (C) Serous drainage.

At pin insertion locations, a minimal quantity of serous drainage is suspected. Infection symptoms such as discomfort, purulent discharge, and inflammation should be reported to the doctor.

(41) (B) Slurred speech.

10–20 mcg/mL of phenytoin are considered therapeutic levels. Nystagmus develops at a concentration greater than 20 mcg/mL. At levels greater than 30 mcg/mL, ataxia and slurred speech develop.

(42) (A) Voluntary movement impairment.

With high levodopa doses, reduced voluntary movement and dyskinesia are side effects. Other adverse effects include akinesia, bradycardia, orthostatic hypotension, dizziness, and anorexia.

(43) (A) Intervention planning.

Intervention planning requires clinical judgment and knowledge to design procedures or treatments to satisfy the requirements of patients.

(44) (D) Play a role in emergency rooms.

This is false. Interprofessional teams play a major role in the emergency room. They can change their viewpoints when given new information. They have an openness to learning, understand others' roles and responsibilities, and are vital to decision-making. They share goals, keep patients as their primary focus, communicate clearly, and have mutual respect.

(45) (A) Flaccid paralysis.

Flaccid paralysis is a sign of persistent spinal shock after a spinal cord injury. Spinal shock refers to the temporary loss of reflexes below the level of the injury. During this period, muscles are flaccid, and reflex activity is absent, which includes a lack of motor and sensory functionality.

(46) (A) Task-based conflict.

Task-based conflicts occur when two medical experts disagree on a particular method.

(47) (C) It uses fictitious or real-life clinical scenarios.

Case-based learning uses fictitious or real-life clinical scenarios. Feedback gives the students information about performance. Passive teaching methods include reading or lectures. The facilitator decides on the topic, organization, and speed of delivery.

(48) (D) Endotracheal suction.

Basic skills support a patient's activities of feeding, cleanliness, and daily living, as well as those that assist expert nursing evaluations. They do not include endotracheal suctioning, which is a more advanced skill. The secondary skills rely on each state's practice legislation and need extra training and proof of proficiency before they are carried out by the assistive nursing staff.

(49) (B) You should talk at a normal volume.

It is important to speak to a patient who is hard of hearing directly, in a regular tone, face-to-face with the patient. The nurse should change the volume only if the patient does not understand what is stated.

(50) (C) Put ice on the eye.

A contusion is treated right away. Ice is quickly administered. The patient should see a doctor and have a comprehensive eye examination to rule out potential injuries.

(51) (C) It is permissible to share patient information with any family member.

Unless a nurse has the patient's permission or has a legal or ethical need, patient information should not be shared with unauthorized individuals, such as the media, friends, or family members.

(52) (C) Increase the physical distance between rooms.

A lack of physical distance is a significant issue in privacy observance.

(53) (D) Chocolate, soda, and coffee.

A methylxanthine bronchodilator is a theophylline. The patient must be instructed to avoid too many xanthine-containing foods while this medicine is taken. These include chocolate, coffee, and soda.

(54) (B) Pharmacists.

Pharmacists should follow up with patients on their medications.

(55) (C) Gloves, gown, and particulate respirator.

When there is a chance that the nurse may come into contact with a patient who has TB, they should wear a gown, gloves as per normal procedures, and individually fitted particulate respirators.

(56) (B) Bronchospasm.

Bronchospasm is a serious complication that can occur after a bronchoscopy and indicates an urgent need to inform the doctor. There is a narrowing of the bronchial tubes, which can cause difficulty breathing and potentially life-threatening respiratory distress.

(57) (C) Diminished air entry and breath sounds.

Shortness of breath and chest discomfort are the main signs of a closed pneumothorax. Subcutaneous emphysema, reduced breath sounds, cyanosis, and tachypnea are symptoms of a bigger pneumothorax. An open chest injury would produce a suction sound where it occurred.

(58) (C) Relief of epigastric pain.

A patient who takes NSAIDs regularly may damage their stomach mucosa. Misoprostol, a gastric protectant, is used to stop this from happening and will provide relief from epigastric pain. Diarrhea is not an intended side effect.

(59) (B) Diarrhea.

Loperamide is used as an antidiarrheal. It may lessen the discharge from an ileostomy and treat acute and chronic diarrhea in inflammatory bowel disease.

(60) (D) Low protein.

Hepatocytes are diffusely degenerated and destroyed in cirrhosis, a chronic and progressive liver disease. Ammonia is produced as a by-product as the liver breaks down protein. A low-protein diet would be advised if the patient has hepatic encephalopathy.

(61) (B) Decrease the patient's fluid intake with meals.

The vasomotor symptoms known as dumping syndrome occur after food consumption, particularly after a Billroth II operation. Early symptoms, such as palpitations, pallor, sweating, syncope, tachycardia, and vertigo, often appear within half an hour after meals. The patient should be advised to use antispasmodic medications, lie down for half an hour after eating to delay stomach emptying, avoid foods rich in carbohydrates, and consume fewer liquids with meals.

(62) (D) A decrease in oxygen supply to the brain.

Significant blood loss can lead to decreased oxygen supply to the brain. This can cause mental status changes, which include confusion, as the brain is susceptible to changes in oxygen supply.

(63) (D) Vital signs.

A change in vital signs from baseline during the transfusion may indicate a transfusion response. Because of this, the nurse must check vital signs 15 minutes before and after.

(64) (D) Pork.

Cirrhosis patients should consume foods rich in thiamine, especially products made from pork. Legumes, whole grain cereals, and nuts are other healthy dietary sources. Folic acid and vitamins K, E, and C are in broccoli, niacin is in chicken, and vitamins B2, D, and A are in milk.

(65) (A) It is a normal value.

Between 150,000 to 400,000 cells/mm^3 is the common platelet count.

(66) (B) Pinch the tube to interrupt the flow.

When colostomy irrigation causes cramps, stop the solution flow and instruct the patient to take a deep breath. The tube does not need to be removed. A different position will not stop the cramps, and if you increase the flow of the solution, this will make the cramps worse.

(67) (A) You should put the patient in a recumbent position.

A pressure dressing should have been put on the biopsy location, and the patient should lie in bed in a recumbent position on top of the dressing. Before the surgery, an analgesic may be prescribed. Pressure should be applied to the area for several minutes.

(68) (B) Gown and gloves.

Contact precautions should be taken, which call for the carer to put on gloves and a gown to protect against wound drainage and bandages that could be contaminated. After the gloves are removed, the nurse should wash their hands with antibacterial soap before leaving the patient's room.

(69) (C) Give directions as simply as possible.

The patient may understand simple directions. Too much information may confuse them. In-depth care instructions might lead to further misunderstanding. The patient may not be able to understand what is written.

(70) (A) Upon admission.

The end of care from a healthcare organization is referred to as discharge. Planning for discharge starts at the time of admission when patient data is gathered and recorded.

(71) (A) Hypoglycemia.

The mother's hyperglycemia could cause the infant's pancreas to produce more insulin, which could rapidly deplete his sugar reserves. He has no motherly sugar after birth and is thus in danger of hypoglycemia.

(72) (D) All of the above.

Nursing reports include the patient's wounds or pressure injuries and their care, specific medical tests the next nursing shift should oversee, discharge instructions, whether the patient needs help to get up or use the restroom, the type and rate of the IV fluids received, the use of a catheter, isolation to stop the spread of illness or disease, and oxygenation needs if any are present.

(73) (B) Flexion of the knees while the patient lies on his side.

A position that opens the gaps between the vertebrae, such as on the side with the knees bent or semi-seated with the knees bent, will help the patient be most comfortable.

(74) (D) Decreased urine output.

Nephrotoxicity, a common side effect of gentamicin, and decreased urine production are signs of kidney injury. Gentamicin does not cause hypertension, orange sputum, or impaired vision. With rifampin, orange-colored secretions might appear.

(75) (D) Nourishment.

Safety and psychological needs include comfort, emotional support, low-level stress and anxiety, emotional and physical security, and environmental and medical safety. They do not include nourishment. That is a biological need.

(76) (D) Use dressings or sterile towels to cover the intestines.
To avoid infection and to keep the exposed intestines from drying and adhering, the first recommended action is to cover the intestines with a sterile cloth and hydrate with sterile normal saline.
(77) (D) Lung auscultation.
Before hygienic care is provided, the nurse should auscultate the lungs. The nurse might suggest the patient cough and breathe deeply if the patient has crackles.
(78) (D) Fidelity.

Fidelity is the obligation to fulfill one's promises.

(79) (C) Train for aseptic technique.
Peritonitis is a common side effect for those getting peritoneal dialysis. Teaching aseptic techniques is vital because the patient oversees the daily care of continuous ambulatory dialysis.
(80) (C) Decrease carbohydrate and sodium consumption.
The patient is susceptible to dumping syndrome after a gastrectomy and should have a diet rich in protein and low in simple carbs and salt. After a meal, the patient should lie down.
(81) (A) Fecal impaction.
An oil retention enema should be administered to the fecal impaction patient to soften the stool, and an hour later, a cleaning enema should be used to remove the feces. Oil retention and cleaning enemas are not indicated for straining. Melena is blood in the feces and does not require an enema. Patients with ulcerative colitis should not use enemas.
(82) (C) Special consent.
Special consent is required for the use of shackles, patient photographs, disposal of body parts after surgery, donation of organs after death, and autopsies. Admission consent is obtained at admission and outlines the healthcare agency's obligations to the patient. Surgical consent is obtained for surgical or invasive operations or diagnostic tests. Research consent is required to participate in a research project.

(83) (C) Give oxygen at a high level.

Before and after tracheostomy suction, the nurse should provide the patient with hyperoxygenation.

(84) (C) Personal attention.

Personal attention requires a person to examine ideas, feelings, strengths, weaknesses, and emotions that may impact their overall well-being and relationships with others.

(85) (D) All of the above.

Older adults in poor physical condition, with functional limitations, or who live in nursing facilities are in danger of being abused by staff, other residents, and family members.

(86) (B) Decreased platelet count.

A decreased platelet count could make it difficult for the body to form clots, which puts the patient at an increased risk for further blood loss.

(87) (D) Fraud.

Fraud is purposeful deceit designed to create illegal profits.

(88) (D) Diarrhea.

Due to its ability to reduce gastrointestinal motility and propulsion, diphenoxylate hydrochloride with atropine sulfate is given for diarrhea. It can cause hypertension and tachycardia. It can also increase depression.

(89) (D) All of the above.

Quality improvement initiatives are a methodical way to identify quality concerns, implement quality improvement activities, and monitor outcomes to guarantee that the intended results are obtained.

(90) (B) A preference for warmth.

As people age, they need a warmer atmosphere. They often have constipation. Knee and foot pain are symptoms of severe arthritis. Halos around lights might be a sign of glaucoma, which is not a normal symptom of aging.

(91) (B) Audible gurgles or high-pitched clicks in all four quadrants.

Normal bowel noises are generally high-pitched clicks or gurgles. However, the intensity and frequency of bowel sounds vary based on the stage of digestion. Loud gurgles indicate hyperperistalsis. When the intestines are under strain, such as a blockage in the digestive tract, bowel noises become louder and higher pitched.

(92) (D) Demonstrate confidence in the patient's ability to deal with stressors.

It is important for the nurse to demonstrate confidence in the patient's ability to cope with stressors. This approach helps to empower the patient and can foster a sense of self-efficacy and hope. It is important to establish a therapeutic relationship based on trust, understanding, and support. The nurse should actively listen to the patient's concerns, validate their feelings, and encourage them to express and work through their emotions in a safe environment.

(93) (A) Case studies.

Case studies are considered Level 4 evidence-based rankings.

(94) (B) That intestinal sounds are audible.

A nurse should assess the patient for audible intestinal sounds. Signs of intestinal blockage include stomach discomfort, vomiting, and distention. Nasogastric tubes may be used to relieve vomiting and abdominal distention as well as to drain the stomach of gas and liquid. As the blockage is removed and regular bowel function is resumed, bowel sounds become audible.

(95) (A) Urinary incontinence.

Skin deterioration may result from traction. Constipation may happen because of immobility, and the evaluation process may include an assessment of bowel movements. Skin traction is not associated with urinary incontinence.

(96) (D) Respiratory distress.

Rapid pulse, rashes, respiratory distress, laryngeal edema, hypotension, and the severe collapse of venules and arterioles in the circulatory system all indicate anaphylaxis and anaphylactic shock.

(97) (D) They should be taken on an empty stomach.

Iron is required for the fetus and the mother's RBC count. Iron may induce constipation and is better absorbed on an empty stomach. A great source of iron is meat.

(98) (C) PTT of 61 seconds.

PTT (normal values are 20 to 36 seconds) should be 1.5 to 2.5 times the common value. Therefore, if the patient's activated partial thromboplastin time were 61 seconds, it would be considered therapeutic.

(99) (A) Tuberculin skin test.

A mild cough that produces mucoid sputum is one of the initial lung signs of tuberculosis. The tuberculin skin test is the most accurate way to diagnose Mycobacterium tuberculosis.

(100) (B) Normal saline administration.

The main objective is to restore the patient's fluid volume and address any electrolyte deficiencies. An IV infusion of regular saline is the first step in intravenous fluid replacement, which is done similarly to DKA.

(101) (D) Acute pain.

Acute pain is the patient's top nursing diagnosis. Most patients have some pain in the first few weeks after giving birth. No information in the question suggests the existence of an unbalanced fluid volume, urine elimination, or a problem with body image.

(102) (B) 300 units/L.

Serum amylase levels should range from 25 to 151 units/L. The increase in blood amylase levels in chronic pancreatitis often doesn't exceed three times the normal amount. The value may be five times higher in cases of acute pancreatitis. Options C and D are normal, but option A represents the highly increased amount seen in acute pancreatitis.

(103) (B) Scissors.

One of the risks associated with the Sengstaken-Blakemore tube is that it might move and exert pressure on the trachea, which can lead to an emergency case of acute dyspnea. If this happens, the nurse must immediately cut the tube so the balloons deflate and the pressure on the trachea is reduced. Therefore, scissors must be close to the patient and easily accessible.

(104) (D) Maalox should be taken after meals, cimetidine with meals, and omeprazole before meals.

Omeprazole (Prilosec) should be administered before meals. Antacids like Maalox should be taken after meals. Cimetidine (Tagamet) is best taken with meals.

(105) (C) Cystitis.

An ascending urinary tract infection is pyelonephritis, as the ureters carry cystitis into the renal pelvis. Uric acid kidney stones (urolithiasis) are linked to a high uric acid diet. Acute glomerulonephritis is preceded by pharyngitis.

(106) (A) Abdominal pain in the lower right quadrant.

Abdominal discomfort in the lower right quadrant of a patient may indicate appendicitis. Someone with appendicitis should not use laxatives since they might cause colon rupture.

(107) (C) Lie on the side.

When a patient exhibits the opisthotonos position, the torso is arched forward, and the head and heels are cocked in the opposite direction. The only position that is feasible is for the patient to lie on the side.

(108) (A) CN VI.

Watch the patient's eyes follow a moving finger to determine if cranial nerve VI, also known as the abducens nerve, is appropriate. The trochlear nerve, or cranial nerve IV, controls inward and downward eye movements. The optic nerve, or CN II, controls vision.

(109) (D) The first baby will not be affected.

The mother may be exposed to the Rh factor and produce antibodies to Rh when the first Rh-positive fetus is born. The first child will be unaffected. Unless the mother receives RhoGam to prevent the production of anti-Rh antibodies after each potential exposure to Rh-negative pregnancies or losses, subsequent infants are in danger. Although intrauterine transfusions are possible, the first child will not need one.

(110) (C) HCO_3 = 10, pCO_2 = 31, and pH = 7.31.

The patient with diabetic ketoacidosis is in metabolic acidosis. Option C's low HCO_3 indicates a metabolic cause, and pH indicates acidosis. Low CO_2 levels suggest the patient's attempts to compensate by deep breathing.

(111) (D) Antiviral.

The signs and symptoms suggest shingles, which are treated with an antiviral such as acyclovir. An analgesic might also be prescribed. The other drugs are not appropriate.

(112) (D) Bismuth subsalicylate.

Black stools and a black tongue are side effects of bismuth subsalicylate chewable pills. Red meat does not make the feces black, but it tests positive for occult blood. Iron supplements cause black stools but not a black tongue. Beets may cause feces to become red, but neither broccoli nor beets will cause stools to turn black.

(113) (D) Take on an empty stomach.

This is false. Diphenhydramine is utilized as a sedative-hypnotic, anti-dyskinetic, antitussive, and antihistaminic. Use hard candies, sugarless gum, or mouth rinses to reduce dry mouth. To lessen gastrointestinal disturbance, take the medication with food or milk. Avoid activities that require mental alertness, such as driving a vehicle or using CNS depressants.

(114) (A) Chemotherapy-associated vomiting.

Metoclopramide is both an antiemetic and digestive stimulant. It is contraindicated in cases of perforation, hemorrhage, or gastrointestinal blockage since it is a gastrointestinal stimulant.

(115) (A) Electrolyte and fluid imbalance.

Fluid and electrolyte imbalance is a common post-ileostomy problem that must be constantly monitored and treated with intravenous infusions. Later in the postoperative phase, issues include folate insufficiency and fat malabsorption.

(116) (A) Check the gag reflex.

The patient's airway is examined to determine if the gag reflex has returned. The nurse must also monitor the patient's vital signs, discomfort, and temperature fluctuations, which can indicate a GIT perforation.

(117) (B) Increase the NPH insulin dose.

Blood glucose levels rise because of glucocorticoid use. During glucocorticoid treatment, patients with diabetes mellitus may need to have their insulin or oral hypoglycemic drug doses raised.

(118) (D) Decreased urinary output.

Desmopressin acts on the collection ducts of the kidney to improve their permeability to water, which leads to an increase in water reabsorption, hence the promotion of renal water conservation. The medication's therapeutic impact will be seen as reduced urine production.

(119) (A) At room temperature.

An open vial of insulin can be stored at room temperature. Most types of insulin remain stable and effective for about 28 days when kept at room temperature, which is generally considered to be between 20°C to 25°C (68°F to 77°F). Storing insulin at room temperature can also make injections more comfortable compared to administering cold insulin from the refrigerator.

(120) (D) Potassium is not restricted.

A diet high in potassium and protein and low in salt and carbs is recommended for a Cushing's syndrome patient. This diet helps rebuild wasted tissue, control hypokalemia, and reduce hypertension, edema, and weight loss.

(121) (D) Vital signs.

A tumor that produces catecholamines is a pheochromocytoma. The defining feature of pheochromocytoma is hypertension. The nursing priority is to monitor vital signs, especially blood pressure.

(122) (C) Maintain a patent airway.

Maintenance of a patent airway and oxygen administration is the first nursing intervention. Then IV fluids and thyroid hormones can be administered, vital signs can be checked, and the patient can be kept warm.

(123) (A) Low plasma bicarbonate and high glucose level.

Ketones are found in the blood and urine. In DKA, RBS is more than 250, bicarbonate is less than 15, and arterial pH is less than 7.3. If untreated, the patient may have polyuria and Kussmaul respirations.

(124) (B) Help the patient get out of bed.

During the first eight hours after delivery, orthostatic hypotension may be visible. A sensation of faintness or dizziness is a warning indicator.

(125) (A) Fetal HR.

Following amniotomy, the fetal HR is monitored to detect compression or cord prolapse. Due to the infection risk, a minimal vaginal exam will be performed once the membranes have burst. The mother's BP or bladder distention are not the first things to check after an amniotomy.

(126) (B) A gravida 2 who has dead fetus syndrome.

The DIC triggers a clotting cascade, which causes clots to develop in the microcirculation. DIC risk factors include dead fetus syndrome. A risk factor for DIC is hemorrhage. 300 mL is not a hemorrhage. Mild preeclampsia is not a risk factor for DIC.

(127) (B) Hypervolemia.

Rapid or excessive fluid administration, such as from parenteral nutrition, may cause hypervolemia. Patients who suffer from renal, cardiac, or hepatic failure are vulnerable. The signs and symptoms of the patient described in the question are consistent with hypervolemia. The increased intravascular volume raises blood pressure and pulse rate as the heart works harder to pump the excess fluid. This causes fluid to move into the alveoli, which causes lung crackles and neck vein enlargement.

(128) (D) Open the airway.

The first nursing intervention is to open the airway. Once ventilation and an open airway are established, chest compressions are initiated. Without the airway being opened, ventilation cannot be started.

(129) (C) Hemoglobin is 7.5.

All these laboratory test results fall within the normal range except for the hemoglobin. Surgery may be delayed if a patient has a low hemoglobin level.

(130) (A) Sensorineural hearing loss.

Presbycusis is a progressive sensorineural loss brought on by auditory nerve or inner ear nerve deterioration.

(131) (C) Clean the eye with water.

It is vital to flush the eye with running water for at least 20 minutes as soon as possible. The preferred cleaning solution in the emergency room is often regular saline. Never use hydrogen peroxide for eyes.

(132) (D) Osteoporosis.

Cortisol levels are elevated in Cushing's syndrome, which leads to osteoporosis. Due to elevated aldosterone levels, which promote salt and fluid retention, a patient with Cushing's syndrome will be at risk for hypertension and fluid volume excess. They also have the risk of being hot rather than cold.

(133) (B) Contractures of the hip flexor.

An extended hip in the pronated position is less likely to develop hip flexor contractures, which are a side effect after amputation of the lower limbs.

(134) (A) Down syndrome children have heart disorders associated with murmurs.

Down syndrome children are often diagnosed with heart problems.

(135) (D) Calcium gluconate.

Calcium gluconate is the antidote for magnesium poisoning. It must be immediately available to treat the respiratory depression brought on by excessive magnesium levels.

(136) (B) Hypertension.

A patient who uses cyclosporine may develop hypertension, and because this patient complains of a headache, blood pressure must be checked. Hirsutism, nephrotoxicity, and infection are among other adverse side effects.

(137) (B) CBC.

Anemia and leukopenia are two of zidovudine's frequent adverse effects. The nurse must keep an eye out for these changes in the CBC results.

(138) (A) Asbestos exposure.

An AIDS indication, Kaposi's sarcoma is vascular cancer that manifests as a skin condition. The development of Kaposi's sarcoma is unrelated to asbestos exposure. Immunosuppression is dangerous for patients who undergo antineoplastic therapy and kidney transplant recipients.

(139) (B) Bradycardia.

Methocarbamol administered intravenously has the potential to result in bradycardia and hypotension. These adverse effects need to be monitored by the nurse.

(140) (A) Blurred vision.

The main clinical symptom of a cataract is a painless progressive blurring of central vision. Early signs include a decline in color perception and mild visual haziness.

(141) (B) Increased BUN level.

Cyclosporine usage may result in nephrotoxicity, indicated by serum creatinine levels and increased BUN. The bone marrow is not suppressed by cyclosporine.

(142) (B) Monitor for bleeding signs.

The patient should be kept under observation for bleeding. Tissue plasminogen activator is a thrombolytic, and hemorrhage is a side effect of all thrombolytic drugs. The patient's psychological state and renal failure should be monitored, but these are not the most critical issues.

(143) (C) Chest X-ray shows a hyperinflated chest.

The use of respiratory accessory muscles, oxygen desaturation during exercise, dyspnea at rest and activity, hypercapnia, and hypoxemia are all clinical signs of COPD. A flattened diaphragm and a hyperinflated chest are shown on chest X-rays.

(144) (A) Cervical upward tap.

A floating structure is palpable via the ballottement method. This involves a gentle push on the object, which then rebounds. The fetus rises when the examiner softly taps up from the vagina with a finger. The examiner then feels a slight touch on the finger as the fetus sinks.

(145) (B) After administration of the medication, clamp the NG tube for half an hour.

When administering medication through a nasogastric tube that is connected to suction, it is appropriate to clamp the tube for about 30 minutes post-administration. This allows time for the medication to be absorbed in the stomach without being immediately removed by the suction.

Test 5: Questions

(1) A gastroenteritis patient has diarrhea and nausea. What treatment option is most appropriate?

(A) Administer a prochlorperazine suppository.

(B) Administer loperamide and prochlorperazine orally.

(C) Administer loperamide.

(D) Administer prochlorperazine orally.

(2) Which statement about a routine blood glucose test is accurate?

(A) You should collect blood in a vial after the finger puncture.

(B) You should use the antecubital vein in the arm to draw blood.

(C) You should use the side of the finger as the preferred puncture site.

(D) You should use the side of the thumb as the preferred puncture site.

(3) For a patient with an NG tube, which side effect would concern the nurse?

(A) Nose irritation.

(B) Sore throat.

(C) Muscle weakness.

(D) Mouth dryness.

(4) Which characteristic is most associated with an abuser?

(A) Physical ailment.

(B) Substance abuse.

(C) Positive self-esteem.

(D) Financial stability.

(5) What is the best result after a pancrelipase drug is administered?

(A) Relief from abdominal pain.

(B) Reduction in steatorrhea.

(C) Relief from heartburn.

(D) Weight loss.

(6) Who cannot serve as the executor of an advance directive?

(A) Family member.

(B) Friend.

(C) Patient's adult child.

(D) Patient's 12-year-old child.

(7) What is a side effect of desmopressin acetate?

(A) Increased urination.

(B) Weight loss.

(C) Drowsiness.

(D) Insomnia.

(8) A diabetic patient takes glimepiride. Which substances should he not consume?

(A) Carbonated beverages.

(B) Whole-grain cereals.

(C) Organ meats.

(D) Alcohol.

(9) Who is the best advocate for a patient?

(A) Family members.

(B) Doctors.

(C) Nurses.

(D) Patient's child.

(10) What is the best communication approach to tell a patient about his condition?

(A) Practitioner-centered communication.

(B) Patient-centered communication.

(C) Doctor-centered communication.

(D) None of the above.

(11) What can Rho (D) immune globulin administered to a pregnant woman after delivery protect a baby from?

(A) Rh incompatibility.

(B) Physiological jaundice.

(C) Rubella infection.

(D) Having Rh-positive blood.

(12) During a cesarean delivery assessment, which results will prompt the nurse to inform the doctor?

(A) WBC count = 13,000.

(B) Maternal heart rate = 89 bpm.

(C) Fetal heart rate = 190 bpm.

(D) Hemoglobin level = 12.5.

(13) Which course of action should a nurse take if a tracheostomy tube is accidentally dislodged?

(A) Close the tracheostomy tube site with a sterile dressing.

(B) Reinsert the tracheostomy tube with the assistance of the respiratory therapy department.

(C) Grasp the retention sutures and spread the opening.

(D) Reinsert the tracheostomy tube with the assistance of the doctor.

(14) Which statement about the administration of aspirin before surgery is false?

(A) You should check with the physician to see if aspirin should be discontinued before surgery.

(B) The patient should take aspirin until the day of surgery.

(C) Aspirin affects blood clotting.

(D) Aspirin can cause bleeding.

(15) Before a blood transfusion, a nurse checked the patient's temperature and found it to be 39°C. What is the proper course of action?

(A) Administer acetaminophen and start the transfusion.

(B) Administer antihistamine and start the transfusion.

(C) Notify the physician and delay hanging the blood.

(D) Start the transfusion.

(16) What are the side effects of IUD contraceptives?

(A) Diarrhea, decrease in breast size, and increased libido.

(B) Sleepiness.

(C) Increased activity.

(D) Weight gain, fluid retention, and nausea.

(17) When developing a nursing care plan, which of these goals is not effective?

(A) Goals should have specific time frames.

(B) Goals should be realistic.

(C) Goals should be achievable.

(D) Goals should be broad and vague.

(18) A patient is being treated for Russell's leg traction. Which area requires thorough examination?

(A) The inner side of the thigh.

(B) The popliteal area.

(C) The femoral area.

(D) The pedal area.

(19) Which management strategy is most appropriate when it is difficult to insert an indwelling catheter into a male urethra?

(A) Discontinue the indwelling catheter insertion.

(B) Use a smaller catheter.

(C) Use a straight catheter.

(D) Try another position.

(20) Which statement does not describe the function of nurses in interprofessional teams?

(A) They should report their observations on patients' current health state to colleagues.

(B) They should refuse to care for stroke patients.

(C) They should offer direct care to assigned patients throughout the day.

(D) They should learn about patients' living environment at home.

(21) An alcoholic patient arrives with confusion and tremors three days after a surgery. Which statement best describes this presentation?

(A) The patient is in severe pain.

(B) The patient is in alcohol withdrawal.

(C) This is a narcotic reaction.

(D) The patient has resumed alcohol consumption after surgery.

(22) What is a conflict that happens when two nurses have different personal values?

(A) Task-based conflict.

(B) Value-based conflict.

(C) Interpersonal-based conflict.

(D) None of the above.

(23) Which information should be given first to a diabetes mellitus type 2 patient?

(A) Diabetes complications.

(B) Insulin reaction signs.

(C) Diabetes-specific diet.

(D) Insulin self-injection information.

(24) Which statement is true about feedback methods?

(A) It gives the students information about their performance.

(B) It involves active interaction between the facilitator and the learner.

(C) It uses fictitious or real-life clinical scenarios.

(D) It gives students information through lectures or educational materials without active participation.

(25) A patient is addicted to hallucinogens. Which symptom is most likely to occur?

(A) Convulsions.

(B) Respiratory distress.

(C) Violent behavior.

(D) Severe depression.

(26) Which discharge instruction is most important for a patient with recurrent kidney uric acid stones?

(A) Take allopurinol.

(B) Stop exercise.

(C) Increase fluid intake.

(D) Increase organic meat and chicken intake.

(27) Which statement is true about secondary nursing skills?

(A) They support a patient's feeding.

(B) They support a patient's hygiene.

(C) They support a patient's daily activities.

(D) They require additional training and proof of proficiency in accordance with state practice legislation before being performed.

(28) Which statement is false about sensitivity?

(A) You should protect patients' privacy.

(B) You should establish new hospital wards or departments.

(C) You should provide information to patients in clear and intelligible language.

(D) You should allow family visits at any time.

(29) A patient was involved in a motor vehicle accident. What is a contraindication of shock position?

(A) Thrombophlebitis.

(B) Head injury.

(C) Air embolus.

(D) Long bone fractures.

(30) What is the most reliable indicator of fluid restoration?

(A) Input and output.

(B) Thirst sensation.

(C) Weight gain.

(D) Skin turgor.

(31) A patient has an appointment for a cleaning enema and an oil retention enema. Which of these statements is true?

(A) An oil retention enema should be administered after a cleansing enema for two days.

(B) They are given at the same time.

(C) A cleansing enema is given after an oil retention enema on the same day.

(D) An oil retention enema is given after a cleansing enema on the same day.

(32) Which healthcare provider should follow up on blood pressure and glucose levels?

(A) Nurses.

(B) Pharmacists.

(C) Primary care doctors.

(D) Office personnel.

(33) What best defines the movement of a patient from one unit to another within a healthcare facility?

(A) Transfer.

(B) Discharge.

(C) Follow-up.

(D) Nursing care plan.

(34) Which procedure should be performed prior to the paracentesis procedure?

(A) Administer diazepam.

(B) Empty the patient's bowels.

(C) Empty the patient's bladder.

(D) Drink enough water.

(35) Which position should a patient be placed in if they have suffered a head injury?

(A) Upright.

(B) 20-degree head elevation.

(C) Supine.

(D) Prone.

(36) What should be avoided when someone takes lovastatin?

(A) Ibuprofen.

(B) Aspirin.

(C) Grapefruit juice.

(D) Apples.

(37) A male patient receives IV fluids and complains of pain in his arm. The IV fluids were not administered, and the IV site appears blanched and cold. Which statement best describes the situation?

(A) The patient has experienced phlebitis.

(B) The patient has experienced IV fluid infiltration.

(C) The patient has experienced a common situation.

(D) The patient needs to be administered normal saline to flush the IV line.

(38) Which laboratory test should be performed before divalproex sodium is prescribed?

(A) Liver function.

(B) CBC.

(C) Pregnancy test.

(D) Urinalysis.

(39) Which haloperidol side effects demand immediate attention?

(A) Drooling.

(B) Leg cramps.

(C) Erectile dysfunction.

(D) Weight gain.

(40) Which situation requires greater attention in the postpartum unit?

(A) A woman who gave birth 20 hours ago and now has large amounts of urine and profuse sweating.

(B) A woman who asks the nurse not to bring her baby in for breastfeeding during the night.

(C) A woman with her uterine fundus 4 cm above the umbilicus after giving birth 14 hours ago.

(D) A woman with red vaginal drainage after giving birth three hours ago.

(41) A patient with a chest tube has the drainage system checked, and the nurse observes the water seal chamber is bubbling. Which course of action is appropriate?

(A) Inform the doctor.

(B) Look for air leaks.

(C) Write up the results.

(D) Modify the drainage system for the chest tube.

(42) Which statement is not necessary to prepare a nursing report?

(A) Use a structured format that helps the next nurse find the required patient information.

(B) Ensure documentation and communication of specific orders from the patient's healthcare provider.

(C) Gather relevant data throughout the shift.

(D) Craft concise reports with precise language and brief phrases.

(43) Which term best describes an individual's fundamental need for affection, a sense of community, and acceptance from others?

(A) Self-actualization.

(B) Self-esteem.

(C) Love.

(D) Safety.

(44) What is the term that represents a commitment to speak the truth?

(A) Truthfulness.

(B) Fidelity.

(C) Nonmaleficence.

(D) Paternalism.

(45) What is required for any surgical or invasive procedure?

(A) Research consent.

(B) Admission consent.

(C) Special consent.

(D) Surgical consent.

(46) When NPH insulin and normal insulin are combined, a nurse should not:

(A) Inject an air amount with the insulin dose.

(B) Inject air into NPH insulin first.

(C) Withdraw the regular insulin first.

(D) Withdraw the NPH insulin first.

(47) What is the most appropriate management step for a postpartum patient with cystitis?

(A) Hematocrit and hemoglobin tests.

(B) Perineum ice.

(C) Increased fluid intake.

(D) Sitz baths.

(48) A patient has been issued an NPO. Which medication should still be given to the patient prior to surgery?

(A) Conjugated estrogen.

(B) Cyclobenzaprine.

(C) Ferrous sulfate.

(D) Prednisone.

(49) Which parameters should be evaluated during home parenteral feeding?

(A) Blood pressure and temperature.

(B) Blood pressure and pulse.

(C) Weight and temperature.

(D) Weight and pulse.

(50) Which statement about vasectomy surgery is correct?

(A) It is associated with intermittent impotence.

(B) The procedure usually lasts around two hours.

(C) It is permanent contraception.

(D) It is not a tubal ligation surgery.

(51) What is a complication of myelomeningocele repair?

(A) Hydrocephalus.

(B) Hypertension.

(C) Hypoxemia.

(D) Hyperactive bowel sounds.

(52) What is not a complication of chlamydial infection during pregnancy?

(A) Congenital anomalies.

(B) Pregnancy-induced hypertension.

(C) Neonatal ophthalmia.

(D) Transplacental infection

(53) Which metric is used to analyze how long it takes for a doctor to visit a patient?

(A) Balance metric.

(B) Outcome metric.

(C) In-process metric.

(D) Structural metric.

(54) What is the best activity to prevent venous stasis in immobile patients?

(A) Turn the patient often.

(B) Anti-embolism stockings.

(C) ROM exercises.

(D) Coughing and deep breathing exercises.

(55) Which of these areas should you clean first in elderly individuals?

(A) Hands.

(B) Upper torso.

(C) Face.

(D) Perineal area.

(56) An eight-year-old boy displays symptoms of increased eating, drinking, and frequent urination without fever. What is the first step in his case management?

(A) Urine culture and sensitivity.

(B) IV pyelogram.

(C) Fingerstick and urine glucose test.

(D) CBC.

(57) The patient has a dark complexion. Which diagnostic step is most accurate for assessing jaundice?"

(A) Check the fingers.

(B) Examine the nail beds.

(C) Examine the sclera.

(D) Examine the stool for color change.

(58) Which suggestion is helpful for nurses to overcome barriers and problems they face while providing care?

(A) Seek assistance.

(B) Work on self-compassion.

(C) Create a plan to enhance self-care.

(D) All of the above.

(59) A patient has a ventricular pacemaker. Which of these cases should concern the nurse?

(A) The patient does not feel his heartbeat.

(B) Before the QRS complex, there is a spike.

(C) The heart rate is 53 beats/minute.

(D) The blood pressure is 124/75.

(60) Which healthcare behavior is not a cause for complaint?

(A) Disrespect.

(B) Failure to provide the patient with adequate information.

(C) The provision of inadequate care.

(D) Failure to provide the patient's family with adequate information.

(61) A 60-year-old widowed female patient displays anxiety and fear during an examination. She has bruises and mentions that she fell down. Which types of abuse best characterizes her situation or behavior?

(A) Physical abuse.

(B) Social abuse.

(C) Financial abuse.

(D) Psychological abuse.

(62) An HIV-positive patient's menstrual blood is on the floor. Which chemical must the nurse use to mop the floor?

(A) Ammonia.

(B) Betadine.

(C) Hydrogen peroxide.

(D) Chlorine bleach.

(63) Which therapeutic strategies are most effective to prevent the risk of pulmonary emboli and DVT?

(A) Restrict fluid intake.

(B) Place cushions below the knee.

(C) Perform ROM exercises.

(D) Apply a heating pad to the lower limbs.

(64) What is the desired outcome of levothyroxine?

(A) Relieve depression.

(B) Increased blood glucose levels.

(C) Thyroid hormones return to normal levels.

(D) Increased energy levels.

(65) A patient will undergo a transsphenoidal hypophysectomy. Which directive is the most important?

(A) Inform the patient about spinal anesthesia.

(B) Tell the patient to postpone teeth brushing until 15 days after surgery.

(C) Emphasize the importance of coughing and deep breathing after surgery.

(D) Shave the patient's hair.

(66) What word describes a dangerous or offensive touch?

(A) Assault.

(B) Battery.

(C) Defamation.

(D) Fraud.

(67) What is an indication of a proper therapeutic level of buspirone?

(A) Delusions.

(B) Symptoms of alcohol withdrawal.

(C) Anxiety or tachycardia.

(D) Paranoia.

(68) Which instruction is most appropriate for a patient who takes Risperidone?

(A) Move slowly when positions are changed.

(B) Drive with caution.

(C) Avoid high-potassium foods.

(D) Limit exposure to sunlight.

(69) What is a benefit of hospital quality improvement initiatives?

(A) It satisfies regulatory standards.

(B) It simplifies operations.

(C) It enhances patient care.

(D) All of the above.

(70) Which statement is correct when a nurse applies eye ointment and eye drops?

(A) He should wait for 15 minutes after the eye ointment and then use the eye drops.

(B) He should wait for 15 minutes after the eye drops and then use the eye ointment.

(C) He should immediately administer the eye drops after the eye ointment.

(D) He should immediately administer the eye ointment after the eye drops.

(71) What is a potential side effect of betaxolol hydrochloride eye drops for a glaucoma patient?

(A) Hyperglycemia.

(B) Sleepiness.

(C) Hypotension.

(D) Fever.

(72) What is the recommended position for a patient with hyphemia after an automobile accident?

(A) Laterally on the unaffected side.

(B) Laterally on the affected side.

(C) The semi-Fowler’s position.

(D) Flat.

(73) What is an evidence-based Level 5 ranking?

(A) Expert judgment.

(B) Case-control studies.

(C) Cohort studies.

(D) Meta-analysis.

(74) What is the primary purpose of pursed-lip breathing in COPD patients?

(A) Elimination of carbon dioxide.

(B) Strengthen intercostal muscles.

(C) Strengthen the diaphragm.

(D) Increased oxygen intake.

(75) A well-controlled diabetic patient takes a daily dose of glyburide. Which medication can lead to a sudden increase in the FBS (fasting blood sugar) level to 220 mg/dL?

(A) Allopurinol.

(B) Atenolol.

(C) Phenelzine.

(D) Prednisone.

(76) Which statement about adult cardiopulmonary resuscitation is correct?

(A) You should check for visible chest rise after each rescue breath that is given over one second.

(B) You should administer two rapid breaths.

(C) You should provide two quick breaths for every 15 compressions.

(D) You should deliver two breaths for every 15 compressions.

(77) Which statement is associated with HSV-1 in a male patient with nose and mouth lesions?

(A) It can be transmitted through sneezes and coughs.

(B) If the patient has a fever, fever blisters will occur.

(C) It can be transmitted through kisses.

(D) It is not infectious.

(78) Which reason will prompt a doctor to prescribe IV mannitol after a cerebrovascular accident?

(A) Decreased muscle spasms.

(B) Decreased blood pressure.

(C) Clot dissolution.

(D) Increased urine output.

(79) Which suggestion could help a sleep-deprived patient?

(A) Drink warm milk.

(B) Watch television.

(C) Drink a cup of soda.

(D) Exercise before bedtime.

(80) Which activity is most effective to prevent muscle atrophy in a bedridden patient?

(A) Active exercises.

(B) Frequent position changes.

(C) Patient turning.

(D) ROM exercises.

(81) Which condition should be evaluated after a complete thyroidectomy?

(A) Mental confusion.

(B) Reflex loss.

(C) Hypercalcemia signs.

(D) Hoarseness.

(82) Which nursing care practice is not correct for a patient with dentures and a hearing aid?

(A) Use a wet cloth to wipe the hearing aid's exterior surface.

(B) Use alcohol to wipe the hearing aid's exterior surface.

(C) Clean the dentures with toothpaste.

(D) Brush the dentures and put them in a washcloth by the sink.

(83) A five-month-old baby has a fever and a non-itchy, blanchable skin rash. Which medication is recommended?

(A) Antibiotics.

(B) Acetaminophen.

(C) Ibuprofen.

(D) Aspirin.

(84) Which statement about the drainage color of postoperative thoracic surgery patients with chest tubes is correct?

(A) Small clots and blood.

(B) Bloody.

(C) Serosanguineous.

(D) Serous.

(85) What is the correct position for a lumbar puncture?

(A) Face up on an incline between 15 and 30 degrees to raise the legs higher than the head.

(B) Flat on the abdomen with the feet extended.

(C) On one side, with a pillow placed under the hip.

(D) On one side with the legs pulled up and the head bent.

(86) What is a side effect of fluoxetine?

(A) Excessive perspiration.

(B) Dry mouth.

(C) Gastrointestinal dysfunction.

(D) Cardiovascular problems.

(87) Which statement about oxazepam administration is correct?

(A) The patient should take an antidiarrheal drug if diarrhea occurs.

(B) The patient should rest if tachycardia develops.

(C) The patient should increase dietary fiber and fluid intake.

(D) The patient should consume more low-fiber foods.

(88) Which elevated laboratory test indicates that an HIV patient should discontinue didanosine?

(A) Serum creatinine level.

(B) Serum amylase level.

(C) Blood glucose level.

(D) Serum protein level.

(89) Which statement about Lyme disease is correct?

(A) It is transmitted through the inhalation of bird droppings.

(B) It is transmitted through direct skin contact with an infected person.

(C) It is transmitted through cat feces.

(D) It is transmitted through deer ticks.

(90) What is a sign of SLE?

(A) Cheek and nose bridge rash.

(B) Increased RBC count.

(C) Subnormal temperature.

(D) Weight gain.

(91) Which laboratory test result indicates gout?

(A) Phosphorus level = 4 mg/dL.

(B) Potassium level = 3.6 mEq/L.

(C) Uric acid level = 9.5 mg/dL.

(D) Calcium level = 10.2 mg/dL.

(92) What statement is not true about crutch safety?

(A) The tips of the crutch should be inspected for wear.

(B) Spare crutches should be available.

(C) The tips of the crutch can be wet and still not slip.

(D) Never use anyone else’s crutches.

(93) Which laboratory values represent acetaminophen toxicity after daily use?

(A) Platelet count= 350,000/mm3.

(B) Direct bilirubin level = 3.1 mg/dL.

(C) Prothrombin time = 11 seconds.

(D) Sodium level = 139 mEq/L.

(94) What symptom may manifest during limbic system neurological deficit assessment?

(A) The patient cannot subtract or add.

(B) The patient cannot remember what he ate today for breakfast.

(C) The patient has emotional lability and flat affect.

(D) The patient is disoriented to time, place, and person.

(95) What should a myasthenia gravis patient do to avoid cholinergic and myasthenic crises?

(A) Take the drugs on time to maintain therapeutic blood levels.

(B) Do all daily tasks early before fatigue happens.

(C) Do daily muscle-strengthening exercises.

(D) Eat large, well-balanced meals.

(96) What medical condition warrants the discontinuation of oxytocin labor induction?

(A) Fetal HR early deceleration.

(B) Uterine hyperstimulation.

(C) Drowsiness.

(D) Fatigue.

(97) Which therapeutic action is appropriate if fetal distress occurs during cesarean birth preparation?

(A) Administer oxygen via face mask at a rate of 8–10 L/min.

(B) Administer oxytocin intravenously.

(C) Place the patient in a high Fowler's position.

(D) Reduce the IV flow rate.

(98) What is the correct course of action when a patient develops dyspnea and cough during NG tube insertion?

(A) Pull back the NG tube and attempt insertion after the dyspnea resolves.

(B) Remove the NG tube and attempt insertion after the dyspnea resolves.

(C) Notify the doctor.

(D) Proceed with the NG tube insertion immediately.

(99) Why would a nurse place a post-myelogram patient in a semi-reclined position?

(A) To facilitate dye excretion.

(B) To prevent seizures.

(C) To prevent headaches.

(D) To prevent infection.

(100) A patient with urolithiasis has a:

(A) Risk of infection.

(B) Risk of ineffective health maintenance.

(C) Diarrhea.

(D) Acute pain.

(101) Which factor causes the urine output of a postoperative cardiac surgery patient to become 18 L?

(A) Diuresis.

(B) Inadequate fluid replacement.

(C) Inadequate cardiac output.

(D) Hyperkalemia.

(102) A 12-year-old boy's left knee swells due to hemophilia. What should be included in his care plan?

(A) Prevent hemarthrosis with 500 mL of fluid hourly.

(B) Use a bed cradle to decrease the pain.

(C) Do frequent ambulation.

(D) Do ROM exercises.

(103) To assess a newborn with a low-positioned ear, which action is appropriate?

(A) Inform the doctor.

(B) Conduct hearing tests.

(C) Record the findings.

(D) Apply gauze pads to cover the ear.

(104) A patient with schizophrenia who is on antipsychotic medication exhibits symptoms like grimaces, tongue protrusion, and mouth movements. What is a probable diagnosis?

(A) Neuroleptic malignant syndrome.

(B) Hypertensive crisis.

(C) Tardive dyskinesia.

(D) Parkinsonism.

(105) Which laboratory test is utilized to identify side effects of clozapine in a schizophrenia patient?

(A) Liver function tests.

(B) WBC count.

(C) Blood glucose level.

(D) Platelet count.

(106) A patient with AIDS treated with pentamidine for a Pneumocystis jirovecii infection presents with a body temperature of 39°C. What is a probable reason for this elevated temperature?

(A) Pentamidine may cause leukopenia, which leads to another infection.

(B) It could be a result of inadequate thermoregulation.

(C) There might be pentamidine toxicity involved.

(D) The dosage of pentamidine may be insufficient.

(107) Which test is the most appropriate to monitor the potential side effects of dantrolene sodium?

(A) Liver function test.

(B) BUN tests.

(C) CBC.

(D) Serum creatinine level.

(108) Which symptom will not occur with trimethoprim-sulfamethoxazole treatment?

(A) Sore throat.

(B) Headache.

(C) Diarrhea.

(D) Nausea.

(109) What is an indication of stoma prolapse after colostomy?

(A) Bluish-colored and dark stoma.

(B) Flattened and narrowed stoma.

(C) Hidden and sunken stoma.

(D) Stoma that protrudes.

(110) What could be a complication found during an assessment of a pheochromocytoma patient?

(A) Irregular heart rate.

(B) BUN= 19.

(C) Urinary output= 60 mL/hour.

(D) Coagulation time of six minutes.

(111) What should be monitored during the care of a placenta previa case?

(A) DIC.

(B) Chronic hypertension.

(C) Hemorrhage.

(D) Infection.

(112) What is the primary long-term goal in the management of a woman who has experienced domestic violence?

(A) Make the abuser accountable.

(B) Discuss her behavior.

(C) Empower her to feel like a survivor.

(D) Establish a long-term support network.

(113) What is the best explanation for a non-bubbled underwater seal compartment three hours after chest tube insertion?

(A) No suction has been applied.

(B) The drainage system has an air leak.

(C) The tube from the pleural cavity is blocked.

(D) The lung has re-expanded again.

(114) Which symptom will appear in a diabetic ketoacidosis patient?

(A) Red rash.

(B) Constipation.

(C) Foul breath.

(D) Deep respirations.

(115) Which site is the most suitable to assess jaundice?

(A) Ear canal.

(B) Sacral area.

(C) Abdominal area.

(D) Nail bed.

(116) Which sign suggests that a patient has bupropion toxicity?

(A) Dizziness.

(B) Increased weight.

(C) Seizures.

(D) Diarrhea.

(117) Which statement correctly describes the administration of sertraline?

(A) It can be taken as needed for depression.

(B) It should be divided into three doses.

(C) It should be taken in the evening at the same time.

(D) It should be taken on an empty stomach.

(118) Which instruction is given for the use of saquinavir in an HIV patient?

(A) Take on an empty stomach.

(B) Consume a low-fat diet.

(C) Consume a low-calorie diet.

(D) Avoid exposure to direct sunlight.

(119) Which group is at the greatest risk of a latex allergy?

(A) Group home residents.

(B) Children at day cares.

(C) Homeless individuals.

(D) Hairdressers.

(120) Which evaluation should be done after post-spinal fusion surgery?

(A) Pain during deep-breathing exercises or coughing.

(B) Observation of surgical dressing for signs of old blood.

(C) Assessment of discomfort when the patient is repositioned.

(D) Monitor for a temperature of 39°C.

(121) What is recommended for multiple trauma patients with plaster casts on their leg fractures?

(A) Continuously elevated the leg for two days.

(B) Elevate the legs for three hours.

(C) Elevate the legs for five hours, then keep them in a flat position.

(D) Keep the legs in a flat position.

(122) Which measure is recommended for postoperative knee arthroscopy patients to prevent complications?

(A) Don't eat until the end of the day after surgery.

(B) Inform the doctor if inflammation or fever occurs.

(C) Avoid putting weight on the affected leg until the day after surgery.

(D) Begin regular exercises the day after surgery.

(123) Which of these could be used for patient identity verification?

(A) Two-factor authentication.

(B) Driver's license.

(C) ID photos.

(D) All of the above.

(124) Which medication can cause a “roar” heard by a gastrointestinal bleeding patient?

(A) Diltiazem hydrochloride.

(B) Atropine sulfate.

(C) Acetylsalicylic acid.

(D) Doxycycline.

(125) What is the first step in care management for a patient who presents with a wooden piece stuck in the eye?

(A) Use a sterile clamp to remove the wood from the eye.

(B) Clean the eye with water.

(C) Conduct tests for visual acuity.

(D) Cover the eye with a patch.

(126) Which condition is an indication for the use of propylthiouracil?

(A) Cushing’s syndrome.

(B) Addison’s disease.

(C) Graves’s disease.

(D) Myxedema.

(127) What is true about pheochromocytoma?

(A) Excessive release of catecholamines occurs.

(B) A complete cure depends on the symptoms.

(C) It is associated with severe hypoglycemia.

(D) It is associated with severe hypotension.

(128) Which PPE precaution can be taken to reduce the risk of hepatitis B transmission from a positive mother to her fetus?

(A) Use gloves before mealtime and wash hands before and after perineum self-care.

(B) Check the formula temperature before starting feeding.

(C) Hold the infant properly during feeding.

(D) Close the window before feeding.

(129) What is the reason a nurse would check an infant's nose for patency after delivery?

(A) To detect increased respirations.

(B) To detect apnea.

(C) Because infants are obligate nose breathers.

(D) Because infants are unable to sneeze.

(130) A patient arrives at the ER hyperventilating, shaking, and anxious after being assaulted. What should a nurse do first?

(A) Initiate relaxation techniques.

(B) Stay with the patient until his anxiety levels drop.

(C) Provide the patient with a quiet, solitary environment to reduce stimulation.

(D) Prompt the patient to talk about the attack.

(131) Amikacin is prescribed for a bacterial infection. What is a possible side effect?

(A) Muscle aches.

(B) Hearing loss.

(C) Lethargy.

(D) Nausea.

(132) What should be assessed during etanercept administration for the treatment of rheumatoid arthritis?

(A) Loss of appetite and a metallic taste in the mouth.

(B) Joint pain and fatigue.

(C) Platelet and WBC count.

(D) Edema and itching at the site of injection.

(133) What is the appropriate action in cases of a suspected limb fracture?

(A) Do not move the affected limb.

(B) Discharge the patient from the ER and advise them to follow up in the clinic.

(C) Assist the patient to walk.

(D) Attempt manual reduction of the fracture.

(134) What is true about cerebrospinal fluid?

(A) It tests positive for glucose and separates into concentric rings.

(B) It has a pH of 7 and clumps together on the dressing.

(C) It has a pH of 6 and is bloody.

(D) It tests negative for glucose and is clear.

(135) What best describes the mechanism of action of cyclopentolate eye drops?

(A) Pupil constriction.

(B) Eye lubrication.

(C) Pupil dilation.

(D) Miosis.

(136) Which symptom is associated with rib fracture?

(A) Pain during inspiration.

(B) Paradoxical respirations.

(C) Deep rapid respirations.

(D) Deep slow respirations.

(137) A post-hypophysectomy patient has a clear nasal discharge. Which action is the most appropriate for the nurse to take?

(A) Monitor the discharge.

(B) Culture the discharge.

(C) Test the discharge for glucose.

(D) Lower the head of the bed.

(138) A patient has undergone a lumbar laminectomy. What should the nurse evaluate?

(A) Abdominal muscle strength.

(B) Ability to swallow.

(C) Foot strength.

(D) Hand grips.

(139) Which precaution is most appropriate when a patient takes phenobarbitals?

(A) Avoid alcohol consumption.

(B) Use a pill container to prevent missed doses.

(C) Take at consistent times each day.

(D) Take the medication with meals.

(140) A diabetic patient has undergone a below-knee right leg amputation. Which aspect of their history should be assessed?

(A) Separation of wound edges.

(B) Incision redness.

(C) Stump edema.

(D) Hemorrhage.

(141) What is the best way to minimize the systemic effects of eye drops?

(A) Have the patient close the nasolacrimal duct at the inner canthus with a finger for a minute after administration of the drops.

(B) Have the patient blink repeatedly after administration of the eye drops.

(C) Have the patient swallow repeatedly after administration of the eye drops.

(D) Have the patient administer the eye drops before a meal.

(142) A patient takes levothyroxine. He should monitor himself for:

(A) Dry skin.

(B) Cold intolerance.

(C) Tremors.

(D) Fatigue.

(143) A patient has been physically abused. What is a nursing care priority?

(A) Have his family member begin treatment.

(B) Remove the patient from the abusive situation.

(C) Check to see if the abuser is a family member.

(D) Report the abuse.

(144) What is an acetaminophen antidote?

(A) Acetylcysteine.

(B) Fludarabine.

(C) Auranofin.

(D) Pentostatin.

(145) What is a contraindication for the use of terbutaline?

(A) Polycystic ovary disease.

(B) Diabetes mellitus.

(C) Hypothyroidism.

(D) Osteoarthritis.

Test 5: Answers and Explanations

(1) (B) Administer Loperamide and prochlorperazine orally.

Prochlorperazine, an antiemetic drug, is commonly used to treat nausea and vomiting. In this case, since the patient has nausea and diarrhea, it is important to address both symptoms. The patient should be advised to take Prochlorperazine orally for the nausea. To address diarrhea, the doctor will prescribe Loperamide, an antidiarrheal medication that helps reduce symptoms because it slows down bowel movements and promotes better absorption of fluids.

(2) (C) You should use the side of the finger as the preferred puncture site.

To measure blood glucose levels, the side of the finger is recommended due to its fewer pain receptors compared to the thumb and its suitability for collecting a small drop of blood for the test strip.

(3) (C) Muscle weakness.

An NG tube is connected to a drainage system that removes potassium and salt from the body. Common side effects of an NG tube include nose irritation, sore throat, dry mouth, and muscle weakness. Muscle weakness could be indicative of a more serious issue, such as hypokalemia.

(4) (B) Substance abuse.

People who display aggression and mistreat others often have a tendency to struggle with substance abuse, which can exacerbate the issue. Other factors are not as strongly associated with abusers. Typically, abuse manifests in individuals who face financial stress and have low self-esteem. There is generally no direct connection between abusers and specific health problems.

(5) (B) Reduction in steatorrhea.

Pancrelipase is a medication used to treat pancreatitis. It assists in the digestion and absorption of nutrients in the digestive system, which leads to a reduction in steatorrhea and an improvement in nutritional status. It is not intended for the alleviation of heartburn or gastrointestinal discomfort, nor is it associated with weight loss. In fact, it may even contribute to weight gain due to improved nutrient absorption.

(6) (D) Patient's 12-year-old child.
In the absence of an advance directive, the patient's state-of-residence laws will determine who has the authority to make medical decisions. The designated person must be of legal age or have the legal capacity to make such decisions. The patient's 12-year-old child wouldn't qualify. If the patient's children are adults, this authority may fall to their parents, partners, or spouses based on the specific laws and regulations in that state.

(7) (C) Drowsiness.
Desmopressin acetate is commonly used to treat illnesses characterized by excessive fluid. It can also cause overhydration in some situations, particularly if not taken as prescribed. Early signs of overhydration include headache, drowsiness, seizures, rapid weight gain, and decreased urine production.

(8) (D) Alcohol.
Glimepiride may cause a disulfiram-like response when taken with alcohol. This reaction can include symptoms such as nausea, palpitations, flushing, and an overall feeling of discomfort. Furthermore, alcohol can enhance the hypoglycemic (low blood sugar) effects of glimepiride, which leads to a more significant drop in blood sugar levels. This can be dangerous for individuals with diabetes.

(9) (C) Nurses.
Regardless of their position, everyone in the medical industry must advocate for the rights of patients. However, since they spend so much time with their patients, nurses are often seen as patients' primary advocates.

(10) (B) Patient-centered communication.
In a hospital, expressed consent occurs when written or spoken approval is granted for a specific medical procedure or operation. The patient is informed about their medical condition and presented with treatment options. The patient can either choose to proceed with the recommended therapy or decline it. This process ensures that patients are fully informed and have the autonomy to make choices about their treatment.

(11) (A) Rh incompatibility.

Sensitization occurs when an Rh-negative mother becomes pregnant with an Rh-positive fetus. Fetal Rh-positive blood cells can enter the mother's circulation during pregnancy, especially during childbirth. If this exposure occurs, the mother's immune system may produce antibodies against the Rh-positive blood cells. To prevent Rh incompatibility in future pregnancies, Rho (D) immune globulin, commonly known as Rhogam, is administered to a woman after delivery.

(12) (C) Fetal heart rate = 190 bpm.

A fetal heart rate of 190 bpm is unusually high, and it could be a cause for concern. The nurse should promptly inform the doctor so that further evaluation and appropriate intervention can be initiated to ensure the health of both the mother and the baby.

(13) (C) Grasp the retention sutures and spread the opening.

If a tracheostomy tube is dislodged, it is important for a nurse to respond appropriately. The nurse should gently grasp the retention sutures and stabilize the aperture to temporarily help maintain the airway. If agency policy allows, the nurse should then attempt to replace the tube as soon as possible.

(14) (B) The patient should take aspirin until the day of surgery.

This is false. Anticoagulants, such as aspirin, interfere with natural clotting mechanisms and can increase the risk of postoperative bleeding. It is generally recommended to stop aspirin at least 48 hours before surgery to allow the effects of the medication to wear off and reduce the risk of excessive bleeding during and after the surgical procedure.

(15) (C) Notify the physician and delay hanging the blood.

The doctor is likely to prescribe the administration of blood, regardless of the patient's temperature. However, it is important to note that this decision is beyond the nurse's scope of practice. The nurse must always obtain a doctor's prescription before proceeding with a blood transfusion.

(16) (D) Weight gain, fluid retention, and nausea.

IUDs are long-term contraceptive methods. Common side effects associated with certain types of IUDs can include weight gain, fluid retention, and nausea. Some IUDs that release hormones might cause these symptoms. The other options listed are not usually associated with IUDs.

(17) (D) Goals should be broad and vague.

Broad and ambiguous goals can be less effective because they may not provide the necessary specificity to achieve the desired patient outcomes.

(18) (B) The popliteal area.

The popliteal area is vital to examine in Russell's traction due to the band around it, which can impact circulation if not monitored. It is important to ensure proper blood flow to the lower leg. Though it's generally important to assess all areas mentioned (inner side of the thigh, femoral area, and pedal area) as part of a comprehensive patient assessment, the popliteal area demands particular attention due to the traction mechanism's placement.

(19) (A) Discontinue the indwelling catheter insertion.

If there is trouble during catheter insertion, it is essential to discontinue the procedure and inform the doctor. This approach prioritizes patient safety and ensures that the healthcare provider can assess the situation and determine the best course of action. The other options may not only be ineffective but could also potentially harm the patient.

(20) (B) They should refuse to care for stroke patients.

This is false. Individuals with complicated physical challenges, limited mobility, or neurological disorders, such as stroke patients, must be moved frequently to prevent pressure ulcers. Specific instructions and training are provided to nurses to execute safe moving and handling procedures.

(21) (B) The patient is in alcohol withdrawal.

Alcohol withdrawal symptoms, such as confusion and tremors, can occur in individuals who are dependent on alcohol and abruptly stop or reduce their alcohol intake. It is important to recognize these symptoms and provide appropriate care and support to manage alcohol withdrawal safely.

(22) (B) Value-based conflict.

Value-based conflict in a healthcare setting often occurs when two healthcare professionals have different personal values, beliefs, or ethical principles. These differences can lead to disagreements or conflicts in patient care approaches and decision-making.

(23) (C) Diabetes-specific diet.

The dietary guidelines are often the first step in the management of Type 2 diabetes and can be addressed with all patients, regardless of their specific treatment plan. Other options, like diabetes complications, insulin reaction signs, and insulin self-injection, may be important, but they are more relevant to patients with Type 1 diabetes or those with advanced Type 2 diabetes who require insulin therapy.

(24) (A) It gives the students information about their performance.

Feedback provides students with information about their performance. Case-based learning involves the use of fictitious or real-life clinical scenarios. The active teaching method involves interaction, discussion, collaboration, and hands-on activities. The passive teaching method, on the other hand, gives information to the students with the use of reading materials and lectures without active participation.

(25) (C) Violent behavior.

People who use hallucinogens are more prone to exhibit violent behavior. For instance, if they are confined to a bed, they might display violent tendencies due to the belief that they possess the ability to fly. These behaviors are characteristic of hallucinogen use, whereas other options are not usually associated with it.

(26) (C) Increase fluid intake.

The best advice for patients with uric acid nephrolithiasis is to increase their fluid intake. This recommendation aims to dilute the urine and reduce the risk of uric acid stone formation.

(27) (D) They require additional training and proof of proficiency in accordance with state practice legislation before being performed.

The secondary skills are those that depend on state-specific practice regulations and require additional training and evidence of competence before assistive nursing staff can perform them.

(28) (D) You should allow family visits at any time.

This is false. Sensitivity refers to the ability to interact with empathy, respect, and understanding. In a hospital setting, it is of utmost importance.

(29) (B) Head injury.

The shock position should not be used in patients with head injuries since it raises intracranial pressure.

(30) (A) Input and output.

The most reliable indicator of fluid restoration is the measurement of input and output. This refers to closely monitoring the amount of fluid a patient takes in (input) and the amount they excrete (output), including urine, vomit, and other forms of fluid loss. Maintaining a balance between these two is necessary for assessing fluid restoration.

(31) (C) A cleansing enema is given after an oil retention enema on the same day.

An oil retention enema is initially administered to soften the feces, and approximately an hour later, a cleansing enema is given to aid in feces elimination. Other answer options are not standard procedures in this context.

(32) (A) Nurses.

Nurses and medical assistants measure blood pressure and blood glucose levels, provide education on healthy habits, and evaluate medication compliance. Pharmacists monitor and communicate with patients about their medication regimens. In situations that involve sensitive issues, the primary care doctor may be called upon to provide additional follow-up and care. This collaborative approach ensures comprehensive patient care.

(33) (A) Transfer.

In this context, “transfer” refers to the movement of a patient from one unit or department to another within the same healthcare facility, such as from a general medical unit to a surgical unit or from the emergency department to an intensive care unit, without the patient being discharged and sent home.

(34) (C) Empty the patient’s bladder.

Prior to a paracentesis procedure, it is important to empty the patient’s bladder. This helps ensure the comfort of the patient during the procedure and reduces the risk of accidental bladder puncture during the paracentesis.

(35) (B) 20-degree head elevation.

The ideal position for a patient with a head injury is a 20-degree head elevation, often referred to as the "head-up" position. This position can help reduce intracranial pressure (ICP) and improve cerebral perfusion in patients with head injuries. Other positions may not be suitable for patients with head injuries as they could potentially worsen ICP or interfere with proper airway management.

(36) (C) Grapefruit juice.

Grapefruit juice can interfere with the metabolism of certain statin medications, such as lovastatin. This can lead to elevated levels of the medication in the bloodstream, which increases the risk of side effects. As for apples, aspirin, and ibuprofen, these substances do not usually have significant interactions with lovastatin. They are not known to interfere with the metabolism of this medication.

(37) (B) The patient has experienced IV fluid infiltration.

Fluids have leaked into the surrounding tissue, which causes the IV site to appear blanched and cold. Phlebitis involves inflammation of the vein and may present with redness and pain at the IV site but not necessarily blanching or coldness.

(38) (C) Pregnancy test.

Depakote (divalproex sodium) is contraindicated during pregnancy due to the significant risk of fetal harm. Liver function tests may be performed during treatment if there are signs of toxicity, but they are not usually required. The choice of tests may depend on the patient's specific medical history and clinical circumstances.

(39) (B) Leg cramps.

Leg cramps, which can be a manifestation of extrapyramidal symptoms (EPS) associated with medications like haloperidol, demand immediate attention and notification to healthcare providers. EPS can be uncomfortable and require management, often with medications like benztropine. Drooling, weight gain, and erection disorders can occur as side effects of medications like haloperidol, but they are generally not considered as immediately concerning as EPS.

(40) (C) A woman with her uterine fundus 4 cm above the umbilicus after giving birth 14 hours ago.

A uterine fundus that is 4 cm above the umbilicus, especially 14 hours after giving birth, can be a sign of uterine atony or incomplete contraction of the uterus. This can lead to postpartum hemorrhage. This is a potentially serious medical condition and demands immediate attention and intervention.

(41) (B) Look for air leaks.

Bubbling in the water seal chamber of a chest tube drainage system may indicate an air leak. The nurse should first inspect the system to determine the source of the leak, starting at the patient and working down the tubing to the drainage system. If a leak is found, it should be corrected. Continuous bubbling is a cause for concern, while intermittent bubbling can be normal, especially if it's associated with inspiration. If the nurse cannot identify or rectify the source of the leak, then the doctor should be informed.

(42) (B) Ensure documentation and communication of specific orders from the patient's healthcare provider.

It is important to use a structure for nursing reports that makes it simple for the nurse on duty to locate the patient data they want, collect pertinent information during their shift, and write reports with accurate language and short phrases. Only document and communicate specific orders from the patient's healthcare provider when it is necessary for the patient's care.

(43) (C) Love.

This need for love and belonging is one of the psychological needs identified in Maslow's hierarchy of needs. It is a theory that categorizes human needs in a hierarchical manner, with love and belonging situated just above physiological and safety needs. It encompasses the desire for social connections, affectionate relationships, and a sense of belonging within a community or among peers.

(44) (A) Truthfulness.

Truthfulness is the quality of being honest in one's actions.

(45) (D) Surgical consent.

Surgical consent is the formal agreement or authorization provided by a patient or their legally authorized representative for a specific surgical procedure. Research consent patients are asked to participate in medical research. Admission consent is acquired at the time of admission, which outlines the healthcare agency's obligations to the patient. Special consent is required to use physical restraints like shackles. These are separate and distinct forms of consent that serve their own purpose.

(46) (D) Withdraw the NPH insulin first.

It is not recommended to withdraw the NPH insulin first, as it can lead to contamination and inaccurate dosing. NPH insulin is cloudy in appearance. If you withdraw it first, there is a risk of residual NPH insulin left in the syringe or needle. When you then withdraw the regular (clear) insulin, it may become contaminated with the cloudy NPH insulin, which affects the accuracy of the dose.

(47) (C) Increase fluid intake.

An infection of the bladder is known as cystitis. Patients are advised to increase fluid intake or drink 3,000 mL of fluids each day. It helps flush out the urinary tract and alleviate symptoms of cystitis. Hematocrit and hemoglobin tests are done to assess blood levels and are not directly related to the treatment of cystitis. Perineum ice and sitz baths are more commonly used to manage discomfort or pain in the perineal area, which may be necessary after childbirth but not specifically for cystitis.

(48) (D) Prednisone.

Prednisone is a corticosteroid. An abrupt discontinuation of this medication can have adverse effects, especially for patients who are on long-term treatment. It is necessary to continue for specific medical reasons, even when the patient is NPO.

(49) (C) Weight and temperature.

The patient who receives parenteral nutrition at home is more susceptible to infection and sepsis because the catheter is in a blood vessel. Therefore, it is important to monitor temperature. Additionally, weight is regularly monitored to determine the efficacy of nutritional treatment and to spot hypervolemia.

(50) (C) It is permanent contraception.

Vasectomy is a surgical procedure performed on males to achieve permanent contraception, but it does not affect a man's ability to have an erection. The procedure usually lasts around 15 to 30 minutes and involves cutting or sealing the vas deferens. Its purpose is to prevent the release of sperm during ejaculation.

(51) (A) Hydrocephalus.

After a repair of myelomeningocele, hydrocephalus commonly develops in infants. Hydrocephalus, which is an abnormal accumulation of cerebrospinal fluid in the brain, is a common complication associated with myelomeningocele. The presence of hydrocephalus is indicated by a larger head circumference.

(52) (B) Pregnancy-induced hypertension.

Pregnancy-induced hypertension is a medical condition related to high blood pressure that can occur during pregnancy but is not specifically linked to chlamydia. Chlamydia during pregnancy can lead to congenital anomalies in the baby and neonatal ophthalmia if the infection is transmitted to the newborn's eyes during delivery. Fetal infection through transplacental transmission is a potential complication of Chlamydia infection during pregnancy. This infection can affect the developing baby and lead to various complications.

(53) (C) In-process metrics.

In-process metrics are measurements or data collected during the ongoing process to assess its efficiency, quality, and timing. In this case, it would involve tracking the time it takes for a doctor to visit a patient as part of the healthcare process. Balance measurements, outcome metrics, and structural metrics may be relevant in healthcare contexts but are not specifically used to analyze the timing of a doctor's visit to a patient.

(54) (B) Anti-embolism stockings.

Anti-embolism stockings, also known as compression stockings, are used to prevent venous stasis and DVT in immobile patients. Although other options can play a role in the prevention of venous stasis and are often used together in clinical practice, anti-embolism stockings are specifically designed for this purpose and are highly effective when fitted and used in conjunction with other measures.

(55) (C) Face.

The nurse first cleans the face and eyes during a patient's bed bath. After the hands are cleaned, the arms and underarm area are washed, followed by the upper body. Finally, the perineum is washed. Throughout the procedure, it is essential to prioritize the patient's comfort, privacy, and dignity.

(56) (C) Finger stick and urine glucose test.

The boy's symptoms, which include polyphagia, polydipsia, and polyuria, are indicative of type 1 diabetes mellitus. The first step is to test for glucose in the urine and on a finger stick. This test can help determine if hyperglycemia is present and if further evaluation and management are needed.

(57) (C) Examine the sclera.

In individuals with darker skin tones, it is difficult to detect jaundice. In that situation, the sclera (the white of the eye) is the ideal area to look for jaundice since it becomes yellow in all people, regardless of skin tone.

(58) (D) All of the above.

Nurses should integrate self-care into their daily routines to establish healthy habits. All of the listed suggestions can be valuable strategies for nurses to address and overcome challenges they encounter.

(59) (C) The heart rate is 53 beats/minute.

A heart rate of 53 beats per minute in a patient with a ventricular pacemaker may signal a potential problem with the pacemaker's function or a need for a re-evaluation of the pacemaker settings. In such cases, the nurse must conduct a thorough assessment and closely monitor the patient's cardiac rhythm. Any observed abnormalities or concerns should be promptly reported to the healthcare provider for further evaluation and intervention.

(60) (D) Failure to provide the patient's family with adequate information.

Although it is important to keep the patient's family informed to the extent allowed by patient privacy and consent, there may be situations where certain information cannot be disclosed due to patient confidentiality or legal considerations.

(61) (A) Physical abuse.

The presentation of bruises and the patient's explanation that she fell down, coupled with her display of anxiety and fear during the examination, suggests the possibility of physical abuse.

(62) (D) Chlorine bleach.

Chlorine bleach effectively kills many pathogens, such as the HIV virus. This means it is the best chemical to clean and remove the bloodstain. The other options will not effectively disinfect and decontaminate the floor.

(63) (C) Perform ROM exercises.

Immobilized patients are most at risk for pulmonary emboli and DVT. Patients should engage in active ROM exercises to help maintain their blood circulation and prevent stagnation. This can reduce the risk of DVT and PE in immobile or bedridden patients. It is a recommended practice in healthcare settings to promote vascular health.

(64) (C) Thyroid hormones return to normal levels.

Levothyroxine is a medication used to treat hypothyroidism. This medication will provide synthetic thyroid hormone to the body. The goal is to normalize and maintain appropriate levels of thyroid hormones in the bloodstream, which help to regulate metabolism and energy levels.(65) (D) Shave the patient's hair.

The preparation of the surgical site is of utmost importance to prevent infection and complications.

(66) (A) Assault.

Assault involves the threat of harm, even if physical contact does not occur. Battery, on the other hand, involves actual physical contact. Defamation and fraud are different legal concepts unrelated to physical harm.

(67) (C) Anxiety or tachycardia.

Buspirone is an anxiolytic medication used to treat anxiety disorders. A proper therapeutic level of buspirone should lead to a reduction in anxiety symptoms and tachycardia (rapid heart rate).

(68) (A) Move slowly when positions are changed.

Risperidone is an antipsychotic medication that can cause orthostatic hypotension. Orthostatic hypotension causes dizziness and falls when changing positions. The patient must move slowly when changing positions to prevent this potential side effect.

(69) (D) All of the above.

Hospital quality improvement initiatives aim to achieve various goals. These initiatives aim to satisfy regulatory standards, streamline operations for efficiency, and ultimately enhance patient care outcomes. Therefore, all of the listed options are potential benefits of such initiatives.

(70) (D) He should immediately administer the eye ointment after the eye drops.

If the patient uses both eye drops and eye ointment, it is generally recommended to begin with the application of eye drops before eye ointment. This sequence is preferred because it promotes a more effective distribution of the medication.

(71) (C) Hypotension.

Betaxolol is a beta-blocker used to reduce intraocular pressure in glaucoma. Although it mostly affects the eyes, some systemic absorption can occur. The occurrence of systemic absorption leads to potential side effects like tachycardia (rapid heart rate) and hypotension (low blood pressure).

(72) (C) The Semi-Fowler's position.

The Semi-Fowler's position is the recommended position for a patient with hyphemia after an automobile accident. The head of the bed is elevated at a 30- to 45-degree angle. This position helps gravity maintain the hyphemia away from the cornea's optical center and minimizes pressure inside the eye. This can reduce the risk of complications and further damage to the eye.

(73) (A) Expert judgment.

In the hierarchy of evidence-based research, expert judgment is considered the lowest level of evidence. It relies on the expertise and knowledge of individuals in a particular field but does not involve empirical data from clinical studies or systematic research.

(74) (D) Increase oxygen intake.

The primary purpose of pursed-lip breathing in COPD patients is to increase the intake of oxygen. Pursed-lip breathing is a breathing technique where the patient inhales through the nose and exhales slowly through pursed lips. This technique helps improve the exchange of oxygen and carbon dioxide in the lungs.

(75) (D) Prednisone.

Prednisone is a corticosteroid medication known to cause hyperglycemia (high blood sugar) as a side effect. It can significantly affect blood glucose levels, particularly in individuals with diabetes.

(76) (A) You should check for visible chest rise after each rescue breath that is given over one second.

Deliver two breaths for every 15 chest compressions for CPR. This is the recommended ratio for CPR in adults, often referred to as "30:2," where 30 chest compressions are followed by two rescue breaths.

(77) (C) It can be transmitted through kisses.

HSV-1 is an infectious virus, and it is commonly associated with oral herpes. HSV1 may be spread by direct touch, which includes kisses but not coughs or sneezes.

(78) (D) Increased urine output.

IV mannitol is prescribed after a stroke to increase urine output. This could reduce brain swelling and intracranial pressure. It doesn't address muscle spasms, blood pressure, or clot dissolution.

(79) (A) Drink warm milk.

Warm milk before bedtime is a common home remedy that may promote relaxation and help some individuals fall asleep. It is a mild and nonstimulating option compared to caffeine-containing drinks like soda or activities that involve screen time.

(80) (D) ROM exercises.

ROM exercises are the most effective activity to prevent muscle atrophy in a bedridden patient. These exercises help maintain muscle flexibility, joint function, and circulation in the absence of weight-bearing activity or regular movement.

(81) (D) Hoarseness.

Hoarseness should be evaluated after a complete thyroidectomy because it can be a sign of damage or injury to the recurrent laryngeal nerve during the surgery. This nerve controls the movement of the vocal cords, and damage to it can lead to hoarseness.

(82) (B) Use alcohol to wipe the hearing aid's exterior surface.

Alcohol is not recommended for cleaning hearing aids. It can potentially damage the delicate components of the hearing aid, such as the microphone and the receiver.

Instead, a dry or slightly damp cloth is usually used to clean the exterior of the hearing aid.

(83) (B) Acetaminophen.

Acetaminophen is the recommended medication since the symptoms suggest a viral illness. Antibiotics would only be appropriate if the baby's fever was caused by a bacterial infection, which cannot be determined solely based on the symptoms described. Ibuprofen and aspirin are generally not recommended for infants of this age without specific guidance from a healthcare provider due to potential safety concerns. Aspirin, in particular, should be avoided in children with fever due to the risk of Reye's syndrome.

(84) (C) Serosanguineous.

Serosanguineous drainage, a mixture of clear or slightly yellow fluid (serous) and blood, is common after surgery. It may contain small blood clots. Bloody drainage can also occur initially. Serous drainage is clear and does not contain blood, and it is less common after thoracic surgery with chest tubes.

(85) (C) On one side, with a pillow placed under the hip.

The correct position for a lumbar puncture is usually on one's side, with knees drawn toward the chest in a fetal position, with a pillow under the hip. This position helps create the necessary space between the vertebrae for the procedure.

(86) (B) Dry mouth.

Dry mouth is a common side effect of fluoxetine, which is often used to treat conditions like depression and anxiety. Other potential side effects of fluoxetine include gastrointestinal issues, cardiovascular problems, and excessive perspiration. Individual responses to medications can vary.

(87) (C) The patient should increase dietary fiber and fluid intake.

Oxazepam is a medication used to manage anxiety and is a benzodiazepine. It can cause constipation as a side effect. Therefore, the patient should increase dietary fiber intake and fluid consumption.

(88) (B) Serum amylase level.

An elevated serum amylase level can be an indication of pancreatitis, which is a potential side effect of didanosine. If an HIV patient on didanosine experiences an elevated serum amylase level, discontinuation of the drug may be necessary to prevent further complications.

(89) (D) It is transmitted through deer ticks.

Lyme disease is mostly transmitted through the bite of infected black-legged ticks, often referred to as deer ticks (Ixodes scapularis or Ixodes pacificus). These ticks can carry the bacterium Borrelia burgdorferi.

(90) (A) Cheek and nose bridge rash.

A characteristic sign of SLE is a butterfly-shaped rash that usually appears on the cheeks and the bridge of the nose. This rash is known as a “malar rash” or “butterfly rash.”

(91) (C) Uric acid level = 9.5 mg/dL.

A uric acid level of 9.5 mg/dL is elevated and can be indicative of gout, a condition characterized by the deposition of urate crystals in the joints that leads to pain and inflammation.

(92) (C) The tips of the crutch can be wet and still not slip.

This is false. The tips of crutches should not be wet, as wet surfaces can be slippery and increase the risk of falls or accidents. Crutch tips should be dry and in good condition to provide stable support.

(93) (B) Direct bilirubin level = 3.1 mg/dL.

A high level of direct bilirubin in the blood, such as 3.1 mg/dL, can be indicative of acetaminophen toxicity, especially in cases of severe liver damage caused by acetaminophen overdose.

(94) (C) The patient has emotional lability and flat affect.

The limbic system plays a significant role in the regulation of emotions and emotional responses. A limbic system neurological deficit can manifest as emotional lability and flat effects.

(95) (A) Take the drugs on time to maintain therapeutic blood levels.

To avoid cholinergic and myasthenic crises in myasthenia gravis patients, it is essential to maintain therapeutic blood levels of medications, such as acetylcholinesterase inhibitors. Dose adjustments should be made under medical supervision.

(96) (B) Uterine hyperstimulation.

Uterine hyperstimulation is characterized by excessive or prolonged contractions. It is a reason to discontinue oxytocin administration during labor induction. It can lead to fetal distress and other complications.

(97) (A) Administer oxygen via a face mask at a rate of 8–10 L/min oxygen.

If fetal distress occurs during cesarean birth preparation, one appropriate therapeutic action is to administer oxygen to the mother via a face mask at a rate of 8–10 L/min. This can help improve oxygen delivery to the fetus.

(98) (A) Pull back the NG tube and attempt insertion after the dyspnea resolves.

If the patient starts to cough or suffer dyspnea, the nurse should gently remove the tube, halt the tubing's progress, and wait until the discomfort passes. It is not advisable to insert the tube quickly in this circumstance since the tube may enter the bronchus.

(99) (C) To prevent headaches.

The primary purpose of placing a post-myelogram patient in a semi-reclined position is to prevent headaches. A myelogram involves the injection of contrast dye into the spinal canal, which can sometimes lead to CSF leakage and subsequent headaches, especially when the patient assumes an upright position. Seizures are not a common or expected complication of myelograms, and the position is not related to seizure prevention in this context.

(100) (D) Acute pain.

When you assess a patient with urolithiasis (kidney stones), one of the primary concerns is the presence of acute pain. Kidney stones can cause severe pain, often referred to as renal colic.

(101) (A) Diuresis.

An extremely high urine output of 18 liters from a postoperative cardiac surgery patient is most likely caused by diuresis. This can occur due to the administration of diuretic medications, which are often used after cardiac surgery to manage the balance of fluids and prevent fluid overload. Diuretics increase urine production to eliminate excess fluids from the body.

(102) (B) Use a bed cradle to decrease the pain.

The nursing care plan for a 12-year-old boy with left knee swelling due to hemophilia should include ROM exercises. Hemophilia is a bleeding disorder, and it's essential to maintain joint mobility to prevent stiffness and long-term joint damage. ROM exercises can help keep the joint mobile and reduce the risk of hemarthrosis (bleeding into the joint).

(103) (C) Record the findings.

When you assess a newborn with a low-positioned ear, it is appropriate to record the findings as part of the physical examination. This information can be important for the baby's medical records and may prompt further evaluation or intervention if necessary.

(104) (C) Tardive dyskinesia.

The symptoms of grimacing, tongue protrusion, and involuntary mouth movements in a patient with schizophrenia who is on antipsychotic medication are indicative of tardive dyskinesia. Tardive dyskinesia is a side effect of long-term antipsychotic use and involves involuntary, repetitive movements of the face, tongue, and mouth.

(105) (B) WBC count.

A schizophrenia patient who is on clozapine is monitored by healthcare providers with regular WBC counts to identify potential side effects, particularly agranulocytosis.

(106) (A) Pentamidine may cause leukopenia, which leads to another infection.

Pentamidine may cause leukopenia, which can increase the risk of other infections and fever. Inadequate thermoregulation can be compromised in individuals with advanced HIV/AIDS, which can result in an elevated body temperature. Pentamidine toxicity can lead to various side effects, such as fever, as it may indicate a reaction to the medication. An insufficient dosage of pentamidine is not a probable reason for the elevated temperature. Although under-dosing can affect the effectiveness of treatment, it is not a direct cause of fever or elevated body temperature.

(107) (A) Liver function test.

Dantrolene sodium can have hepatotoxic (liver-damaging) side effects, so liver function tests should be carried out both before and after therapy to lower the risk of liver damage.

(108) (A) Sore throat.

Sore throat is not usually associated with trimethoprim-sulfamethoxazole (TMP-SMX) treatment. The more common side effects include gastrointestinal symptoms like diarrhea and nausea, as well as headache and other potential adverse reactions.

(109) (D) Stoma that protrudes.

An indication of prolapse after a colostomy is a stoma that protrudes. Stoma prolapse occurs when the stoma extends outward beyond the level of the skin around it. This can lead to various issues and complications, and it may require medical attention or surgical intervention. Prolapsed stomas can become edematous or discolored, but the key feature is the protrusion of the stoma itself.

(110) (A) Irregular heartbeat.

A complication during the assessment of a pheochromocytoma patient can include irregular and elevated heart rates. Pheochromocytoma is a rare tumor that can cause excessive secretion of adrenaline and noradrenaline (catecholamines). This can lead to symptoms such as high blood pressure, rapid heartbeat (tachycardia), and irregular heart rhythms (arrhythmias) due to the effect of these hormones on the cardiovascular system.

(111) (C) Hemorrhage.

Monitoring for hemorrhage is essential in the care of a placenta previa case. Placenta previa is a condition in which the placenta partially or completely covers the cervix, which increases the risk of bleeding during pregnancy and childbirth.

(112) (C) Empower her to feel like a survivor.

The long-term purpose of the management of a woman who has been abused by her husband is to help her feel like a survivor. Domestic violence survivors often go through a healing process where they learn to rebuild their self-esteem, regain their sense of control, and address the psychological and emotional effects of the abuse.

(113) (B) The drainage system has an air leak.

The underwater seal is mostly used to visualize and monitor air leaks, not blockages in the tube. Although it is possible that a blocked tube from the pleural cavity could result in decreased or no drainage, it would not usually be associated with the absence of bubbling in the underwater seal compartment.

(114) (D) Deep respirations.

Deep, rapid respirations, known as "Kussmaul respirations," are a characteristic symptom of diabetic ketoacidosis (DKA). DKA is a serious complication of diabetes characterized by high blood sugar levels, metabolic acidosis, and ketone production, which leads to rapid and deep breathing as the body tries to compensate for the acidosis. Ketoacidosis is not characterized by rash or constipation.

(115) (C) Abdominal area.

The most suitable site to assess jaundice (yellowing of the skin and mucous membranes) is the abdominal area. Jaundice is often first noticeable in the abdominal region and can then be assessed in other areas of the body, such as the sclera (white part of the eyes) and mucous membranes.

(116) (C) Seizures.

Seizures are a sign of bupropion toxicity. Bupropion is an antidepressant medication that can lower the seizure threshold. Excessive doses can lead to seizures.

(117) (C) It should be taken in the evening at the same time.

Sertraline, an antidepressant medication, should be taken consistently, usually in the evening at the same time each day. It is usually not taken as needed, and there is no requirement to divide it into three doses or take it on an empty stomach.

(118) (A) Taken on an empty stomach.

Saquinavir, an antiretroviral medication used in the treatment of HIV, is often recommended to be taken on an empty stomach at least one hour before or two hours after a meal. This helps improve the absorption of the medication.

(119) (D) Hairdressers.

Hairdressers are at the greatest risk of developing a latex allergy. This is because they often come into close contact with latex-containing gloves and other latex products. Latex allergies can develop due to repeated exposure to latex proteins.

(120) (C) Assessment of discomfort when the patient is repositioned.
After spinal fusion surgery, the assessment of discomfort during repositioning is a standard evaluation. This helps determine how the patient is healing and if there are any complications with the fusion site. It is important to ensure that the spine is stable, and that movement doesn't cause undue pain or harm.
(121) (C) Elevate the legs for five hours, then keep them in a flat position.
For multiple trauma patients with plaster casts on leg fractures, it is recommended to elevate the legs for a specified period (often around five hours) to reduce swelling and then keep them in a flat position to prevent complications. This approach helps promote circulation and healing.
(122) (B) Inform the doctor if inflammation or fever occurs.
It is important to monitor postoperative knee arthroscopy patients for any signs of infection or complications. If there is any inflammation or fever, it should be reported to the doctor promptly.
(123) (D) All of the above.
Two-factor authentication, driver's license, and ID photos can be used for identity verification, which depends on the specific circumstances and the facility's protocols.
(124) (C) Acetylsalicylic acid.
Aspirin can potentially cause a roar or ringing sound in the ears, a condition known as tinnitus. This side effect can occur with aspirin use, especially at higher doses. It is important to note that tinnitus is not directly related to gastrointestinal bleeding.
(125) (D) Cover the eye with a patch.
Cover the eye with a protective patch when a patient has eye-penetrating trauma. This helps prevent further injury or contamination. After that, a healthcare professional can assess visual acuity and proceed with appropriate treatment.
(126) (C) Graves's disease.
Propylthiouracil is commonly used to treat hyperthyroidism, especially in cases of Graves's disease, where there is an overproduction of thyroid hormones. It helps to reduce the production of thyroid hormones.
(127) (A) Excessive release of catecholamines occurs.

Pheochromocytoma is a rare tumor of the adrenal glands that leads to the excessive release of catecholamines, such as adrenaline and noradrenaline, into the bloodstream. This can result in a range of symptoms related to increased sympathetic nervous system activity, such as hypertension, palpitations, and anxiety.

(128) (A) Use gloves before mealtimes and wash hands before and after perineum self-care.

Some of the important precautions to reduce the risk of hepatitis B transmission from a positive mother to her newborn are the use of gloves before meals and the performance of regular hand hygiene before and after perineum self-care. These hygienic measures help prevent direct contact with potentially infectious body fluids.

(129) (C) Because infants are obligate nose breathers.

Healthcare providers usually assess a child's nose for patency after birth delivery. It is important because newborns are obligate nose breathers.

(130) (B) Stay with the patient until his anxiety levels drop.

When the patient suffers from hyperventilation and anxiety after being assaulted, the nurse should stay and provide emotional support and reassurance. This can help the patient feel safe.

(131) (B) Hearing loss.

Amikacin, an antibiotic from the aminoglycoside class, is associated with potential side effects. These side effects include loss of hearing and kidney damage. The nurse should regularly monitor the hearing and kidney functions while the patient takes this medication.

(132) (D) Edema and itching at the site of injection.

Etanercept may cause pancytopenia and infection. A potentially fatal infection may be identified when abnormal platelets and WBC develop. Although these blood counts may be monitored during the overall management of rheumatoid arthritis, the primary focus during etanercept administration is usually the patient's response to the medication and local reactions at the injection site, such as edema and itching.

(133) (A) Do not move the affected limb.

If there is a suspicion of a fracture, the nurse should not move the patient to prevent further injury or displacement of the fracture.

(134) (A) It tests positive for glucose and separates into concentric rings.

Cerebrospinal fluid is a transparent liquid that can exhibit a characteristic separation into concentric rings when collected in a test tube. It usually tests positive for glucose. When a patient blows their nose, sneezes, coughs, performs the Valsalva maneuver, or engages in isometric exercises, this could elevate intracranial pressure.

(135) (C) Pupil dilation.

Cyclopentolate is a mydriatic and cycloplegic drug that causes pupil dilation. This leads to an increase in the size of the pupil. This effect is often used during eye examinations to allow better visualization of the interior of the eye.

(136) (A) Pain during inspiration.

Falls or violent accidents are common causes of rib fractures. Rib fractures cause sharp, localized pain, especially during deep breathing or inspiration. The other options are not usually associated with rib fractures but may be seen in other respiratory or chest-related conditions.

(137) (C) Test the discharge for glucose.

After hypophysectomy, monitor for nasal discharge, as it can be a sign of CSF leakage. If rhinorrhea occurs, obtain a sample of the discharge and conduct a CSF exam to confirm the diagnosis and initiate appropriate treatment.

(138) (C) Foot strength.

A lumbar laminectomy is a surgical procedure performed on the lower back to relieve pressure on the spinal nerves. After this procedure, it is essential to evaluate foot strength and function because the surgery can affect the nerves and muscles in the lower back and legs. An assessment of foot strength helps determine if there are any neurological or muscular deficits related to the surgery.

(139) (A) Avoid alcohol consumption.

Phenobarbital has hypnotic and anticonvulsant properties. Patients should not use other CNS depressants like alcohol with phenobarbital. Patients are advised to take phenobarbital at consistent times each day to ensure the medication's effectiveness and minimize the risk of potential issues like breakthrough seizures.

(140) (A) Separation of wound edges.

All of the options are important factors during the assessment. Stump edema refers to swelling of the remaining limb, which can affect the fit and function of prosthetics, hinder wound healing, and potentially lead to further complications. It is an important consideration for post-amputation care, especially in diabetic patients, because they are particularly vulnerable to complications due to impaired circulation and healing.

(141) (A) Have the patient close the nasolacrimal duct at the inner canthus with a finger for a minute after administration of the eye drops.

When you close the nasolacrimal duct at the inner canthus with a finger for a short duration after the administration of eye drops, this is known as punctal occlusion. This technique is used to prevent the absorption of the medication and reduce the risk of systemic side effects.

(142) (C) Tremors.

Tremors can be a sign of hyperthyroidism, which can occur if the dose of levothyroxine is too high. It is important to monitor tremors to ensure that the patient is on the correct dose of medication.

(143) (B) Remove the patient from the abusive situation.

The immediate priority is to ensure the safety of the patient. Remove the patient from the abusive environment and protect them from further harm. Other possibilities are important, but they are not the priority.

(144) (A) Acetylcysteine.

Acetylcysteine is the acetaminophen antidote because it helps to replenish glutathione levels in the body, which helps neutralize the toxic effects of acetaminophen overdose. Fludarabine is an anticancer drug used to treat certain types of leukemia and lymphoma. Auranofin is a medication used for the treatment of rheumatoid arthritis. Pentostatin is a chemotherapy medication used to treat certain types of cancer.

(145) (B) Diabetes mellitus.

Terbutaline should be used with caution in patients with diabetes mellitus because it can affect blood glucose levels. It may lead to hyperglycemia, and adjustments to the diabetes management plan may be necessary when terbutaline is used. Patients with diabetes should be closely monitored when prescribed this medication. However, in polycystic disease, terbutaline is contraindicated because it can exacerbate this condition. It should not be used in individuals with polycystic disease.

Made in the USA
Middletown, DE
21 October 2024